Crohn's Disease

Giuseppe Lo Re • Massimo Midiri
Editors

Crohn's Disease

Radiological Features
and Clinical-Surgical Correlations

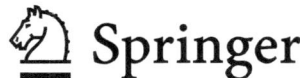 Springer

Editors
Giuseppe Lo Re
Radiology Department
Policlinico Paolo Giaccone
Palermo
Italy

Massimo Midiri
University of Palermo
Radiology Department
Policlinico Paolo Giaccone
Palermo
Italy

ISBN 978-3-319-23065-8   ISBN 978-3-319-23066-5   (eBook)
DOI 10.1007/978-3-319-23066-5

Library of Congress Control Number: 2015956406

Springer Cham Heidelberg New York Dordrecht London

Printed on acid-free paper

Springer International Publishing AG Switzerland is part of Springer Science+Business Media (www.springer.com)

Foreword

Crohn's disease is a chronic pathology that is very difficult to understand and to diagnose especially in the early stages, resulting in a significant deterioration in the patients' quality of life.

In the past, this disease had a higher incidence in the northern Europe countries. Recently we have seen an increase of cases in the Mediterranean area, probably due to environmental factors and changes in lifestyle, becoming increasingly challenging not only for radiologists but also for clinicians.

This book deals thoroughly with Crohn's disease, analyzing the different clinical, diagnostic, and therapeutic aspects. The purpose is to provide a global view of the pathology, necessary to understand the disease in its entirety and in its complexity. In fact these patients cannot be approached in "watertight compartments," but the partnership between the clinician, the radiologist, and the surgeon is more necessary than ever, in order to achieve the most appropriate treatment for each case.

Because of the different presentations, often treacherous and misleading, and the complexity of the several extraintestinal manifestations, only an integrated clinical-radiological approach can lead to proper patient management.

In this scenario, radiological imaging plays an important role, providing various diagnostic options based on the most modern technology. Every diagnostic modality can be exploited differently depending on the various stages of the disease.

The authors involved in this project can boast an internationally recognized expertise, arising from years of research focused on to the study of Crohn's disease. The result of their contribution brings to a complete and integrated text, containing the latest knowledge in this field, providing an extremely useful tool for anyone who decides to tackle this disease.

Dott. Gian Andrea Rollandi
Direttore S.C. Radiodiagnostica
Coordinatore Scientifico
E.O. Ospedali Galliera
Via Volta 8, 16132 Genova, Italy

Acknowledgments

To my wife Maria Cristina, my daughter Roberta Maria, and to my parents.

Giuseppe Lo Re

To my wife Anna and to my sons Federico and Mauro.

Massimo Midiri

Contents

Epidemiological Aspects of Crohn's Disease

Francesco Vitale

1.1 Epidemiology

Crohn's disease (CD) is considered a result of multifactorial interplay between genetic, immune-related, environmental, and infectious triggers all contributing into evolution of clinical disease [1, 2].

The age of onset of Crohn's disease has a bimodal distribution. The first peak occurs between the ages of 15 and 30 years (late adolescence and early adulthood), and the second occurs mainly in women between the ages of 60 and 70 years [3].

In general, the frequency of CD is similar in males and females, with some studies showing a very slight female predominance.

The rate of Crohn's disease is 1.1–1.8 times higher in women than in men. This pattern is reversed with pediatric CD, which has a higher incidence in boys than in girls (pediatric male-to-female ratio, ~1.6:1) [3, 4].

Crohn's disease is reported to be more common in white patients than in black patients and rare in Asian and Hispanic children. Approximately 20 % of all CD patients are of black descent. Rates are higher in people of

Jewish descent, particularly in Ashkenazi Jews and Jews of middle European origin as compared with Sephardic or eastern European Jews [4].

Although there are few epidemiologic data from developing countries, the incidence and prevalence of CD are increasing with time and in different regions around the world, indicating its emergence as a global disease [3].

The incidence of Crohn's disease (CD) differs depending on the region studied. Epidemiologic studies conducted during the last decade has mostly supported the idea of a disease of the developed world, with a typical north to south gradient observed in Europe [4].

Overall, the United Kingdom, North America, and the northern part of Europe are the areas with the highest incidence [5].

In North America, the most notable example of long-term surveillance for CD incidence evolution is the Olmsted County, Minnesota, database, encompassing registries from the 1930s onward [6]. A gradual increase has been continuously observed, with the median annual incidence for the 1990–2001 period reaching 7 cases per 100,000 population, compared to 6.6 per 100,000 for the 1965–1975 period. An inversion of the usual female predominance has been observed in recent years, with more male than female patients diagnosed. The typical patients are young and of urban origin.

Studies on pediatric CD in the USA offer less information, describing an annual incidence of 4.5 per 100.000, while the incidence in children

F. Vitale, MD
Department of Sciences for Health Promotion and Mother to Child care "G.D'Alessandro"- University of Palermo, Preventive Medicine and Public Health – University of Palermo, Palermo, Italy
e-mail: francesco.vitale@unipa.it

© Springer International Publishing Switzerland 2016
G. Lo Re, M. Midiri (eds.), *Crohn's Disease: Radiological Features and Clinical-Surgical Correlations*,
DOI 10.1007/978-3-319-23066-5_1

of Afro-American origin in Georgia was much higher ($7.1/10^5$/year) [7].

In Canada, the district of Manitoba consistently reports one of the highest incidences of CD worldwide, reaching $14.6/10^5$ for the 1987–1994 period: the disease predominates in young females and exhibits a significant variability between smaller geographical regions, and the incidence is characteristically lower in Indian aboriginals, raising the question about a possible different genetic profile. Nevertheless, even in this population, a recent increase has been noted, especially in the 30–40 age group [8, 9].

On the other hand, reports from the 1980s from Quebec and Ontario exhibited significantly low rates: incidence of $0.7/10^5$ and prevalence of 33/105 (reflecting a low incidence), respectively [9].

In Central America, the incidence of the disease was recently investigated for the 1996–2000 period, and an increase from 0.49 to $1.96/10^5$ was observed in Puerto Rico where CD predominates in young males [10].

The disease seems to be scarce in Latin America: a study from a region of Panama and a region of Argentina showed a practically non-existent disease in the 1987–1993 period, [11] while the cumulative cases reported from Chile in the 1990–2002 period account to a very low incidence also [12].

A Brazilian study from the region of Janeiro also showed low incidence in the 1980–1999 period, although the total new CD cases reported in the 1995–1999 timeframe exhibited an increase of 166 % compared to the 1980–1984 cases [13].

In Europe, epidemiological dynamics of CD can be drawn by the development and continuing evolution of the European Crohn's and Colitis Organization (ECCO) and the European Collaborative study of IBD (EC-IBD) [14].

Overall, incidence data describes a North-South Europe gradient of CD incidence (7 versus $3.9/10^5$).

The EC-IBD study showed an high annual incidence rate in adult population in Iceland ($8/10^5$), in Norway ($5.8/10^5$), in Sweden ($8.9/10^5$), and in Denmark ($8.6/10^5$), whereas reports on the incidence of pediatric CD are contradicting showing a huge increase in CD in children in Stockholm (1.7 to $8.4/10^5$ from 1990 to 2001) [15] and a relatively stable annual incidence rates

of $2.5/10^5$ and $2/10^5$ in two studies focusing on pediatric IBD in Norway [16].

In the Baltic former Soviet republics, the only study from this area, Estonia, showed a low incidence ($1.4/10^5$) compared to Scandinavia [17].

The United Kingdom represents, in Europe, the typical model of North-South gradient, with a potentially higher incidence in Scotland compared to England and Wales. The city of Aberdeen, located in Northern Scotland, demonstrated one of the highest incidences worldwide ($11.7/10^5$/year) in 1985–1987, with a young urban female predominance. Increasing trends have also been observed in numerous reports on pediatric CD, with the incidence doubling in the 1990s, reaching a median annual rate of $4.4/10^5$ in the region of Aberdeen [18].

Other English studies have focused on the racial trends of CD incidence, showing lower prevalence in Southeast Asian residents compared to Europeans or West Indians compared to Caucasians [19].

The incidence rates for Ireland reported in the EC-IBD study are roughly similar to the British ones ($6/10^5$/year).

Also in Northern France, the EC-IBD study showed high incidence rate of CD ($9/10^5$/year) [14].

A gradual increase was observed during the 1990s in North France, with the median annual incidence per 100,000 rising from 5.2 to 6.4 from 1988–1990 to 1997–1999, with a female predominance.

A study from the mid-southern French area showed rates comparable to those of Northern France. In the Netherlands, a study from Maastricht had shown annual incidence rates of $6.9/10^5$, and in Belgium, a minimal but stable increase was observed through time, with annual rates of 4.5 new cases per 10^5 [20].

In Germany, a study showed a moderate increase in 1991–1995 compared to 1980–1984 (5.2 versus $4.9/10^5$/ year), although the median age of the patients increased by almost a decade; the overall German rates reported in the EC-IBD study were slightly lower though [14].

The incidence rates in Southern Europe were invariably low in the EC-IBD study: A North-South gradient was observed in Portugal, where previous studies from Oporto in the north confirmed a steady incidence rise during the 1975–1990 period.

Numerous studies from Spain have failed to reproduce this gradient though: A prospective 1991–1993 study from four regions showed an overall annual incidence of $5.5/10^5$, which was actually higher in the southern region ($6.5/10^5$/year) and the island of Mallorca compared to the northern participating regions [21].

Italy exhibits a typical southern European profile in having low CD rates, but, like Spain, there exists no North-South gradient in the country as such, with a study for eight cities from 1989 to 1992 showing homogenous incidence rates. However, a recent Italian administrative database study on IBD, covering a wide area in central Italy, demonstrated incidence rates during the years 2008–2009 of 7.4 and 6.5 for Crohn's disease for males and females, respectively [22]. The lowest European incidence was reported initially from Northwest Greece, although an increasing trend observed recently and a significantly higher incidence reported from the southern island of Crete [23] (data for both areas until mid-1990s, rates 0.1 and 3/105, respectively).

Traditionally, the incidence has been low in Asia and Africa. However, studies from these areas suggest that the incidence of CD is increasing.

The prevalence of CD in Europe varies from less than 10 to about 150 per 100,000 inhabitants.

An adjusted prevalence of 133 per 100,000 was found in Minnesota, United States, in 1991. One study from South Korea indicated prevalence of 11.2 per 100,000 [24].

Population-based studies have demonstrated that the incidence and prevalence of CD have increased over the last three decades. CD is most common in northern Europe and North America, and there is a slight predominance of women diagnosed with the disease.

1.2 Risk Factors

Genetic, microbial, immunologic, environmental, dietary, vascular, and psychosocial factors, as well as smoking, the use of oral contraceptives and nonsteroidal anti-inflammatory agents (NSAIDs) have been associated with increasing risk to develop Crohn's disease. However, interaction between the predisposing genetic factors, environmental factors, host factors, and triggering event is likely necessary for the disease to develop. Most of the genes thought to be involved in the development of the disease play a role in mucosal immunity, and their products are found on the mucosal barrier epithelium [25].

The first gene clearly identified as a susceptibility gene for Crohn's disease was the NOD2 gene (now called CARD15), in which were identified 3 single nucleotide polymorphisms (SNPs), 2 missense, and 1 frameshift. These variations in NOD2/CARD15, which is a polymorphic gene involved in the innate immune system, play a role in 27 % of patients with Crohn's disease, with CARD15 genotype being associated not only with the onset of disease but also with its natural history. A study in a German and Norwegian cohort showed that patients with 1 of the 3 identified risk alleles for CARD15 were more likely to have either ileal or right-colon disease [26].

An early genome-wide association study (GWAS) looked at Jewish and non-Jewish case-control cohorts and identified 2 SNPs in the IL23R gene, which encodes 1 subunit of the IL-23 receptor protein. Interestingly, this study also described the promising nature of certain therapies that block the function of IL-23. Further research suggested that one particular polymorphism in the IL23R gene showed the strongest association in a German population [27].

In a meta-analysis of 3 GWASs, 526 SNPs from 74 distinct genomic loci were found including the genes CCR6, IL12B, STAT3, JAK2, LRRK2, CDKAL1, and PTPN22 [28]. Most of these genes are involved in signal transduction in certain immune function, as well as genes involved more directly with immune function. Other GWASs found associations between susceptibility to Crohn's disease and polymorphisms, and one large study involving nearly 20,000 SNPs in 735 individuals with Crohn's disease found an association in the ATG16L1gene, which encodes the autophagy-related 16-like protein involved in the autophagosome pathway that processes intracellular bacteria [29]. A large genomic study of multiple diseases confirmed many of the findings found in earlier studies and identified several additional loci of interest for Crohn's disease located within the BSN gene, which encodes a brain-specific scaffold protein involved in neurotransmitter release and in the NKX2-3 gene, which is a homeodomain-containing transcription factor [30].

Infectious agents such as *Mycobacterium paratuberculosis*, *Pseudomonas* species, and *Listeria* species have all been implicated in the pathogenesis of Crohn's disease, suggesting that the inflammation seen with the disease is the result of a dysfunctional, but appropriate, response to an infectious source [25].

Also interleukins and TNF-α have been suggested to play a role in the disease process, which is characterized by a Th1 cellular immune response pattern that leads to production of IL-12, TNF-α, and interferon gamma with increased concentrations of TNF-α in the stool, blood, and mucosa [31].

Environmental influences such as tobacco use seem to have an effect on Crohn's disease. Smoking has been shown to double the risk of Crohn's disease [32].

It has also been suggested that a diet high in fatty foods may increase the risk of Crohn's disease, whereas concerns about the measles vaccine and the development of the disease have proved to be unfounded [33, 34]. Finally, the relationship between appendectomy and the risk of developing CD has been debated, and in 2009, a systematic review found a relative risk (RR) of 6.69 (95 % CI: 5.42–8.25), for having CD diagnosed following an appendectomy, significantly elevated within the first year after the surgery [35].

References

1. Duerr RH. Update on the genetics of inflammatory bowel disease. J Clin Gastroenterol. 2003;37(5): 358–67.
2. Gaya DR, Russell RK, Nimmo ER, et al. New genes in inflammatory bowel disease: lessons for complex diseases? Lancet. 2006;367:1271–84.
3. Molodecky NA, Soon IS, Rabi DM, et al. Increasing incidence and prevalence of the inflammatory bowel diseases with time. Based on systematic review. Gastroenterology. 2012;142:46–54.
4. Binder V. Epidemiology of I BD during the twentieth century: an integrated view. Best Pract Res Clin Gastroenterol. 2004;18:463–79.
5. Hovde Ø, Moum BA. Epidemiology and clinical course of Crohn's disease: results from observational studies. World J Gastroenterol. 2012;18(15):1723–31.
6. Jess T, Loftus Jr EV, Harmsen WS, et al. Survival and cause specific mortality in patients with inflammatory bowel disease: a long term outcome study in Olmsted County, Minnesota, 1940-2004. Gut. 2006;55:1248–54.
7. Ogunbi SO, Ransom JA, Sullivan K, et al. Inflammatory bowel disease in African-American children living in Georgia. J Pediatr. 1998;133:103–7.
8. Mendelhoff AI, Calkin BM. The epidemiology of inflammatory bowel disease. In: Kirsner JB, Shorter RG, editors. Inflammatory bowel disease. 3rd ed. Philadelphia: Lea and Febriger; 1988. p. 3–34.
9. Depew WT. Clinical presentation and course of Crohn's disease in south-eastern Ontario. Can J Gastroenterol. 1988;2:107–16.
10. Appleyard CB, Hernandez G, Rios-Bedoya CF. Basic epidemiology of inflammatory bowel disease in Puerto Rico. Inflamm Bowel Dis. 2004;10:106–11.
11. Linares de la Cal JA, Canton C, Pajares JM, et al. Inflammatory bowel disease in Argentina and Panama (1987-1993). Eur J Gastroenterol Hepatol. 1997;9:1129.
12. Figueroa CC, Quera PR, Valenzuela EJ, et al. Inflammatory bowel disease: experience of two Chilean centers. Rev Med Chil. 2005;133:1295–304.
13. Souza MH, Troncon LE, Rodrigues CM, et al. T rends in the occurrence (1980-1999) and clinical features of Crohn's disease and ulcerative colitis in a university hospital in southeastern Brazil. Arq Gastroenterol. 2002;39:98–105.
14. Shivananda S, Lennard-Jones J, Logan R, et al. Incidence of inflammatory bowel disease across Europe: is there a difference between north and south? Results of the European Collaborative Study on Inflammatory Bowel Disease (ECIBD). Gut. 1996;39:690–7.
15. Ekbom A, Helmick C, Zack M, et al. The epidemiology of inflammatory bowel disease: a large, population-based study in Sweden. Gastroenterology. 1991;100:350–8.
16. Moum B, Vatn MH, Ekbom A, et al. Incidence of Crohn's disease in four counties in southeastern Norway, 1990-93. A prospective population- based study. The Inflammatory Bowel South-Eastern Norway (IBSEN) Study Group of Gastroenterologists. Scand J Gastroenterol. 1996;31:355–61.
17. Sepp E, Julge K, Vasar M, et al. Intestinal microflora of Estonian and Swedish infants. Acta Paediatr. 1997;86:956–61.
18. Armitage EL, Aldhous MC, Anderson N, et al. Incidence of juvenile-onset Crohn's disease in Scotland: association with northern latitude and affluence. Gastroenterology. 2004;127(4):1051–7.
19. Fellows IW, Freeman JG, Holmes GK. Crohn's disease in the city of Derby, 1951-85. Gut. 1990;31:1262–5.
20. Economou M, Zambeli E, Michopoulos S, et al. Incidence and prevalence of Crohn's disease and

its etiological influences. Ann Gastroenterol. 2009;22(3):158–67.

21. Mate-Jimenez J, Munoz S, Vicent D, et al. Incidence and prevalence of ulcerative colitis and Crohn's disease in urban and rural areas of Spain from 1981 to 1988. J Clin Gastroenterol. 1994;18:27–31.

22. Di Domenicantonio R, Cappai G, Arcà M, et al. Occurrence of inflammatory bowel disease in central Italy: a study based on health information systems. Dig Liver Dis. 2014;46:777–82.

23. Economou M, Filis G, Tsianou Z, et al. Crohn's disease incidence evolution in North-western Greece is not associated with alteration of NOD2/CARD15 variants. World J Gastroenterol. 2007;13:5116–20.

24. Ahuja V, Tandon RK. Inflammatory bowel disease in the Asia-Pacific area: a comparison with developed countries and regional differences. J Dig Dis. 2010;11:134–47.

25. Thoreson R, Cullen JJ. Pathophysiology of inflammatory bowel disease: an overview. Surg Clin North Am. 2007;87(3):575–85.

26. Hampe J, Grebe J, Nikolaus S, et al. Association of NOD2 (CARD 15) genotype with clinical course of Crohn's disease: a cohort study. Lancet. 2002;359(9318):1661–5.

27. Glas J, Seiderer J, Wetzke M, et al. rs1004819 is the main disease-associated IL23R variant in German Crohn's disease patients: combined analysis of IL23R, CARD15, and OCTN1/2 variants. PLoS One. 2007;2(9):e819.

28. Barrett JC, Hansoul S, Nicolae DL, Cho JH, Duerr RH, Rioux JD, et al. Genome-wide association

defines more than 30 distinct susceptibility loci for Crohn's disease. Nat Genet. 2008;40(8):955–62.

29. Hampe J, Franke A, Rosenstiel P, Till A, Teuber M, Huse K, et al. A genome-wide association scan of nonsynonymous SNPs identifies a susceptibility variant for Crohn disease in ATG16L1. Nat Genet. 2007;39(2):207–11.

30. Wellcome Trust Case Control Consortium. Genome-wide association study of 14,000 cases of seven common diseases and 3,000 shared controls. Nature. 2007;447(7145):661–78.

31. Sandborn WJ, Hanauer SB, Rutgeerts P, et al. Adalimumab for maintenance treatment of Crohn's disease: results of the CLASSIC II trial. Gut. 2007;56(9):1232–9).

32. Lindberg E, Järnerot G, Huitfeldt B. Smoking in Crohn's disease: effect on localisation and clinical course. Gut. 1992;33(6):779–82.

33. D'Souza S, Levy E, Mack D, Israel D, Lambrette P, Ghadirian P. Dietary patterns and risk for Crohn's disease in children. Inflamm Bowel Dis. 2008;14(3):367–73.

34. Davis RL, Kramarz P, Bohlke K, Benson P, Thompson RS, Mullooly J, et al. Measles-mumps-rubella and other measles-containing vaccines do not increase the risk for inflammatory bowel disease: a case-control study from the Vaccine Safety Datalink project. Arch Pediatr Adolesc Med. 2001;155(3):354–9.

35. Kaplan GG, Jackson T, Sands BE, Frisch M, Andersson RE, Korzenik J. The risk of developing Crohn's disease after an appendectomy: a meta-analysis. Am J Gastroenterol. 2008;103:2925–31.

Clinical Presentation of Crohn's Disease

Marta Mazza, Maria Giovanna Cilluffo, and Maria Cappello

Crohn's disease is an idiopathic chronic inflammatory disease of the gut, which may involve the entire gastrointestinal tract from the mouth to the perianal area, though preferring in most cases the distal small bowel and the proximal large bowel. Its heterogeneous nature is reflected in a number of different phenotypes [1]. Approximately 80 % of patients have small bowel involvement, usually in the distal ileum, with one-third of patients having exclusively ileitis. Approximately 50 % of patients have ileocolitis which refers to involvement of both the ileum and colon. From 20 to 25 % of patients have disease confined to the colon. Involvement of the esophagus, stomach, or duodenum is rare and almost always seen in association with disease of the more distal small bowel or large bowel. Approximately one-third of patients have perianal disease [2].

Accurate classification of the disease is of fundamental importance to predict the prognosis and to plan the most appropriate therapy. In 1998, the Vienna classification stratified patients with Crohn's disease according to age at diagnosis (A), disease location (L), and disease behavior (B) [3]. This classification was later revised at the 2005 Montreal World Congress of Gastroenterology

[4]. The Montreal revision of the Vienna classification has not changed the three predominant parameters of age at diagnosis, location, and behavior, but modifications within each of these categories have been made (Table 2.1).

These classifications identify 24 potential subgroups. We must also take account of the fact that the disease phenotype may change during its course [5].

Symptoms at presentation vary depending on the location, behavior, and severity of disease, as well as extraintestinal manifestations and medication. Also often the symptoms can be subtle and require differential diagnosis with other pathologies. For these reasons a long duration of symptoms before a definite diagnosis of inflammatory bowel disease is thought to be common [6]. In the past, a mean delay in diagnosis of 3.3 years from the onset of symptoms was reported [7], but more recent series have reported diagnostic delays of 1 year or less [8]. This change is to be attributed to improved diagnostic techniques and to a greater knowledge of the disease in the last decade. The pattern of penetrating disease was most associated with the risk of late diagnosis [9].

Symptoms of Crohn's disease usually begin in the teens and twenties; however, one-sixth of patients present before the age of 15. More than 90 % of patients have symptoms before the age of 40 and less than 5 % are diagnosed after the age of 60 years. Misdiagnosis at the

M. Mazza • M.G. Cilluffo • M. Cappello (✉)
Department of Integrative Virology,
Gastroenterology Section,
DiBiMis, University of Palermo, Palermo, Italy
e-mail: cmarica@tin.it

© Springer International Publishing Switzerland 2016
G. Lo Re, M. Midiri (eds.), *Crohn's Disease: Radiological Features and Clinical-Surgical Correlations*,
DOI 10.1007/978-3-319-23066-5_2

initial presentation is more common in elderly IBD patients (60 % compared with 15 % of the younger population), because in this age group the symptoms are more subtle and must perform differential diagnosis with most clinical conditions (e.g., ischemic colitis, diverticulitis, NSAID enterocolitis) [10]. Some reports have documented a less severe course of disease in the elderly [11, 12]. In a recent study, at the end of follow-up, only 30 % of the elderly patients had complications (stricturing or penetrating) compared with more than 50 % of the children [13]. With respect to the location, colon disease is the most common form in elderly CD patients, and inflammatory disease was the most frequent phenotype. A change in the behavior of CD is rare in the elderly patients [14].

Signs and symptoms of Crohn's disease can range from mild to severe. They usually develop gradually but sometimes will come on suddenly, without warning. You may also have periods of time when you have no signs or symptoms (remission). A study on the natural history and activity of the disease performed in Copenhagen County described a different behavior of the disease in several years after diagnosis: in the first year after diagnosis, 80 % of patients had high disease activity, 15 % had low activity, and 5 % were in remission. After the first year, 30 % had high activity, 15 % had low activity, and 55 % were in remission during any given year [15]. A subsequent study from Copenhagen County reported that the cumulative probability of operation 15 years after the diagnosis of Crohn's disease was 70 % [16].

The most typical symptoms include abdominal pain and diarrhea. Crampy or steady right lower quadrant or periumbilical pain may develop; the pain precedes and may be partially relieved by defecation. Diarrhea is usually not grossly bloody and is often intermittent. If the colon is involved, patients may report diffuse abdominal pain accompanied by mucus, blood, and pus in the stool. Systemic symptoms may also be present such as malaise, anorexia and weight loss, fever, anemia, malnutrition, and consequently delayed growth (in prepubescent patients). Crohn's disease may cause also intesti-

nal complications such as obstruction due to strictures, fistulas (often perianal), or abscesses [17–19].

Each subtype has a distinct clinical presentation and typical course; thus, the clinical picture of Crohn's disease depends on the areas of the bowel that are involved.

Patients with inflammation of the *jejunum and ileum* often present with cramping abdominal pain 1–2 h after meals and eventually develop diarrhea. Patients lose weight because they eat less to avoid discomfort.

Disease of the *ileum*, often accompanied by involvement of the cecum, may present insidiously. Some patients may present initially with a small bowel obstruction. Many years of subclinical inflammation may progress to fibrotic stenosis, with the subsequent onset of sub-occlusive symptoms characterized by intermittent colicky pain accompanied by nausea and vomiting. Physical examination may reveal fullness or a tender mass in the right lower quadrant. For many patients with ileal Crohn's disease, the predominant complaint is right lower quadrant pain, often exacerbated by eating. Other localizations of pain may be reported in rough proximity to the localization of disease. History provides useful clues to differentiate organic from functional causes of altered bowel habit and abdominal pain. Patients with an active inflammatory disease more often present with anorexia, diarrhea, and weight loss. Examination may reveal fever or evidence of malnutrition. Occasionally, a patient may present with a more acute onset of right lower quadrant pain, mimicking appendicitis. Most patients with small bowel Crohn's disease have an increase in the number of bowel movements, although rarely more than 5 per day, with soft and unformed stools. About 80 % of patients with ileal disease have diarrhea.

Colonic disease may involve primarily the right colon or may extend distally to involve most or all of the colon, although most patients with Crohn's colitis have relative or complete sparing of the rectum; for this reason tenesmus is a less frequent complaint than in patients with ulcerative colitis. The typical presenting symptom is diarrhea, occasionally with passage of obvious blood. Alternating diarrhea and constipation more strongly suggests irritable bowel syndrome than IBD, whereas nocturnal diarrhea is rarely noted in functional disorders of the bowel. The severity of the diarrhea tends to correlate with both the extent of colitis and the severity of inflammation, and the presentation may range from minimally altered bowel habits to fulminant colitis. Abdominal pain may be present to a greater extent than is seen in ulcerative colitis. The most common systemic manifestations are weight loss and malaise.

Perianal disease is another hallmark presentation. In some series it is described that perianal disease may precede the intestinal manifestations of Crohn's disease with a mean lead time of 4 years in 24 % of patients [20]. More often, the onset of perianal disease occurs concomitantly with or after the onset of the symptoms of luminal disease. Perianal disease can occur in various forms: skin lesions, anal canal lesions, and perianal fistulas [21]. Skin lesions include maceration, superficial ulcers, and abscesses. Anal canal lesions include fissures, ulcers, and stenosis. Perianal fistulas are common, estimated to occur among 15–35 % of patients. The patients may have debilitating perirectal pain and malodorous discharge from the fistula. Perianal fistulas are divided into simple and complex, depending on their location in the anal canal, and often represent the manifestation of a deep abscess. In some cases, perianal fistulization may be extensive, forming a network of passages and extending to multiple openings that may include not only the perianal region but also the labia or scrotum, buttocks, or thighs. Patients with rectovaginal fistula present with persistent vaginal discharge and may also complain of dyspareunia or perineal pain.

The involvement of the *upper gastrointestinal* tract in Crohn's disease is uncommon in the absence of disease beyond the ligament of Treitz. It is described in the literature that about one-third of patients with proximal Crohn's disease do not have evidence of distal disease at the time of diagnosis, but virtually all develop distal disease in time [22]. Patients with proximal disease tend to be younger at the time of diagnosis; both

are predictors of a more aggressive disease course [23, 24]. The most common symptoms of this type of localization of the disease are abdominal pain and malaise; often gastroduodenal involvement presents as *Helicobacter pylori*-negative peptic ulcer disease, with dyspepsia or epigastric pain as the primary symptoms. Early satiety, nausea, vomiting, and weight loss may predominate when there is the formation of stenosis.

The involvement of the *esophagus* is rare, occurring in less than 2 % of patients. The presenting symptoms may include dysphagia, odynophagia, substernal chest pain, and heartburn. These symptoms may be progressive and lead to profound weight loss [25].

Aphthous ulcers may sometimes be found in the *mouth and posterior pharynx*. Esophageal stricture and even esophagobronchial fistula may complicate the course [26].

Complications from ulcerations and strictures can result in abdominal or perianal fistulous tracts and abscesses, gastrointestinal (GI) bleeding, or intestinal obstruction.

Fistulas from one segment of the gastrointestinal tract to another also occur frequently. Enteroenteric, enterocolonic, and colocolonic fistulas are often asymptomatic. In patients with coloduodenal or cologastric fistula, fecaloid vomiting may occur, but this is a rare clinical manifestation. Enterovesical or colovesical fistulas may present as recurrent polymicrobial urinary tract infection or as frank pneumaturia and fecaluria. Enterocutaneous fistulas to the anterior abdomen often occur after surgery.

Development of fistulas into the mesentery or luminal microperforation may result in intra-abdominal or retroperitoneal *abscess* formation. It has been estimated that as many as one-fourth of all patients with Crohn's disease will present with an intra-abdominal abscess at some time in their lives [27]. The classic presentation of an intra-abdominal abscess is fevers and focal abdominal pain or localized peritoneal signs.

Obstruction is a common complication of Crohn's disease and one of the major indications for surgical intervention. Strictures represent long-standing inflammation and may occur in any segment of the gastrointestinal tract in which inflammation has been active but are more frequent in the small intestine. Initially, the obstruction is secondary to inflammatory edema and spasm of the bowel and manifests as postprandial bloating, cramping pains (lower right quadrant), and borborygmi. Once the bowel lumen becomes chronically narrowed from fibrosis, patients may complain of constipation and obstipation. These symptoms generally do not improve with anti-inflammatory agents. The stenosis may be asymptomatic until the residual bowel caliber is enough to cause the typical sub-occlusive symptoms characterized by postprandial abdominal pain, nausea, and vomiting. Complete obstruction may sometimes be caused by impaction of undigested foods. The clinician may find it extremely difficult to differentiate a fibrostenotic from an inflammatory stricture because the symptoms are the same.

Microperforation typically occurs into other segments of the bowel, leading to fistulas, or into areas such as the retroperitoneum, resulting in abscess formation.

Frank perforation is more uncommon, but it is one of the most serious complications of Crohn's disease if it occurs. The presenting features of frank perforation are those of classic peritonitis, although these features can sometimes be masked by high-dose corticosteroid or immunosuppressant therapy.

Colonic malignancy is a clinically significant complication of Crohn's disease with colonic involvement, like ulcerative colitis; the risk of colonic neoplasia in patients with Crohn's disease is a recognized complication of the disease. A meta-analysis revealed that the cumulative risk of colon cancer in Crohn's disease approaches 3 % at 10 years and 8 % at 30 years [28]. The risk of colon cancer appears to be related to the severity and the duration of the disease, the age at disease onset, stricture formation, and the presence of primary sclerosing cholangitis. It is widely known that individuals diagnosed at a younger age have a long disease duration (>8 years) and that those with concomitant primary sclerosing cholangitis are at an increased risk for colorectal cancer [29]. Chronic inflammation is the conjectured etiology for the development of dysplasia followed by cancer. Most cases of colorectal cancer develop from early histologic lesions referred

to as low-grade dysplasia (LGD) or dysplasia-associated lesion or mass (DALM). Sporadic adenomas can also progress to colon cancer. These are premalignant or precancerous lesions that progress to cancer via a pathway of inflammation and genetic mutations. In those patients with Crohn's disease for 8–10 years, colonoscopic surveillance should be undertaken at 2–3 year intervals and at 1–2 year intervals for patients with a disease history of over 20 years. Increased risks of small bowel cancer have been also reported [30], and an excess risk of lymphoproliferative disorders in IBD associated with immunosuppressive treatment has been demonstrated [31].

Extraintestinal manifestations of CD include musculoskeletal engaging peripheral or axial joints (arthritis, sacroiliitis), dermatologic (pyoderma gangrenosum, erythema nodosum), ocular (iritis, episcleritis), hepatobiliary, vascular, and renal complications [32]. About 25–46 % of the patients with CD will experience extraintestinal manifestations [33].

The most common EIMs are arthritis and arthralgia. Colitic arthritis is usually a migratory arthritis that affects the large joints knees, ankles, hips, wrists, and elbows that may accompany Crohn's disease (although it is uncommon when Crohn's is confined to the small intestine). Often, joint pain, swelling, and stiffness parallel the course of the bowel disease. Successful treatment of the bowel disease results in improvement in the arthritic symptoms [34].

Pericholangitis, usually associated with primary sclerosing cholangitis (PSC), is the most reported hepatic complication of inflammatory bowel disease. Primary sclerosing cholangitis has prevalence of 1.4–3.5 % in CD, potentially causing liver failure or cholangiocarcinoma [35]. Recent literature has reported however that the most common hepatic complications in Crohn's are steatosis and drug-induced cholestasis [36].

Kidney stones (calcium oxalate stones) and renal failure are seen in patients with small intestine Crohn's disease. Inflammation from the bowel can result in urinary tract complications. Occlusion of the ureters, leading to obstruction and hydronephrosis, usually involves the right ureter in Crohn's patients. Fistula can form between the inflamed bowel and the urinary bladder leading to infection.

Malnutrition, micronutrient deficiencies, and metabolic bone disease are reported in 20–50 % of CD outpatients [37]. Short bowel syndrome with intestinal failure as a result of extensive disease or bowel resection is rare but highly influential on morbidity and mortality. CD patients are also liable to functional GI disorders, either idiopathic or secondary to bowel resection [38]. Finally, published data indicate a higher prevalence of psychiatric disorders, especially depression, in CD compared with background population [39]. CD has been associated also with a wide array of diseases, many of which reflect susceptibility to autoimmune disorders (rheumatoid arthritis, psoriasis, diabetes mellitus type 1, thyroid disorders, etc.).

2.1   Physical Examination

The physical examination should focus on temperature, weight, nutritional status, the presence of abdominal tenderness or a mass, perianal and rectal examination findings, and extraintestinal manifestations (EIMs). A patient may have a completely normal physical examination of the right lower quadrant. For months, the only objective evidence of disease may be unexplained low-grade fever, polyarthralgia, iron-deficiency anemia, hypoalbuminemia, guaiac-positive stools, elevated C-reactive protein, or an elevated erythrocyte sedimentation rate. Children and teenagers who present with fever and arthralgia may be given a misdiagnosis of rheumatic fever or juvenile rheumatoid arthritis. Prepubescent patients may have a slowing of growth 1–2 years before weight gain slows or gastrointestinal symptoms begin. Vital signs are usually normal in patients with Crohn's disease, though tachycardia may be present in anemic or dehydrated patients. Chronic intermittent fever is a common presenting sign. Abdominal findings may vary from normal to those of an acute abdomen. Diffuse abdominal tenderness or localized pain may be present. Fullness or a discrete mass may be appreciated, typically in the right lower quadrant of the abdomen (which is usual with ileal

involvement), or a mass may be felt secondary to thickened or matted loops of the inflamed bowel.

The perineum should be inspected in all patients who present with signs and symptoms of Crohn's disease because abnormalities detectable in this region substantially increase the clinical suspicion of inflammatory bowel disease (IBD). Inspection of the perianal region can reveal skin tags, fistulas, ulcers, abscesses, and scarring. A rectal examination can help to determine sphincter tone and aid in detecting gross abnormalities of the rectal mucosa or the presence of hematochezia.

Examination of the skin and oral mucosa may show mucocutaneous or aphthous ulcers, erythema nodosum, and pyoderma gangrenosum. Skin examination may also reveal pallor in patients with anemia or jaundice in those with concomitant liver disease with cholestasis. Eye examination may reveal episcleritis. For the diagnosis of uveitis, a slit-lamp examination by an experienced physician is necessary.

2.2   Clinical Disease Activity Indices

In the absence of a universal benchmark of disease activity in CD, attempts have been made to assemble clinical variables into a single disease activity index. Best et al. devised the Crohn's disease activity index (CDAI) by using the physician's overall appraisal of "how the patient was doing" (very poor, poor, fair to good, very well) as outcome variable in a multiple linear regression analysis of 18 clinical variables and symptoms from the last 7 days, as reported by the patient [40]. Eight independent variables were ultimately chosen to form the index, each weighted by the relative magnitude of its regression coefficient (Table 2.2). The cutoff limits between quiescent/active disease ("very well/fair to good") and active/very severe disease ("poor/very poor") were set to 150 and 450 points, respectively. Subsequently, an additional limit was arbitrarily drawn at 220 points between mild and moderate disease activity, and a reduction of 70–100 points has been deemed to indicate treatment response [41]. The CDAI has been adopted as the "gold standard" for outcome

Table 2.2 Crohn's disease activity index (CDAI)

Variable	Description	Multiplier
Number of liquid stools	Sum of 7 days	×2
Abdominal pain	Sum of 7 days ratings 0 = none 1 = mild 2 = moderate 3 = severe	×5
General well-being	Sum of 7 days ratings 0 = generally well 1 = slightly under par 2 = poor 3 = very poor 4 = terrible	×7
Extraintestinal complications	Number complications: arthritis/arthralgia, iritis/uveitis, erythema nodosum, pyoderma gangrenosum, aphthous stomatitis, anal fissure/fistula/abscess, fever >37.8	×20
Antidiarrheal drugs	Use in the previous 7 days 0 = no 1 = yes	×30
Abdominal mass	0 = no 1 = questionable 5 = definite	×10
Hematocrit	Expected–observed Hct Males: 47 observed Females: 42 observed	×6
Body weight	Ideal/observed ratio $[1-(ideal/observed)] \times 100$	×1 (NOT < −10)

Remission: less than 150
Response: decrease greater than 70 points (greater than 100 points in more recent clinical trials)
Mild disease: 150–220
Moderate disease: 220–450
Severe disease: greater than 450

assessment in clinical trials, its use being a prerequisite for regulatory approval of new therapies by authorities in the USA and Europe. Adapted versions of the CDAI have been constructed for use in children and in patients with perianal fistulizing disease. Concerns were raised against the CDAI as being largely determined by subjective variables [41].

The Harvey-Bradshaw index (HBI) [42] is a derivative of the CDAI, excluding the laboratory variables and only recalling symptoms from the last 24 h (Table 2.3). The HBI correlates strongly ($r > 0.90$) with the CDAI and has been used to simplify disease activity assessment.

Emerging CD concepts emphasize the progressive and irreversible character of the tissue-damaging process. To capture this aspect, a multinational project has been launched to develop a global score of cumulative bowel damage (the Lemann score) [43], taking into account location and extent of stricturing or penetrating lesions and bowel resection. However, the Lemann score has not been introduced yet in clinical practice or randomized clinical trials where the CDAI or HBI is still currently used.

References

1. Silverberg MS, Satsangi J, Ahmad T, Arnott ID, Bernstein CN, Brant SR, et al. Toward an integrated clinical, molecular and serological classification of inflammatory bowel disease: report of a Working Party of the

Table 2.3 Harvey-Bradshaw simple index (HBI)

Variable	Scoring
General well-being	0 = very well 1 = slightly below par 2 = poor 3 = very poor 4 = terrible
Abdominal pain	0 = none 1 = mild 2 = moderate 3 = severe
Number of liquid stools daily	1 per occurrence
Abdominal mass	0 = none 1 = dubious 2 = definite 3 = definite and tender
Complications	1 per item: Arthralgia Uveitis Erythema nodosum Aphthous ulcer Pyoderma gangrenosum Anal fissure New fistula Abscess
Total score	Sum of variable scores

Remission: <5
Mild disease: 5–7
Moderate disease: 8–16
Severe disease: >16

2005 Montreal World Congress of Gastroenterology. Can J Gastroenterol. 2005;19(Suppl A):5–36.

2. Henriksen M, Jahnsen J, Lygren I, et al. Clinical course in Crohn's disease: results of a five-year population-based follow-up study (the IBSEN study). Scand J Gastroenterol. 2007;42:602–10.

3. Gasche C, Scholmerich J, Brynskov J, et al. A simple classification of Crohn's disease: report of the Working Party for the World Congresses of Gastroenterology, Vienna 1998. Inflamm Bowel Dis. 2000;6:8–15.

4. Satsangi J, Silverberg MS, Vermeire S, Colombel JF. The Montreal classification of inflammatory bowel disease: controversies, consensus, and implications. Gut. 2006;55:749–53.

5. Munkholm P. Crohn's disease occurrence, course and prognosis. An epidemiologic cohort-study. Dan Med Bull. 1997;44:287.

6. Pimentel M, Chang M, Chow EJ, et al. Identification of a prodromal period in Crohn's disease but not ulcerative colitis. Am J Gastroenterol. 2000;95:3458–62.

7. Higgens CS, Allan RN. Crohn's disease of the distal ileum. Gut. 1980;21:933.

8. Burgmann T, Clara I, Graff L, Walker J, Lix L, Rawsthorne P, et al. The Manitoba Inflammatory Bowel Disease Cohort Study: prolonged symptoms before diagnosis–how much is irritable bowel syndrome? Clin Gastroenterol Hepatol. 2006;4(5): 614–20.

9. Pellino G, Sciaudone G, Selvaggi F, Riegler G. Delayed diagnosis is influenced by the clinical pattern of Crohn's disease and affects treatment outcomes and quality of life in the long term: a cross-sectional study of 361 patients in Southern Italy. Eur J Gastroenterol Hepatol. 2015;27(2):175–81.

10. Wagtmans MJ, Verspaget HW, Lamers CB, et al. Crohn's disease in the elderly: a comparison with younger adults. J Clin Gastroenterol. 1998;27:129–33.

11. Travis S. Is IBD, different in the elderly? Inflamm Bowel Dis. 2008;14 Suppl 2:S12–3.

12. Piront P, Louis E, Latour P, Plomteux O, Belaiche J. Epidemiology of inflammatory bowel diseases in the elderly in the province of Liege. Gastroenterol Clin Biol. 2002;26:157–61.

13. Gower-Rousseau C, Vasseur F, Fumery M, et al. Epidemiology of inflammatory bowel diseases: new insights from a French population-based registry (EPIMAD). Dig Liver Dis. 2013;45:89–94.

14. Heresbach D, Alexandre JL, Bretagne JF, et al. Crohn's disease in the over-60 age group: a population based study. Eur J Gastroenterol Hepatol. 2004;16:657–64.

15. Munkholm P, Langholz E, Davidsen M, Binder V. Disease activity courses in a regional cohort of Crohn's disease patients. Scand J Gastroenterol. 1995;30: 699–706.

16. Munkholm P, Langholz E, Davidsen M, Binder V. Intestinal cancer risk and mortality in patients with Crohn's disease. Gastroenterology. 1993;105: 1716–23.

17. Kornbluth A, Sachar DB, Salomon P. Crohn's disease. In: Feldman M, Scharschmidt BF, Sleisenger MH, editors. Sleisenger & Fordtran's gastrointestinal and liver disease: pathophysiology, diagnosis, and management, vol. 2. 6th ed. Philadelphia: WB Saunders Co; 1998. p. 1708–34.

18. Thoreson R, Cullen JJ. Pathophysiology of inflammatory bowel disease: an overview. Surg Clin North Am. 2007;87(3):575–85.

19. Friedman S, Blumberg RS. Inflammatory bowel disease. In: Braunwald E, Fauci AS, Kasper DS, et al., editors. Harrison's principles of internal medicine, vol. 2. 15th ed. New York: McGraw-Hill Professional Publishing; 2001. p. 1679–91.

20. Baker WN, Milton-Thompson GJ. The anal lesion as the sole presenting symptom of intestinal Crohns disease. Gut. 1971;12:865.

21. Buchmann P, Alexander-Williams J. Classification of perianal Crohn's disease. Clin Gastroenterol. 1980;9:323.

22. Wagtmans MJ, Verspaget HW, Lamers CB, et al. Clinical aspects of Crohns disease of the upper gastrointestinal tract: a comparison with distal Crohns disease. Am J Gastroenterol. 1997;92:1467.

23. Jess T, Winther KV, Munkholm P, et al. Mortality and causes of death in Crohn's disease: follow-up of

a population-based cohort in Copenhagen County, Denmark. Gastroenterology. 2002;122:1808–14.

24. Loly C, Belaiche J, Louis E. Predictors of severe Crohn's disease. Scand J Gastroenterol. 2008;43: 948–54.

25. DHaens G, Rutgeerts P, Geboes K, et al. The natural history of esophageal Crohns disease: three patterns of evolution. Gastrointest Endosc. 1994;40:296.

26. Oberhuber G, Puspok A, Peck-Radosavlevic M, et al. Aberrant esophageal HLA-DR expression in a high percentage of patients with Crohns disease. Am J Surg Pathol. 1999;23:970.

27. Ribeiro MB, Greenstein AJ, Yamazaki Y, et al. Intra-abdominal abscess in regional enteritis. Ann Surg. 1991;213:32.

28. Canavan C, Abrams KR, Mayberry J. Meta-analysis: colorectal and small bowel cancer risk in patients with Crohn's disease. Aliment Pharmacol Ther. 2006;23(8): 1097–104.

29. Herrinton LJ, Liu L, Levin TR, Allison JE, Lewis JD, Velayos F. Incidence and mortality of colorectal adenocarcinoma in persons with inflammatory bowel disease from 1998 to 2010. Gastroenterology. 2012;143(2):382–9.

30. Jess T, Gamborg M, Matzen P, Munkholm P, Sørensen TIA. Increased risk of intestinal cancer in Crohn's disease: a meta-analysis of population-based cohort studies. Am J Gastroenterol. 2005;100:2724–9.

31. Beaugerie L, Brousse N, Bouvier AM, Colombel JF, Lémann M, Cosnes J, Hébuterne X, Cortot A, Bouhnik Y, Gendre JP, Simon T, Maynadié M, Hermine O, Faivre J, Carrat F, for the CESAME Study Group. Lymphoproliferative disorders in patients receiving thiopurines for inflammatory bowel disease: a prospective observational cohort study. Lancet. 2009;374(7–13):1617–25.

32. Repiso A, Alcántara M, Muñoz-Rosas C, Rodríguez-Merlo R, Pérez-Grueso MJ, Carrobles JM, Martínez-Potenciano JL. Extraintestinal manifestations of Crohn's disease: prevalence and related factors. Rev Esp Enferm Dig. 2006;98:510–7.

33. Ephgrave K. Extra-intestinal manifestations of Crohn's disease. Surg Clin North Am. 2007;87:673–80.

34. Nikolaus S, Schreiber S. Diagnostics of inflammatory bowel disease. Gastroenterology. 2007;133(5): 1670–89.

35. Navaneethan U, Shen B. Hepatopancreatobiliary manifestations and complications associated with inflammatory bowel disease. İnflamm Bowel Dis. 2010;16:1598–619.

36. Cappello M, Randazzo C, Bravatà I, et al. Liver function test abnormalities in patients with inflammatory bowel diseases: a hospital-based survey. Clin Med Insights Gastroenterol. 2014;7:25–31.

37. Lim H, Kim HJ, Hong SJ, Kim S. Nutrient intake and bone mineral density by nutritional status in patients with inflammatory bowel disease. Bone Metab. 2014; 21(3):195–203.

38. De Schepper HU, De Man JG, Moreels TG, Pelckmans PA, De Winter BY. Review article: gastrointestinal sensory and motor disturbances in inflammatory bowel disease – clinical relevance and pathophysiological mechanisms. Aliment Pharmacol Ther. 2008;27(8):621–37.

39. Häuser W, Janke K-H, Klump B, Hinz A. Anxiety and depression in patients with inflammatory bowel disease: comparisons with chronic liver disease patients and the general population. Inflamm Bowel Dis. 2011;17(2): 621–32.

40. Best WR, Becktel JM, Singleton JW, Kern Jr F. Development of a Crohn's disease activity index. Gastroenterology. 1976;70:439–44.

41. Travis SPL, Stange EF, Lémann M, Oresland T, Chowers Y, Forbes A, D' Haens G, Kitis G, Cortot A, Prantera C, Marteau P, Colombel JF, Gionchetti P, Bouhnik Y, Tiret E, Kroesen J, Starlinger M, McM Mortensen NJ, for the European Crohn's and Colitis Organisation (ECCO). European evidence based consensus on the diagnosis and management of Crohn's disease: current management. Gut. 2006;55(1): 16–35.

42. Harvey R, Bradshaw J. A simple index of Crohn's-disease activity. Lancet. 1980;8167:514.

43. Pariente B, Cosnes J, Danese S, et al. Development of the Crohn's disease digestive damage score, the Lémann score. Inflamm Bowel Dis. 2011;17:1415–22.

Laboratory Tests in Crohn's Disease

3

Gaetano C. Morreale, Maria Cappello, and Antonio Craxì

3.1   Introduction

Laboratory tests are useful for diagnosing Crohn's disease, assessing disease activity, identifying complications, and monitoring response to therapy. Their role has been considered limited in the past due to lack of specificity. The introduction of biological therapies in inflammatory bowel disease (IBD) has renewed interest in inflammatory markers, especially C-reactive protein (CRP), given their potential to select responders to these treatments. There are several reasons why laboratory markers have been studied in IBD in the past decades: firstly, to gain an objective measurement of disease activity as symptoms are often subjective; secondly, to avoid invasive (endoscopic) procedures which are often a burden to the patient. An ideal marker should have many qualities. It should be easy and rapid to perform, cheap, and reproducible between patients and laboratories. The ideal laboratory marker should furthermore be able to identify individuals at risk for the disease and should be disease specific; it should be able to detect disease activity and monitor the effect of treatment; and finally, it should have a prognostic value towards relapse or recurrence of the disease. Unfortunately, no

single marker has proven to possess all the above listed qualities although some interesting markers have been identified. The presence of active gut inflammation in patients with IBD is associated with an acute-phase reaction and migration of leucocytes to the gut, and this is translated into the production of several proteins, which may be detected in serum or stools [1–4].

Initial testing often includes white blood cell count, platelet count, measurement of hemoglobin, hematocrit, blood urea nitrogen, creatinine, liver enzymes, CRP, and erythrocyte sedimentation rate (ESR). Stool culture and testing for *Clostridium difficile* toxin should be considered [5]. Presence of antibodies to *Escherichia coli* outer membrane porin and *Saccharomyces cerevisiae* is suggestive of Crohn's disease, whereas perinuclear antineutrophil cytoplasmic antibody is more suggestive of ulcerative colitis [6]. Subsequent testing may include measurement of iron, ferritin, total iron-binding capacity, vitamin B_{12}, folate, albumin, prealbumin, calcium, and vitamin D to monitor common complications (especially malnutrition and selective deficiencies). Fecal lactoferrin and calprotectin are surrogate markers for bowel inflammation and may help distinguish between inflammatory conditions and irritable bowel syndrome [7, 8]. An elevated fecal calprotectin level reliably indicates relapse in patients with Crohn's disease (sensitivity 80 %, specificity 90.7 %; positive likelihood ratio 1.9; negative likelihood ratio 0.04) [7].

G.C. Morreale • M. Cappello (✉) • A. Craxì
Gastroenterology Section,
DiBiMis, University of Palermo, Palermo, Italy
e-mail: cmarica@tin.it

© Springer International Publishing Switzerland 2016
G. Lo Re, M. Midiri (eds.), *Crohn's Disease: Radiological Features and Clinical-Surgical Correlations*,
DOI 10.1007/978-3-319-23066-5_3

3.2   CRP and ESR

CRP level and ESR correlate with disease activity. Unfortunately, a normal ESR or CRP level does not rule out disease activity and should be considered ancillary texts to endoscopic or radiological assessment. This is due, as above-mentioned, to a problem of specificity. CRP is a pentameric protein consisting of five monomers and is one of the most important acute-phase proteins in humans [9]. Under normal circumstances, CRP is produced by hepatocytes in low quantities (0.1 mg/l). However, following an acute-phase stimulus such as inflammation, hepatocytes rapidly increase production of CRP under the influence of interleukin (IL)-6, tumor necrosis factor-α (TNF-α), and IL-1beta and may reach peak levels of 350–400 mg/l. CRP has a short half-life (19 h) compared with other acute-phase proteins and will therefore rise early after the onset of inflammation and rapidly decrease after resolution of the inflammation. The function of CRP in vivo is still incompletely understood. CRP binds to phosphocholine-containing microorganisms or particles which in turn lead to C1q and classical complement activation. CRP also plays a role in the opsonization of infectious agents and damaged cells [10–13]. CD is associated with a strong CRP response, due to serum IL-6 concentrations elevation compared to healthy controls. ESR is the rate at which erythrocytes migrate through the plasma. Inevitably, ESR will depend on the plasma concentration and on the number and size of the erythrocytes. Conditions such as anemia, polycythemia, and thalassemia affect ESR [14]. Compared with CRP, ESR will peak much less rapidly and may also take several days to decrease, even if the clinical condition of the patient or the inflammation is ameliorated. Increases in ESR with age have been described [15].

Only a few studies have investigated the value of laboratory markers in identifying individuals at risk for IBD and furthermore not all studies used the same markers. An early study from St Mark's Hospital, London, UK, investigated 82 adults referred with abdominal symptoms [16]. In all patients, clinical examination as well as a rectal biopsy were performed and ESR, CRP,

and a1-glycoprotein were determined. Of these markers, CRP was increased in all patients who subsequently were diagnosed with CD ($n = 19$), in 50 % of patients diagnosed with UC ($n = 22$), but in none of the 41 patients with functional bowel symptoms. The best laboratory marker in differentiating IBD from normal subjects was CRP. Similar results were reported in the study by Shine and colleagues on a pediatric population undergoing colonoscopy [16], in which 100 % of CD patients had increased CRP compared with none of the children with polyps and none of the children with a normal investigation. ESR proved to be the second best marker, with 85 % of CD positive compared with none of the children with a normal investigation. Finally, a larger study on 203 individuals referred for symptoms suggestive of lower bowel disease also showed that CRP was a good marker in discriminating IBD from irritable bowel syndrome (IBS) [17].

Laboratory tests are useful to monitor disease activity. In general, patients with severe disease more often have abnormal inflammatory markers, compared with patients without or with only low-grade inflammation. This has been shown in a prospective study by Tromm and colleagues [18] who investigated laboratory markers such as ESR, serum albumin, a1 proteinase inhibitor, cholinesterase, CRP, and hematocrit, and correlated these markers with endoscopic activity. A previous study in IBD showed a good correlation between ESR and clinical activity [19]. The correlation was, however, dependent on disease location, and ESR correlated less well with UC restricted to the rectum and with CD restricted to the upper small bowel [19, 20]. The study by Fagan et al. [21] showed that both CRP and ESR correlated well with disease activity but the correlation was better for CRP. This was also the conclusion from various other studies where CRP was either the best marker or the only marker which correlated significantly with clinical activity status [21]. However, a wide range of CRP values was observed and overlap existed between mild to moderate (10–50 mg/l), moderate to severe (50–80 mg/l), and severe disease (.80 mg/l). What is undoubtedly more important than a particular cut off value for CRP is the comparison of the CRP value with previous values in a given patient. Apart from clinical activity, data from the Mayo Clinic have also shown good correlation between CRP and endoscopic and histologic activity in CD.

CRP has been shown to be a good marker for predicting disease course and outcome in a number of diseases. Well known is its association with cardiovascular disease and poor outcome after myocardial infarction [22–24]. Also, in multiple myeloma, serum CRP is a highly significant prognostic factor and high CRP and high beta2 microglobulin levels are associated with worse survival [25]. A number of studies in CD have investigated a panel of laboratory markers in predicting clinical relapse. A prospective study by Brignola et al. monitored 41 CD patients with clinically inactive disease (CDAI <150) for 6 months using a panel of inflammatory markers (ESR, white blood cells, hemoglobin, albumin, a2 globulin, serum iron, CRP, a1 glycoprotein, and a2 antitrypsin) [26]. All patients were followed up until relapse. A total of 17/41 patients relapsed. ESR, a2 globulin, and a1 glycoprotein were best at distinguishing relapsers from non-relapsers. Based on these markers, a prognostic index (PI) was calculated and the threshold of discriminant power was 0.35. Using this threshold, all patients with a PI >0.35 relapsed over a period of 18 months, compared with 5/29 patients with a PI< 0.35. Therefore, although normal values did not guarantee remission in all patients, high values predicted relapse in the following 1–2 years. A few years later, Boirivant et al. prospectively followed 101 outpatients with CD [27]. Half of the patients had a raised CRP and this correlated well with clinical activity. Approximately one third of CD patients presented with active disease despite normal CRP, and one third had raised CRP but clinically inactive disease. The likelihood of relapse after two years was higher in patients with an increased CRP compared with patients with normal CRP. More recently, the GETAID group prospectively followed 71 CD patients with medically induced remission and measured laboratory markers (full blood count, CRP, ESR, a1 antitrypsin, orosomucoid) every 6 weeks [28]. In total, 38 patients relapsed (defined as a CDAI >150 or an increase of .100 points from baseline) after a median of 31 weeks. Only two

laboratory markers were predictive of relapse: CRP (.20 mg/l) and ESR (.15 mm). Patients with both markers positive had an eightfold increased risk for relapse with a negative predictive value of 97 %, suggesting that normal CRP and ESR could almost certainly rule out relapse in the next 6 weeks.

It is clear that we still cannot rely on CRP alone to predict clinical relapse in CD. One of the crucial questions is how early or late CRP and other inflammatory markers start increasing and what the ideal time would be to measure them.

A change in CRP following therapy is a good parameter to assess the effect of the drug on the underlying inflammation. A decrease in CRP in response to therapy is objective evidence that the drug has a beneficial effect on gut inflammation and this holds even in patients with little change in symptoms. On the other hand, persistently raised CRP indicates failure of the therapy to control mucosal inflammation. Introduction of biological therapies in IBD has led to a major improvement in treatment options. Anti-TNF-alpha antibodies are very efficacious in patients with CD. Nevertheless, anti-TNF treatment fails in approximately 25 % of patients. In a Belgian study, in 153 patients treated with infliximab, a baseline CRP >0.5 mg/l before the start of therapy was associated with a higher response (76 %) compared with patients with CRP< 0.5 mg/l (46 %) ($p = 0.004$) [29]. Very similar results have been demonstrated for the humanized anti-TNF molecules CDP-571 and CDP-870 and for the fully human anti-TNF antibodies adalimumab and anti-adhesion molecule strategies [30–32]. Along the same lines, low or normal baseline CRP values have been associated with a high placebo response and remission rate in clinical trials [33].

3.3 Hematologic Tests

The components of the complete blood cell (CBC) count can be useful indicators of disease activity and iron or vitamin deficiency. An elevated white blood cell (*WBC*) count is common in patients with active inflammatory disease and does not necessarily indicate infection. High leukocyte count is common also in patients taking steroids due to drug-induced mobilization of marginated neutrophils. Anemia is common and may be either an anemia of chronic disease (usually normal mean corpuscular volume [MCV]) or an iron deficiency anemia (MCV is often low). Anemia may result from acute or chronic blood loss and malabsorption (iron, folate, and vitamin B_{12}) or may reflect reduced intake or chronic inflammatory burden. Note that macrocytosis (elevated MCV) occurs in patients taking azathioprine or 6-mercaptopurine (6-MP). Generally, the platelet count is normal but may be elevated in the setting of active inflammation or iron deficiency. Given to wide variability of reference value, the use of platelet count to monitor disease activity is low.

Due to the high prevalence of malnutrition in CD, vitamin B_{12} and folic acid level often need to be evaluated. *Vitamin B_{12}* deficiency can occur in patients with CD who have significant terminal ileum disease or in patients who have had terminal ileum resection. The standard replacement dose of vitamin B_{12} is 1000 mg subcutaneously (SC) every month, because oral replacement is often insufficient. Serum *iron* studies should be obtained at the time of diagnosis, because active IBD is a source for GI blood loss, making iron deficiency common. A microcytic hypochromic anemia suggests iron deficiency; if confirmed with serum iron/total iron-binding capacity (TIBC), iron can be replaced either orally or parenterally. For parenteral replacement, intravenous (IV) iron sucrose or, more recently, iron-carboxymaltose, can be used, and dosing is based on the table in the package insert, with a maximum of 30 mL (1500 mg) at once. Although *folate* deficiency is not common in persons with IBD, several concerns have been raised regarding this vitamin. Sulfasalazine (Azulfidine) is a folate reductase inhibitor and may inhibit normal uptake of folate; thus, many practitioners commonly administer folate supplements in patients taking sulfasalazine. Folate supplements are indicated in all women who are pregnant to help prevent neural tube defects; this is particularly true for patients with IBD, and supplementation with 2 mg/day or more (rather than the usual 1 mg/day) should be considered in those on sulfasalazine. Folic acid deficiency is common in patients taking methotrexate and folic acid supplementation the day after methotrexate administration is recommended. Nutritional status can be assessed by serum albumin, prealbumin, and transferrin levels. However, note that transferrin is an acute-phase reactant that can be falsely elevated in persons with active IBD. Hypoalbuminemia may reflect malnutrition because of poor oral intake or because of the protein-losing enteropathy that can coexist with active IBD. *Albumin* is a typical example of a negative acute-phase reactant, and decreased levels may be found during inflammation. However, other conditions such as malnutrition and malabsorption also cause low albumin levels. Other acute-phase reactants include *sialic acid*, alpha-1-acid glycoprotein orosomucoid, fibrinogen, lactoferrin, b2microglobulin, serum amyloid A, a2 globulin, and a1antitrypsin. Most of these markers have not been studied widely in IBD and many have shown conflicting results. Furthermore, their use in IBD has not proved superior to CRP in general, mainly due to the longer half-life of these proteins. Beta2 microglobulin is a low-molecular-weight protein and is released by activated T and B lymphocytes on activation. The estimated half-life is 2 h. Beta2 microglobulin is filtered through the glomeruli, and levels increase with age and also with decreasing kidney function. Orosomucoids have been shown to correlate well with disease activity, but its half-life of 5 days makes this a less useful marker in clinical practice [34, 35]. Finally, some authors showed good correlation between beta2 microglobulin and disease activity [36–38]. However, data were conflicting and not all authors were able to confirm these findings [39].

3.4 Fecal Calprotectin and Other Fecal Marker

Stool samples should be tested for the presence of white blood cells (WBCs), occult blood, routine pathogens, ova, parasites, and *Clostridium difficile* toxin. An obvious reason to search for fecal markers is that stools are easily accessible in IBD patients and because fecal markers would have a higher specificity for IBD in the absence of gastrointestinal infection. Stool samples can also be studied to rule out infectious etiologies during relapses and before the initiation of immunosuppressive agents [40]. A number of neutrophil-derived proteins present in stools have been studied, including fecal lactoferrin, lysozyme, elastase, myeloperoxidase, and calprotectin [4].

Fecal calprotectin has been proposed as a noninvasive surrogate marker of intestinal inflammation in IBD. As colorectal neoplasia and gastrointestinal infection also increase fecal calprotectin, this marker is not in widespread use. Note that relatives of patients with IBD may also have elevated levels of fecal calprotectin (with unknown degrees of inflammation) [41]. Calprotectin, a 36 kDa calcium- and zinc-binding protein, is probably the most promising marker for various reasons. In contrast with other neutrophil markers, calprotectin represents 60 % of cytosolic proteins in granulocytes. The presence of calprotectin in feces can therefore be seen as directly proportional to neutrophil migration to the gastrointestinal tract. Although calprotectin is a very sensitive marker for detection of inflammation in the gastrointestinal tract, it is not a specific marker and increased levels are also found in neoplasia, IBD, infections, and polyps [4]. Fecal calprotectin is a very stable marker (stable for more than 1 week at room temperature) and is resistant to degradation, which makes it attractive. Early studies using fecal calprotectin in IBD have shown a good correlation with indium-labeled leukocyte excretion and intestinal permeability [42]. Increased fecal calprotectin levels have been reported after the use of nonsteroidal anti-inflammatory drugs as well as with increasing age [43]. More recently, fecal calprotectin was shown to predict relapse of CD [44–46]. In the study by Tibble et al., calprotectin levels of 50 mg/g or more predicted a 13-fold increased risk for relapse [44]. A baseline level of calprotectin of 150 mg/g or more was predictive for a relapse in the next year. A study by Henderson et al. indicated that fecal calprotectin has a high sensitivity and modest specificity for diagnosing IBD in children. The researchers conducted a systematic review and meta-analysis of eight studies including 394 pediatric IBD cases and 321 non-IBD controls [47, 48]. The use of fecal calprotectin during the investigation of suspected pediatric IBD was associated with a pooled sensitivity of 97.8 %, a pooled specificity of 68.2 %, a positive likelihood ratio of 3.07, and a negative likelihood ratio of 0.03. *Fecal lactoferrin* is another potential marker derived from feces. It is an iron-binding glycoprotein secreted by most mucosal membranes. It is a major component of the secondary granules of PMNs and is released during inflammation, serving a role in the innate immune response. It is bactericidal, and its level may reflect the degree of neutrophil infiltration into the intestinal epithelium. Lactoferrin is less stable than calprotectin in stool and must be frozen to ensure accuracy over time. Langhorst et al. [50] assessed fecal lactoferrin, fecal calprotectin, fecal PMN-elastase, and serum CRP in patients with IBD. These markers were compared with endoscopic findings and specific activity indices for Crohn's disease and ulcerative colitis (UC). Sensitivity and specificity were measured for each test to distinguish IBD from IBS. Although there was no statistical difference between fecal markers, all three were superior to CRP. However, when any of the three fecal markers were combined with CRP and an activity index, diagnostic accuracy approached 90 %. Schroder et al. [51] compared only fecal markers in identifying established inflammation and found calprotectin to be superior to lactoferrin and PMN-elastase. Any combination of the three markers proved no more effective than the effect with calprotectin alone. Shitrit et al. [52] used calprotectin to predict abnormal colonic pathology of any type in 72 consecutive patients undergoing colonoscopy, including screening. Each patient submitted stool specimens for measurement of fecal calprotectin before colonoscopy. Patients with abnormal colonic findings had calprotectin levels that were significantly higher than in those with normal colonoscopic findings. Using a cutoff of 150 mcg/mL, calprotectin had a sensitivity of 75 %, specificity of 84 %, and positive and negative predictive values of 80 % and 75 %, respectively. Calprotectin proved effective in identifying colorectal neoplasia as well, probably related to PMN infiltration of the tumor. The authors recommended that calprotectin levels be obtained in all patients undergoing colonoscopy. Focusing specifically on its role in IBD, a number of authors have confirmed the accuracy of calprotectin in distinguishing IBD from IBS. In a meta-analysis of 13 studies involving over 1500 patients, von Roon et al. [53] found calprotectin to have a sensitivity of 89–98 % and specificity of 81–91 %. Calprotectin can also be used to assess the level of disease activity in patients with known IBD [54]. This paper demonstrated a significant association of calprotectin levels in patients with UC with clinical disease activity indices, endoscopic findings for disease extent and activity, and CRP. In the same study for patients with Crohn's disease, calprotectin did not correlate with clinical disease activity but did significantly so for both the Vienna classification and endoscopic findings of active inflammation. In another study of patients with UC alone, Schoepfer et al. [55] not only found a significant correlation with the endoscopic activity index but also found that, among CRP, clinical activity index, and leukocytosis, only calprotectin levels were able to reliably discriminate between all levels of clinical activity. It is not surprising that in Crohn's disease, there is no significant correlation between calprotectin and clinical activity index, as clinical activity indices such as Crohn's Disease Activity Index (CDAI) or Harvey-Bradshaw Index correlate poorly with endoscopic findings. This again was demonstrated by Jones et al. [56] who evaluated the relationship between disease activity and fecal biomarkers. With the advent of biological agents, for example, tumor necrosis factor inhibitors, mucosal healing is becoming the gold standard by which therapeutic trials are measured. Serum CRP levels are inconsistent in this regard. Genetic polymorphisms within various regions of the CRP gene may influence the response to inflammation in IBD patients, making a response to Crohn's disease, at best, unpredictable. The authors in this trial measured both serum biomarkers and fecal calprotectin and lactoferrin in 164 patients with Crohn's disease scheduled for colonoscopy. There proved to be no significant association between the CDAI and endoscopic scores, nor between fecal biomarkers and CDAI. However, fecal calprotectin and lactoferrin levels were significantly higher in patients with more severe endoscopic activity.

In the *Journal of Clinical Gastroenterology*, Licata et al. [57] from the University of Palermo have assessed the role of fecal calprotectin in the evaluation of patients with chronic diarrhea. The patients were selected quite carefully after excluding all patients with overt gastrointestinal bleeding, known colorectal or gastric cancer, polyposis syndromes, active nongastrointestinal infections, and recent use of nonsteroidal anti-inflammatory drugs or aspirin. Patients who were pregnant, alcoholics, or had any other prior gastrointestinal history were also excluded. This was essential, as calprotectin may be elevated in association with many of these conditions and separating out the factors contributing to its elevation is difficult. Also, if endoscopic assessment is required regardless of the calprotectin level, the test would be unnecessary. A total of 346 consecutive patients who met these criteria and with diarrhea persisting for >4 weeks were subjected to a thorough investigation including analyses of serum CRP level, sedimentation rate, stool cultures, and ova and parasites. All patients underwent colonoscopy with biopsies. Upper endoscopy and small bowel enteroclysis studies were obtained if Crohn's disease was confirmed. After informed consent, a single stool specimen for calprotectin was submitted before colonoscopy.

Of the 346 patients entering the study, 242 (69.9 %) had normal results in the endoscopic study. IBD was confirmed in 82 patients (23.7 %), ischemic colitis in 1 (0.3 %), polyps in 10 (2.9 %), and simple diverticulosis in 11 (3.2 %). Calprotectin levels were significantly higher in those patients with an abnormal colonoscopy (*P* value <0.0001). When the authors focused on histologic changes alone, 142 (41.0 %) patients had an abnormal histology, 82 patients had IBD, 17 patients had microscopic colitis, and 22 patients had nonspecific colitis. On the basis of clinical findings, 21 of 142 patients were still believed to have IBS despite the mild increase in intestinal lymphocytes, which did not fulfill the criteria for microscopic colitis. Again, calprotectin levels were significantly higher in the patient with histologic inflammation (P value<0.001). On the basis of a multivariate linear regression model, the presence of histologic inflammation was significantly and independently associated with calprotectin levels. Using a cutoff of 150 mcg/g of stool, fecal calprotectin had 75.4 % sensitivity, 88.3 % specificity, and 81 % and 83 % positive and negative predictive values, respectively.

3.5 Other Serological Markers

Perinuclear antineutrophil cytoplasmic antibodies (pANCA) have been identified in some patients with ulcerative colitis, and anti-Saccharomyces cerevisiae antibodies (ASCA) have been found in patients with Crohn's disease. The combination of positive pANCA and negative ASCA has high specificity for ulcerative colitis, whereas the inverse pattern—positive ASCA, negative pANCA—is more specific for Crohn's disease [57]. The World Gastroenterology Organization (WGO) indicates that ulcerative colitis is more likely when the test results are positive for pANCA and negative for ASCA antigen; however, the pANCA test may be positive in Crohn's disease, and this may complicate obtaining a diagnosis in otherwise uncomplicated colitis [58]. It should be noted that both tests are recommended only as an adjunct to clinical diagnosis; the results are not specific and have been found to be positive in other bowel diseases. Patients with Crohn's disease whose condition is ASCA positive have a higher rate of surgery and require surgery earlier in the course of the disease, independent of the area of involvement [39, 59, 60]. Additional serologic markers, such as Escherichia coli anti-ompC (outer membrane porin C), can be found in more than 50 % of Crohn's disease cases. Pseudomonas fluorescens (anti-12) may be found in more than 50 % of Crohn's disease, flagellin-like antigen (anti-Cbir1) is associated independently with small bowel, penetrating, and fibrostenosing disease.

Indeed, serum response to anti-CBir1, an antibody associated with the presence of IBD, has been shown to differentiate pANCA-positive results in ulcerative colitis versus ulcerative colitis-like Crohn's disease [61]. Patients with Crohn's disease who have a greater titer of positive ASCA may be at a greater risk for complications such as strictures and fistulas, and they may also be at a higher risk for surgery. However, serologic markers do not appear to predict response to medical therapy, and there is currently insufficient evidence to recommend the use of antibody testing to predict responses to treatment or surgery in patients with IBD [49].

3.6 Microbiology

Before making a definitive diagnosis of idiopathic inflammatory bowel disease (IBD), perform a stool culture, ova and parasite studies, bacterial pathogen culture, and evaluation for Clostridium difficile infection [62]. At a minimum, a Clostridium difficile toxin assay should be performed on any patient hospitalized with a flare of colitis, because pseudomembranous colitis is commonly superimposed on IBD colitis. Assessment for Cytomegalovirus colitis should be performed in cases refractory to steroids [58]. Amebiasis can be difficult to identify from the stool; therefore, consider serologic testing.

3.7 Laboratory Texts in Screening for Biologics

Opportunistic infections in patients with Crohn's disease (CD) have become an important issue, particularly with the increasing use of immunosuppressants and TNF-α inhibitors [63]. That's why a panel of texts is recommended by current guidelines before starting biologics: hepatitis B and C markers, HIV antibodies, and screening for latent tuberculosis. Viral markers are assessed to prevent viral reactivation, which, in the case of hepatitis B, can lead to fulminant liver failure.

Chronic HBV is the most common chronic viral infection of the liver, affecting 350 million people worldwide. High rates of HBV (HBsAg-prevalence C8 %) are found in some parts of South America and Sub- Saharan Africa. In the Middle East and Indian subcontinent, an estimated 2–7 % of the general population is chronically infected [64]. Therefore, it is particularly important to focus HBV screening efforts on high-risk patient groups, such as immigrants from Sub-Saharan Africa or some parts of South America (HBsAg-prevalence C8 %). In addition, the cost-effectiveness of HBV screening was affected by the HBVR risk and HBVR-related mortality. If the HBVR risk is more than 62 %, HBV screening became cost-effective. Similarly, HBV screening became cost-effective if the HBVR-related mortality is more than 37 %. Comparable thresholds were found in a cost-effectiveness study of HBV screening in patients beginning with chemotherapy for solid tumors (67 % and 41 %, respectively). Although CD patients and cancer patients are not entirely comparable with regard to their clinical and treatment characteristics (infliximab versus chemotherapy), these findings indicate that CD patients that are severely immunocompromised as a result of cotreatment with steroids or other immunosuppressive drugs, malnutrition, or serious comorbidities may benefit from HBV screening prior to initiating infliximab treatment.

Screening for TB using chest X-ray and tuberculin skin test (TST) effectively reduces the occurrence of TB in patients treated with TNF-α inhibitors [65]. Presently, the additive value of the interferon-gamma release assay (IGRA) in TB screening remains unclear. Although the utilization of IGRA may reduce the rate of false-positive results, this comes with higher costs [66]. The cost-effectiveness of TB screening is unclear. Extended TB screening becomes cost-effective if the prevalence of latent TB is above 12 %. This indicates that extended TB screening targeted at populations at risk of latent TB may be more cost-effective than a universal screening strategy. However, ECCO guidelines on opportunistic infections in IBD recommend TB skin text (TST) or, better, interferon-gamma assays (Quantiferon-TB) in all patients candidates to biologics [67, 68] to prevent the reactivation of

TB. In Europe, the estimated incidence of active TB ranges from 10 to 99 per 100,000 inhabitants [69]. Worldwide, one third of the population is infected with latent TB. As reported by various post-marketing surveillance registries and one meta-analysis, CD and rheumatoid arthritis patients treated with TNF-α inhibitors have a 4- to 20-fold increased risk of active TB, with a mortality up to 14 % [70–75].

TST carries a high rate of false-positive tests, which is caused by the nonspecific nature of purified protein derivative (PPD) leading to cross-reactivity with non-tuberculosis mycobacterium and the booster phenomenon of serial TST testing [76, 77]. In a recently published meta-analysis of nine studies comparing TST with different IGRAs, Shahidi et al. [65] showed a modest to strong agreement between TST and IGRA. However, particularly in the immunosuppressive treatment-naive IBD population, this agreement was highly affected by the bacille Calmette-Guérin (BCG) vaccination status. As BCG increases the false-positivity rate of TST, IGRA may have an additive value in IBD patients who are BCG vaccinated. This is further strengthened by a recent cost-effectiveness analysis showing that among multiple screening strategies—including TST alone, IGRA alone, and sequential screening of TST followed by IGRA—using IGRA in BCG vaccinated individuals is the most cost-effective screening strategy [78].

In addition to this, Helwig et al. demonstrate that corticosteroids and immunosuppressive therapy influence the result of QuantiFERON-TB Gold testing in inflammatory bowel disease patients; 45 consecutive patients were enrolled; 24 patients out of 45 (corresponding to 53.3 %) received at least low doses of corticoid treatment and 27 patients out of 45 (corresponding to 60.0 %) received immunosuppressive agents. 13 patients out of 45 (corresponding to 28.9 %) had an indeterminate result of the QuantiFERON test. A correlation between the indeterminate result and combination therapy of corticosteroids was found. The concomitant therapy of immunosuppressive agents lead to a lower IFN release but no significance was found.

3.8 Therapeutic Drug Monitoring in Inflammatory Bowel Disease

Dramatic advances in the treatment of IBD have been seen with the availability of new drugs and our ability to tailor the treatment strategy for each patient. Tumor necrosis factor (TNF)-α inhibitors and thiopurines are among the most important classes of medications utilized in the clinical management of Crohn's disease. Monitoring of drug levels and anti-drug antibodies (for TNF-α inhibitors) and metabolite levels (for thiopurines) can provide valuable insight into the possible etiology of unfavorable outcomes and allow for an appropriate management strategy for these patients. Drug monitoring is relevant not only when trying to achieve treatment efficacy but also when trying to mitigate toxic side effects and optimize costs.

IFX is a chimeric IgG1 (human-constant and murine-variable regions) monoclonal antibody consisting of human-constant and murine-variable regions; it is indicated for induction and maintenance of clinical remission in patients with moderate to severely active CD [79, 80]. ADA is a recombinant fully human IgG1 monoclonal antibody, also approved for the induction and maintenance of remission in patients with CD [81–83].

These biologic therapies are of proven benefit, reducing rates of hospitalization and surgery rates while improving quality of life [84, 85]. Unfortunately, up to 50 % of patients lose response to treatment (secondary nonresponders) and up to 30 % do not respond at all (primary nonresponders) [86]. The rationale for lack or loss of response is multifactorial, but the most important is the development of anti-drug antibodies. One of the proposed strategies when patients lose response to an anti-TNF is switching to another drug in the same or different class. Another strategy is to empirically increase the dose, hoping to overcome increased drug clearance. Unfortunately, this can lead to significant adverse events including hypersensitivity reactions. A third potential tactic is to measure drug levels and antibodies, trying to identify those patients who will benefit from dose escalation and those who will be best served by switching to an alternate drug class. This latter strategy has been proven to be more cost-effective when compared to the former and highlights the importance and usefulness of measuring levels in these patients [87].

Multiple studies have confirmed a correlation between clinical response and trough *serum levels* of anti-TNF medications [88–92]. Currently, there is no clear consensus on the trough level values that correspond to clinical response. Recently, a cutoff trough level of 3 µg/mL has been suggested to have the optimal discriminatory accuracy for response to IFX in [93]. Trough levels of 3–7 µg/mL [94] and 5–10 µg/mL [95] have recently been suggested as target levels for maintenance therapy for CD. In addition, post-induction (week 14) trough levels of IFX were correlated with long-term (week 54) clinical response in a subgroup analysis of the ACCENT 1 study [96]. Moreover, serum levels at non-trough time points have also correlated with clinical response. For example, a serum level of IFX of 12.0 µg/mL at 4 weeks from the last infusion was independently correlated with clinical response [90] For ADA, a cutoff drug level of 5.85 µg/mL yielded optimal sensitivity, specificity, and positive likelihood ratio for prediction of clinical response [97]. Currently, there are several methods to measure IFX and ADA. Most studies have been performed using a solid-phase, double-antigen, enzyme-linked immunosorbent assay (ELISA). Unfortunately, this assay cannot measure the presence of antibodies when there are detectable levels of anti-TNF. Another method is a fluid-phase radioimmunoassay, which can report antibodies irrespective of the presence of drug. A recently developed assay is a homogeneous mobility shift assay using size-exclusion high-performance liquid chromatography, which has a high sensitivity and specificity and can potentially detect all isotypes of immunoglobulin [98]. This modality permits the measurement of antibodies to anti-TNF medications, even in the presence of detectable drug. However, most clinical studies have used the ELISA assay, which could have implications in how we interpret the available data.

ATI directed against the FAB fragment of the molecule [99] develop against both chimeric and fully humanized anti-TNFs. ATI interfere with the biologic activity by inhibiting the binding of the TNF-α inhibitors to both serum and membrane-bound TNF-α molecules and by creating immune complexes that are eliminated by the reticuloendothelial system [100, 101]. Formation of ATIs has been demonstrated to be correlated with decreased levels of anti-TNFs and diminished clinical response, although not all studies support that [88–91, 102]. his discrepancy may result from several factors, such as different sensitivity of the employed assays (see below), nonneutralizing antibodies, non-anti-TNF-driven disease, and alternative methods of elimination of anti-TNFs [103]. Moreover, serum anti-TNF levels and ATI most likely represent a continuous process, which may frequently start with low-titer antibodies that do not hamper the serum levels of the drug significantly, progressing to high-titer antibodies leading to a complete elimination of the drug. Frequently detection of ATI will precede the development of LOR by several weeks or, alternatively, will be detected after LOR has developed [104]. Moreover, transient (appearing on a single measurement without recurrence) ATI are a frequent phenomenon, described in up to 28 % of patients [105]. In contrast to persistent ATI that rarely (<10 %) appear after 1 year of treatment, these transient antibodies may be detected at any point during the treatment without a significant impact on LOR-free survival [104].

Several techniques are available for the purpose of measurement of antibodies. The most common is a solid-phase double-antigen ELISA, in which IFX serves as both the capture antigen and the detection antibody. This technique is relatively simple, reproducible, and inexpensive [105]. This method has some important drawbacks, the main one being an inability to detect ATI in the presence of IFX in the serum. These results, reported as "inconclusive," are very commonly reported. For instance, 72 % of measurements of ATI in the SONIC trial were deemed inconclusive. In addition, this method is also incapable of detection of immunoglobulin 4 (IgG4) ATI. A modified ELISA, employing anti-human λ antigen detection antibody (AHLC), has an improved capacity for detection of ATI in the presence of IFX, a well as for detection of IgG4 ATI [31, 104]. Additional detection methods, including homogenous mobility shift assay [106] and radioimmunoassay [107], are used in clinical practice. Both techniques, despite the presumable superior analytical accuracy, did not demonstrate superior diagnostic value on direct comparison with ELISA techniques [105, 108].

Observations from randomized controlled trials have shown that the concomitant use of immunomodulators (AZA, MP, or methotrexate) and biologic medications increases anti-TNF levels. It is generally believed that this occurs by diminishing immunogenicity (decreasing the formation of anti-TNF antibodies) while simultaneously reducing the amount of systemic inflammation which, as we describe below, will negatively affect IgG levels. The presence of ATI has consistently been associated with lower IFX levels [109] (Fig. 3.1). In an exploratory analysis of a randomized controlled trial looking at efficacy of IFX monotherapy, AZA monotherapy, and the two drugs combined, the authors found that at week 30, the IFX levels were 1.6 μg/mL for patients in the IFX group and 3.5 μg/mL for those in the combination therapy group ($P < 0.001$). They also found that only 1 of 116 patients (0.9 %) receiving combination therapy (compared to 15 of 103 patients (14.6 %) receiving IFX monotherapy) had ATI [110]. Studies looking at the effect of ATA on ADA levels have yielded similar results [91, 107]. The presence of ATI has been associated with treatment failure and lower IFX levels [109]. Even though most studies have shown a clear association between the presence of anti-TNF antibodies and drug levels, some data have failed to support this observation. Lichtenstein et al. looked at the influence that concomitant immunomodulators and IFX therapy had on drug levels. They reviewed the ACCENT I and II trials (effect on induction and maintenance of remission that IFX have in CD) as well as ACT 1 and 2 (effect on induction and maintenance of remission that IFX have in UC). In contrast to the previously mentioned studies, they found that IFX levels were similar when comparing patients who did and did not receive immunomodulators, even though

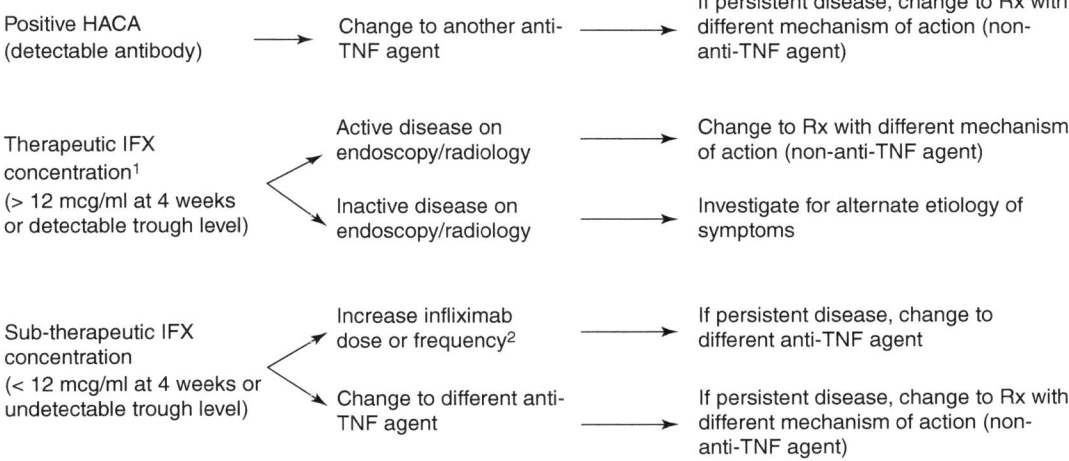

Fig. 3.1 Treatment algorithm based on therapeutic drug monitoring (IFX concentrations and antibody levels). *HACA* human anti-chimeric antibodies (From Afif et al. [112])

those patients that received immunomodulators had a higher incidence of ATI antibodies to infliximab [111]. Of note, this report was based on a post hoc analysis and the results should be interpreted in that context. An algorithm reporting treatment strategies tailored on IFX and ATI levels [112] is shown below in Fig. 3.1.

3.8.1 Thiopurine Metabolites

Thiopurine medications (6-MP and AZA) have long constituted the mainstay of IBD immunomodulator therapy. Once absorbed, AZA is converted to 6-MP by a nonenzymatic pathway. Measuring metabolites has two important applications, increasing the likelihood of treatment efficacy and reducing the risk of treatment-related toxicities. The two metabolites that are commercially available are 6-TGN and 6-MMP. 6-TGN has been the metabolite most associated with treatment efficacy; as such, its measurement has been proposed as a strategy to optimize treatment in patients with IBD receiving AZA/MP. 6-TGN is a metabolite of TIMP, which goes through a series of phosphorylation events resulting in 6-thioguanine diphosphate. A 6-TGN level >230 pmol/8×10^8 RBC has been correlated with clinical remission in both adults and children with IBD [113, 114]. Another study using a different

assay that included only adult patients failed to show a relation between 6-TGN levels and clinical activity [115].

A potential use for metabolite measurement is to assess adherence to medical therapy. Indeed, 6-TGN values have been proposed to optimize therapeutic response [116]. In patients without clinical response and "subtherapeutic" 6-TGN levels, optimization of the levels was significantly associated with improved response rates [117]. An association between TPMT activity and response to thiopurines has been suggested. TPMT activity below 35 pmol/h/mg of hemoglobin correlated with a greater chance of clinical response (81 % vs. 43 %; $P<0.001$). In an additional study, TPMT activity below 15.3 U/mL RBC is associated with a sixfold higher response rate to AZA [119]. The risk of resistance is increased in patients with high TPMT activity (over 14 U/mL RBC) (OR, 0.21; 95 % CI, 0.06–0.71; $P=0.009$) [116].

AZA metabolite measurement can also be used to help prevent drug-related toxicity. 6-MMP is a metabolite produced from MP by TPMT. Higher 6-MMP levels have been found to correlate with a higher risk of hepatotoxicity. Even though patients with 6-MMP levels >5700 pmol/8×10^8 RBC have a threefold increased risk of hepatotoxicity, not all patients with a high 6-MMP level will develop elevated liver enzymes, and having a low 6-MMP level does not preclude the development of hepatotoxicity [112, 119]. As with 6-MMP, some patients with very high 6-TGN levels do not develop myelotoxicity, while some with low 6-TGN levels may still develop this abnormality 118.

Thus, measuring 6-TGN and 6-MMP levels do not replace monitoring liver enzymes and blood counts. 6-TGN level measurements can also be useful to identify those patients who will not experience clinical benefit despite an optimal AZA/MP dose. Patients with normal TPMT activity and 6-TGN levels >400 pmol/8 × 10^8 RBC who do not achieve clinical remission will likely remain refractory to treatment even if the treatment is continued for 6 more months or the dose is increased [120]. CBC and transaminases should be assessed before onset of treatment and at 2, 4, and 8 weeks after initiating therapy, irrespective of TPMT status. Baseline and follow-up pancreatic enzymes should also be followed, as in some cases, elevated amylase and lipase may precede the clinical presentation of pancreatitis. Blood counts should then be repeated every 3 months or 2 weeks after dose adjustment. Thiopurine metabolite levels can be determined after 2–3 weeks on therapy or after dose adjustment; the levels should be reassessed when facing a loss of response, adverse effect, or when a medication with a potential effect on the thiopurine metabolism (such as 5-ASA, allopurinol, furosemide etc) is added. In addition, it is advisable to assess metabolite levels twice yearly for the purposes of routine monitoring and verification of adherence [121].

Despite available evidence, measurement of thiopurine metabolites is not widely used unless in tertiary referral centers.

References

1. Mazlam MZ, Hodgson HJ. Peripheral blood monocyte cytokine production and acute phase response in inflammatory bowel disease. Gut. 1992;33:773–8.
2. Niederau C, Backmerhoff F, Schumacher B, et al. Inflammatory mediators and acute phase proteins in patients with Crohn's disease and ulcerative colitis. Hepatogastroenterology. 1997;44:90–107.
3. Pepys MB, Druguet M, Klass HJ, et al. Immunological studies in inflammatory bowel disease. In: Porter R, Knight J, editors. Immunology of the gut, Ciba Foundation Symposium. Amsterdam: Elsevier/Excerpta Medica/North Holland; 1977. p. 283–97.
4. Tibble J, Teahon K, Thjodleifsson B, et al. A simple method for assessing intestinal inflammation in Crohn's disease. Gut. 2000;47:506–13.
5. Stange EF, Travis SP, Vermeire S, et al. European Crohn's and Colitis Organisation. European evidence based consensus on the diagnosis and management of Crohn's disease: definitions and diagnosis. Gut. 2006; 55(suppl 1):i1–i15.
6. Zholudev A, Zurakowski D, Young W, Leichtner A, Bousvaros A. Serologic testing with ANCA, ASCA, and anti-OmpC in children and young adults with Crohn's disease and ulcerative colitis: diagnostic value and correlation with disease phenotype. Am J Gastroenterol. 2004;99(11):2235–41.
7. Kallel L, Ayadi I, Matri S, et al. Fecal calprotectin is a predictive marker of relapse in Crohn's disease involving the colon: a prospective study. Eur J Gastroenterol Hepatol. 2010;22(3):340–5.
8. Sidhu R, Wilson P, Wright A, et al. Faecallactoferrin–a novel test to differentiate between the irritable and inflamed bowel? Aliment Pharmacol Ther. 2010; 31(12):1365–70.
9. Tillet WS, Francis T. Serological reactions in pneumonia with a non-protein somatic fraction of the pneumococcus. J Exp Med. 1930;52:561–71.
10. Pepys MB. C-reactive protein fifty years on. Lancet. 1981;1:653–7.
11. Ballou SP, Kushner I. C-reactive protein and the acute phase response. Adv Intern Med. 1992;37:313–36.
12. Young B, Gleeson M, Cripps AW. C-reactive protein: a critical review. Pathology. 1991;23:118–24.
13. Mold C, Baca R, Du Clos TW. Serum amyloid P component and C-reactive protein opsonize apoptotic cells for phagocytosis through Fcgamma receptors. J Autoimmun. 2002;19:147–54.
14. Thomas RD, Westengard JC, Hay KL, et al. Calibration and validation for erythrocyte sedimentation tests. Role of the International Committee on Standardization in Hematology reference procedure. Arch Pathol Lab Med. 1993;117:719–23.
15. Gabay C, Kushner I. Acute-phase proteins and other systemic responses to inflammation. N Engl J Med. 1999;340:448–54.
16. Shine B, Berghouse L, Jones JE, et al. C-reactive protein as an aid in the differentiation of functional and inflammatory bowel disorders. Clin Chim Acta. 1985;148:105–9.
17. Poullis AP, Zar S, Sundaram KK, et al. A new, highly sensitive assay for Creactiveprotein can aid the differentiation of inflammatory bowel disorders from constipation- and diarrhoea-predominant functional bowel disorders. Eur J Gastroenterol Hepatol. 2002; 14:409–12.
18. Tromm A, Tromm CD, Huppe D, et al. Evaluation of different laboratory tests and activity indices reflecting

the inflammatory activity of Crohn's disease. Scand J Gastroenterol. 1992;27:774–8.

19. Sachar DB, Smith H, Chan S, et al. Erythrocytic sedimentation rate as a measure of clinical activity in inflammatory bowel disease. J Clin Gastroenterol. 1986;8:647–50.

20. Sachar DB, Luppescu NE, Bodian C, et al. Erythrocyte sedimentation as a measure of Crohn's disease activity: opposite trends in ileitis versus colitis. J Clin Gastroenterol. 1990;12:643–6.

21. Fagan EA, Dyck RF, Maton PN. et al. Serum levels of C-reactive protein in Crohn's disease and ulcerative colitis. Eur J Clin Invest. 1982;12:351–9.

22. Ridker PM, Hennekens CH, Buring JE, et al. C-reactive protein and other markers of inflammation in the prediction of cardiovascular disease in women. N Engl J Med. 2000;342:836–43.

23. Pearson TA, Mensah GA, Alexander RW, Centers for Disease Control and Prevention, Association AH, et al. Markers of inflammation and cardiovascular disease: application to clinical and public health practice: a statement for healthcare professionals from the Centers for Disease Control and Prevention and the American Heart Association. Circulation. 2003;107: 499–511.

24. Danesh J, Wheeler JG, Hirschfield GM, et al. C-reactive protein and other circulating markers of inflammation in the prediction of coronary heart disease. N Engl J Med. 2004;350:1387–97.

25. Bataille R, Boccadoro M, Klein B, et al. C-reactive protein and beta-2 microglobulin produce a simple and powerful myeloma staging system. Blood. 1992;80:733–7.

26. Brignola C, Campieri M, Bazzocchi G, et al. A laboratory index for predicting relapse in asymptomatic patients with Crohn's disease. Gastroenterology. 1986;91:1490–4.

27. Boirivant M, Leoni M, Tariciotti D, et al. The clinical significance of serum C reactive protein levels in Crohn's disease. Results of a prospective longitudinal study. J Clin Gastroenterol. 1988;10:401–5.

28. Consigny Y, Modigliani R, Colombel JF, et al. Biological markers of short term relapse in Crohn's disease (CD). Gastroenterology. 2001;20(suppl):A53.

29. Louis E, Vermeire S, Rutgeerts P, et al. A positive response to infliximab in Crohn disease: association with a higher systemic inflammation before treatment but not with 2308 TNF gene polymorphism. Scand J Gastroenterol. 2002;37:818–24.

30. Rutgeerts P, Colombel J, Enns R, et al. Subanalysis from a phase 3 study on the evaluation of natalizumab in active Crohn's disease. Gut. 2003;52(suppl):A239.

31. Sandborn WJ, Feagan BG, Radford-Smith G, et al. CDP571, a humanized monoclonal antibody to tumour necrosis factor alpha, for moderate to severe Crohn's disease: a randomised, double blind, placebo controlled trial. Gut. 2004;53:1485–93.

32. Schreiber S, Rutgeerts P, Fedorak RN, et al. CDP870 Crohn's Disease Study Group. A randomized, placebo-controlled trial of certolizumab pegol (CDP870)

for treatment of Crohn's disease. Gastroenterology. 2005;129:807–18.

33. Feagan B, Rutgeerts P, Schreiber S, et al. Low baseline CRP correlates with high placebo remission rate in Crohn's disease Clinical trials at 12 weeks. Gastroenterology. 2005;128 suppl 2:A307.431.

34. Jensen KB, Jarnum S, Koudahl G, et al. Serum orosomucoid in ulcerative colitis: its relation to clinical activity, protein loss, and turnover of albumin and IgG. Scand J Gastroenterol. 1976;11:177–83.

35. Andre C, Descos L, Landais P, et al. Assessment of appropriate laboratory measurements to supplement the Crohn's disease activity index. Gut. 1981;22: 571–4.

36. Descos L, Andre C, Beorghia S, et al. Serum levels of beta-2-microglobulin—a new marker of activity in Crohn's disease. N Engl J Med. 1979;301:440–1.

37. Manicourt DH, Orloff S. Serum levels of beta 2-microglobulin in Crohn's disease. N Engl J Med. 1980;302:696.

38. Zissis M, Afroudakis A, Galanopoulos G, et al. B2 microglobulin: is it a reliable marker of activity in inflammatory bowel disease? Am J Gastroenterol. 2001;96:2177–83.

39. Ricci G, D'Ambrosi A, Resca D, et al. Comparison of serum total sialic acid, C reactive protein, alpha 1-acid glycoprotein and beta 2-microglobulin in patients with non-malignant bowel diseases. Biomed Pharmacother. 1995;49:259–62.

40. Takeuchi K, Smale S, Premchand P, et al. Prevalence and mechanism of nonsteroidal anti-inflammatory drug-induced clinical relapse in patients with inflammatory bowel disease. Clin Gastroenterol Hepatol. 2006;4(2):196–202.

41. Gisbert JP, McNicholl AG. Questions and answers on the role of faecal calprotectin as a biological marker in inflammatory bowel disease. Dig Liver Dis. 2009; 41(1):56–66.

42. Roseth AG, Schmidt PN, Fagerhol MK. Correlation between faecal excretion of indium-111-labelled granulocytes and calprotectin, a granulocyte marker protein, in patients with inflammatory bowel disease. Scand J Gastroenterol. 1999;34:50–4.

43. Tibble JA, Sigthorsson G, Foster R, et al. High prevalence of NSAID enteropathy as shown by a simple faecal test. Gut. 1999;45:362–6.

44. Roseth AG, Aadland E, Jahnsen J, et al. Assessment of disease activity in ulcerative colitis by faecal calprotectin, a novel granulocyte marker protein. Digestion. 1997;58:176–80.

45. Tibble JA, Sigthorsson G, Bridger S, et al. Surrogate markers of intestinal inflammation are predictive of relapse in patients with inflammatory bowel disease. Gastroenterology. 2000;119:15–22.

46. Costa F, Mumolo MG, Ceccarelli L, et al. Calprotectin is a stronger predictive marker of relapse in ulcerative colitis than in Crohn's disease. Gut. 2005;54:364–8.

47. D'Inca R, Dal Pont E, Di Leo V, et al. Can calprotectin predict relapse in inflammatory bowel disease? Gastroenterology. 2005;128(suppl):A307.

48. Henderson P, Anderson NH, Wilson DC. The diagnostic accuracy of fecal calprotectin during the investigation of suspected pediatric inflammatory bowel disease: a systematic review and meta-analysis. Am J Gastroenterol. 2014;109:637–45.

49. Prideaux L, De Cruz P, Ng SC, Kamm MA. Serological antibodies in inflammatory bowel disease: a systematic review. Inflamm Bowel Dis. 2012;18(7):1340–55.

50. Langhorst J, Elsenbruch S, Koelzer J, et al. Noninvasive markers in the assessment of intestinal inflammation in inflammatory bowel diseases: performance of fecal lactoferrin, calprotectin, and PMN-elastase, CRP, and clinical indices. Am J Gastroenterol. 2008;103:162–9.

51. Schroder O, Naumann M, Shastri Y, et al. Prospective evaluation of fecal neutrophil-derived proteins in identifying intestinal inflammation: combination of parameters does not improve diagnostic accuracy of calprotectin. Ailment Pharmacol Ther. 2007;26:1035–42.

52. Bar-Gil Shitrit A, Braverman D, Stankiewics H. Fecal calprotectin as a predictor of abnormal colonic histology. Dis Colon Rectum. 2007;50:2188–93.

53. von Roon A, Karamountzos L, Purkayastha S, et al. Diagnostic precision of fecal calprotectin for inflammatory bowel disease and colorectal malignancy. Am J Gastroenterol. 2007;102:803–13.

54. Ricanek P, Brackmann S, Perminow G, et al. Evaluation of disease activity in IBD at the time of diagnosis by the use of clinical, biochemical, and fecal markers. Scand J Gastroenterol. 2011;46:1081–91.

55. Schoepfer A, Beglinger C, Straumann A, et al. Ulcerative colitis: correlation of the Rachmilewitz endoscopic activity index with fecal calprotectin, clinical activity, CRP, and blood leukocytes. Inflamm Bowel Dis. 2009;15:1851–8.

56. Jones J, Loftus E, Panaccione R, et al. Relationships between disease activity and serum and fecal biomarkers in patients with Crohn's disease. Clin Gastroenterol Hepatol. 2008;6:1218–24.

57. Licata A, Randazzo C, Cappello M, et al. Fecal calprotectin in clinical practice: a non-invasive screening tool for patients with chronic diarrhea. J Clin Gastroenterol. 2012;46:504–8.

58. Kornbluth A, Sachar DB. Ulcerative colitis practice guidelines in adults: American College Of Gastroenterology, Practice Parameters Committee. Am J Gastroenterol. 2010;105(3):501–23; quiz 524.

59. World Gastroenterology Organisation (WGO). World Gastroenterology Organisation Global Guideline. Inflammatory bowel disease: a global perspective. Munich: World Gastroenterology Organisation (WGO); 2009.

60. Sandler RS, Loftus EV. Epidemiology of inflammatory bowel disease. In: Sartor RB, Sandborn WJ, Kirsner JB, editors. Kirsner's inflammatory bowel diseases. 6th ed. Edinburgh: Saunders; 2004. p. 245–62.

61. Yu AP, Cabanilla LA, Wu EQ, Mulani PM, Chao J. The costs of Crohn's disease in the United States

62. D' Incà R, Dal Pont E, Di Leo V, Ferronato A, Fries W, Vettorato MG, et al. Calprotectin and lactoferrin in the assessment of intestinal inflammation and organic disease. Int J Colorectal Dis. 2007;22(4):429–37.

63. Rahier JF, Magro F, Abreu C, et al. Second European evidence based consensus on the prevention, diagnosis and management of opportunistic infections in inflammatory bowel disease. J Crohns Colitis. 2014;8:443–68.

64. Alter MJ. Epidemiology of hepatitis B in Europe and in worldwide. J Hepatol. 2003;39(Supp II):S64–9.

65. Shahidi N, Fu Y-T, Qian H, Bressler B, et al. Performance of interferon-gamma release assays in patients with inflammatory bowel disease: a systematic review and meta-analysis. Inflamm Bowel Dis. 2012;18:2034–42.

66. Carmona L, Gómez-Reino JJ, Rodrıguez-Valverde V, et al. Effectiveness of recommendations to prevent reactivation of latent tuberculosis infection in patients treated with tumor necrosis factor antagonists. Arthritis Rheum. 2005;52:1766–72.

67. Kornbluth A, Sachar DB, Practice Parameters Committee of the American College of Gastroenterology. Ulcerative colitis practice guidelines in adults: American College of Gastroenterology Practice Parameters Committee. Am J Gastroenterol. 2010;3:501–23.

68. Mowat C, Cole A, Windsor A, et al. Guidelines for the management of inflammatory bowel disease in adults. Gut. 2011;60:571–607.

69. Dye C, Scheele S, Dolin P, et al. Consensus statement. Global burden of tuberculosis: estimated incidence, prevalence, and mortality by country. WHO Global Surveillance and Monitoring Project. JAMA. 1999;282:677–86.

70. Singh JA, Wells GA, Christensen R, et al. Adverse effects of biologics: a network meta-analysis and Cochrane overview. Cochrane Database Syst Rev. 2011;(2):CD008794.

71. Keane J, Gershon S, Wise RP, et al. Tuberculosis associated with infliximab, a tumor necrosis factor alpha-neutralizing agent. N Engl J Med. 2001;345:1098–104.

72. Gomez-Reino JJ, Carmona L, Valverde VR, et al. Treatment of rheumatoid arthritis with tumor necrosis factor inhibitors may predispose to significant increase in tuberculosis risk—a multicentre active-surveillance report. Arthritis Rheum. 2003;48:2122–7.

73. Askling J, Fored CM, Brandt L, et al. Risk and case characteristics of tuberculosis in rheumatoid arthritis associated with tumor necrosis factor antagonists in Sweden. Arthritis Rheum. 2005;52:1986–92.

74. Wolfe F, Michaud K, Anderson J, et al. Tuberculosis infection in patients with rheumatoid arthritis and the effect of infliximab therapy. Arthritis Rheum. 2004;50:372–9.

75. Ott JJ, Stevens GA, Groeger J, Wiersma ST. Global epidemiology of hepatitis B virus infection: new

and other Western countries: a systematic review. Curr Med Res Opin. 2008;24(2):319–28.

estimates of age-specific HBsAg seroprevalence and endemicity. Vaccine. 2012;30:2212–9.

76. Pal M, Zwerling A, Menzies D, et al. Systematic review: T-Cell-based assays for the diagnosis of latent tuberculosis infection: an update. Ann Intern Med. 2008;149:177–84.

77. Menzies D. Interpretation of repeated tuberculin tests. Boosting, conversion and reversion. Am J Respir Crit Care Med. 1999;159:15–21.

78. Marra F, Marra CA, Sadatsafavi M, et al. Cost-effectiveness of new interferon-based blood assay, QuantiFERON-TB Gold, in screening tuberculosis contacts. Int J Tuberc Lung Dis. 2008;1:1414–24.

79. Hanauer SB, Feagan BG, Lichtenstein GR, Mayer LF, Schreiber S, Colombel JF, Rachmilewitz D, Wolf DC, Olson A, Bao W. Maintenance infliximab for Crohn's disease: the ACCENT I randomised trial. Lancet. 2002;359:1541–9 [PubMed] [DOI].

80. Rutgeerts P, Sandborn WJ, Feagan BG, Reinisch W, Olson A, Johanns J, Travers S, Rachmilewitz D, Hanauer SB, Lichtenstein GR. Infliximab for induction and maintenance therapy for ulcerative colitis. N Engl J Med. 2005;353:2462–76 [PubMed] [DOI].

81. Hanauer SB, Sandborn WJ, Rutgeerts P, Fedorak RN, Lukas M, MacIntosh D, Panaccione R, Wolf D, Pollack P. Human anti-tumor necrosis factor monoclonal antibody (adalimumab) in Crohn's disease: the CLASSIC-I trial. Gastroenterology. 2006;130:323–33; quiz 591.[PubMed] [DOI].

82. Sandborn WJ, Hanauer SB, Rutgeerts P, Fedorak RN, Lukas M, MacIntosh DG, Panaccione R, Wolf D, Kent JD, Bittle B. Adalimumab for maintenance treatment of Crohn's disease: results of the CLASSIC II trial. Gut. 2007;56:1232–9 [PubMed] [DOI].

83. Reinisch W, Sandborn WJ, Hommes DW, D'Haens G, Hanauer S, Schreiber S, Panaccione R, Fedorak RN, Tighe MB, Huang B. Adalimumab for induction of clinical remission in moderately to severely active ulcerative colitis: results of a randomised controlled trial. Gut. 2011;60:780–7 [PubMed] [DOI].

84. Lichtenstein GR, Yan S, Bala M, Blank M, Sands BE. Infliximab maintenance treatment reduces hospitalizations, surgeries, and procedures in fistulizing Crohn's disease. Gastroenterology. 2005;128:862–9 [PubMed] [DOI].

85. Vogelaar L, Spijker AV, van der Woude CJ. The impact of biologics on health-related quality of life in patients with inflammatory bowel disease. Clin Exp Gastroenterol. 2009;2:101–9 [PubMed].

86. Peyrin-Biroulet L, Deltenre P, de Suray N, Branche J, Sandborn WJ, Colombel JF. Efficacy and safety of tumor necrosis factor antagonists in Crohn's disease: meta-analysis of placebo-controlled trials. Clin Gastroenterol Hepatol. 2008;6:644–53 [PubMed] [DOI].

87. Steenholdt C, Brynskov J, Thomsen OO, Munck LK, Fallingborg J, Christensen LA, Pedersen G, Kjeldsen J, Jacobsen BA, Oxholm AS. Individualised therapy is more cost-effective than dose intensification in patients with Crohn's disease who lose response to anti-TNF treatment: a randomised, controlled trial. Gut. 2014;63(6):919–27.

88. Maser EA, Villela R, Silverberg MS, Greenberg GR. Association of trough serum infliximab to clinical outcome after scheduled maintenance treatment for Crohn's disease. Clin Gastroenterol Hepatol. 2006;4:1248–54.

89. Seow CH, Newman A, Irwin SP, Steinhart AH, Silverberg MS, Greenberg GR. Trough serum infliximab: a predictive factor of clinical outcome for infliximab treatment in acute ulcerative colitis. Gut. 2010;59:49–54.

90. Baert F, Noman M, Vermeire S, et al. Influence of immunogenicity on the long-term efficacy of infliximab in Crohn's disease. N Engl J Med. 2003;348:601–8.

91. Karmiris K, Paintaud G, Noman M, Magdelaine-Beuzelin C, Ferrante M, Degenne D, et al. Influence of trough serum levels and immunogenicity on long-term outcome of adalimumab therapy in Crohn's disease. Gastroenterology. 2009;137:1628–40.

92. Colombel JF, Sandborn WJ, Allez M, et al. Association between plasma concentrations of certolizumab pegol and endoscopic outcomes of patients with Crohn's disease. Clin Gastroenterol Hepatol. 2014;12: 423–31.e1.

93. Feagan BG, Singh S, Lockton S, et al. Novel infliximab (IFX) and antibody-to-infliximab (ATI) assays are predictive of diseaseactivity in patients with Crohn's disease (CD). Gastroenterology. 2012;142:S114–S.

94. Vande Casteele N, Compernolle G, Ballet V, et al. Individualised infliximab treatment using therapeutic drug monitoring: a prospective controlled trough level adapted infliXImab treatment (TAXIT) trial. J Crohns Colitis. 2012;6:S6.

95. Vaughn BM-VM, Patwardhan V, et al. Prospective therapeutic drug monitoring to optimizing infliximab (IFX) maintenance therapy in patients with inflammatory bowel disease. Gastroenterology. 2014;146:5, S-54.

96. Cornillie F, Hanauer SB, Diamond RH, et al. Postinduction serum infliximab trough level and decrease of C-reactive protein level are associated with durable sustained response to infliximab: a retrospective analysis of the ACCENT I trial. Gut. 2014;63(11):1721–7. doi:10.1136/gutjnl-2012-304094.

97. Mazor Y, Kopylov U, Ben Hur D, et al. Evaluating adalimumab drug and antibody levels as predictors of clinical and laboratory response in Crohn's disease patients. Gastroenterology. 2013;144:S778–S.

98. Wang SL, Hauenstein S, Ohrmund L, Shringarpure R, Salbato J, Reddy R, McCowen K, Shah S, Lockton S, Chuang E. Monitoring of adalimumab and antibodies-to-adalimumab levels in patient serum by the homogeneous mobility shift assay. J Pharm Biomed Anal. 2013;78–79:39–44 [PubMed] [DOI].

99. Ben-Horin S, Yavzori M, Katz L, et al. The immunogenic part of infliximab is the F(ab′)(2), but measuring antibodies to the intact infliximab molecule is more clinically useful. Gut. 2011;60:41–8.

100. Yamada A, Sono K, Hosoe N, Takada N, Suzuki Y. Monitoring functional serum antitumor necrosis factor antibody level in Crohn's disease patients who maintained and those who lost response to anti-TNF. Inflamm Bowel Dis. 2010;16:1898–904.

101. Rojas JR, Taylor RP, Cunningham MR, et al. Formation, distribution, and elimination of infliximab and anti-infliximab immune complexes in cynomolgus monkeys. J Pharm Exp Ther. 2005; 313:578–85.

102. Vermeire S, Noman M, Van Assche G, Baert F, D'Haens G, Rutgeerts P. Effectiveness of concomitant immunosuppressive therapy in suppressing the formation of antibodies to infliximab in Crohn's disease. Gut. 2007;56:1226–31.

103. Ben-Horin S, Chowers Y. Review article: loss of response to anti-TNF treatments in Crohn's disease. Alimen Pharmacol Ther. 2011;33:987–95.

104. Ungar B, Chowers Y, Yavzori M, et al. The temporal evolution of antidrug antibodies in patients with inflammatory bowel disease treated with infliximab. Gut. 2014;63:1258–64.

105. VandeCasteele N, Gils A, Singh S, et al. Antibody response to infliximab and its impact on pharmacokinetics can be transient. Am J Gastroenterol. 2013;108:962–71.

106. Wang SL, Ohrmund L, Hauenstein S, et al. Development and validation of a homogeneous mobility shift assay for the measurement of infliximab and antibodies-to-infliximab levels in patient serum. J Immunol Methods. 2012;382:177–88.

107. Farrell RJ, Alsahli M, Jeen YT, Falchuk KR, Peppercorn MA, Michetti P. Intravenous hydrocortisone premedication reduces antibodies to infliximab in Crohn's disease: a randomized controlled trial. Gastroenterology. 2003;124:917–24.

108. Steenholdt C, Ainsworth MA, Tovey M, et al. Comparison of techniques for monitoring infliximab and antibodies against infliximab in Crohn's disease. Ther Drug Monit. 2013;35:530–8.

109. Nanda KS, Cheifetz AS, Moss AC. Impact of antibodies to infliximab on clinical outcomes and serum infliximab levels in patients with inflammatory bowel disease (IBD): a meta-analysis. Am J Gastroenterol. 2013;108:40–7; quiz 48.[PubMed] [DOI].

110. Colombel JF, Sandborn WJ, Reinisch W, Mantzaris GJ, Kornbluth A, Rachmilewitz D, Lichtiger S, D'Haens G, Diamond RH, Broussard DL. Infliximab, azathioprine, or combination therapy for Crohn's disease. N Engl J Med. 2010;362:1383–95 [PubMed] [DOI].

111. Lichtenstein GR, Diamond RH, Wagner CL, Fasanmade AA, Olson AD, Marano CW, Johanns J, Lang Y, Sandborn WJ. Clinical trial: benefits and risks of immunomodulators and maintenance infliximab for IBD-subgroup analyses across four randomized trials. Aliment Pharmacol Ther. 2009;30:210–26 [PubMed] [DOI].

112. Afif W LEV, Faubion WA, et al. Clinical utility of measuring infliximab and human anti-chimeric antibody concentrations in patients with inflammatory bowel disease. Am J Gastroenterol. 2010;105:1133–9.

113. Dubinsky MC, Lamothe S, Yang HY, Targan SR, Sinnett D, Théorêt Y, Seidman EG. Pharmacogenomics and metabolite measurement for 6-mercaptopurine therapy in inflammatory bowel disease. Gastroenterology. 2000;118:705–13 [PubMed] [DOI].

114. Osterman MT, Kundu R, Lichtenstein GR, Lewis JD. Association of 6-thioguanine nucleotide levels and inflammatory bowel disease activity: a meta-analysis. Gastroenterology. 2006;130:1047–53 [PubMed] [DOI].

115. Lowry PW, Franklin CL, Weaver AL, Pike MG, Mays DC, Tremaine WJ, Lipsky JJ, Sandborn WJ. Measurement of thiopurine methyltransferase activity and azathioprine metabolites in patients with inflammatory bowel disease. Gut. 2001;49:665–70 [PubMed].

116. Chouchana L, Narjoz C, Beaune P, Loriot MA, Roblin X. Review article: the benefits of pharmacogenetics for improving thiopurine therapy in inflammatory bowel disease. Aliment Pharmacol Ther. 2012;35:15–36.

117. Dubinsky MC, Yang H, Hassard PV, et al. 6-MP metabolite profiles provide a biochemical explanation for 6-MP resistance in patients with inflammatory bowel disease. Gastroenterology. 2002;122:904–15.

118. Lennard L, Van Loon JA, Lilleyman JS, Weinshilboum RM. Thiopurine pharmacogenetics in leukemia: correlation of erythrocyte thiopurine methyltransferase activity and 6-thioguanine nucleotide concentrations. Clin Pharmacol Ther. 1987;41:18–25.

119. Shaye OA, Yadegari M, Abreu MT, Poordad F, Simon K, Martin P, Papadakis KA, Ippoliti A, Vasiliauskas E, Tran TT. Hepatotoxicity of 6-mercaptopurine (6-MP) and Azathioprine (AZA) in adult IBD patients. Am J Gastroenterol. 2007;102:2488–94 [PubMed] [DOI].

120. Roblin X, Peyrin-Biroulet L, Phelip JM, Nancey S, Flourie B. A 6-thioguanine nucleotide threshold level of 400 pmol/8 x 10(8) erythrocytes predicts azathioprine refractoriness in patients with inflammatory bowel disease and normal TPMT activity. Am J Gastroenterol. 2008;103:3115–22 [PubMed] [DOI].

121. Seidman EG. Clinical use and practical application of TPMT enzyme and 6-mercaptopurine metabolite monitoring in IBD. Rev Gastroenterol Dis. 2003;3 Suppl 1:S30–8.

Andrea Affronti, Ambrogio Orlando, and Mario Cottone

Crohn's disease (CD) is an inflammatory bowel disease (IBD) with a chronic course, and it is characterized by different events within time which are in relation to heterogeneity of the disease. This heterogeneity depends on the age of appearance, time elapsed from symptoms to diagnosis, site, extent and behavior of disease, and smoking status.

The initial description of CD by Oppenheimer, Ginzburg, and Crohn [1] still remain valid: "the disease is clinically featured by fever, diarrhea and emaciation, leading eventually to an obstruction of the small intestine; the constant occurrence of a mass in the right iliac fossa usually requires surgical intervention (resection). The terminal ileum is alone involved. The process begins abruptly at and involves the ileocecal valve in its maximal intensity, tapering off gradually as it ascends the ileum orally for from 8 to 12 inches (20 to 30 cm). The familiar fistulas lead usually to segments of the colon, forming small tracts communicating with the lumen of the large intestine; occasionally the abdominal wall, anteriorly, is the site of one or more of these fistulous tracts."

A. Affronti (✉) • A. Orlando, MD. PhD
M. Cottone, MD, PhD
Department of Internal Medicine,
University of Palermo, Ospedali Riuniti Villa-Sofia
Cervello, Via trabucco, 180, Palermo, Italy
e-mail: andrea.affronti@gmail.com
ambrogiorlando@gmail.com;
cottonedickens@gmail.com

Studies evaluating the course of the disease have produced different results according to the adopted methodology. Unselected inception cohort studies are the best ones on which we rely [2–5], in order to avoid the selection bias from referral centers, where patients with more severe disease are usually included. The classical biases of prognostic studies are: (1) prevalence-incidence bias, (2) lead time bias, and (3) length time bias, according to Sackett et al. [6]. The quality of the studies of prognosis depends on: the presence of inception cohort, the correct description of referral pattern, a complete follow-up, and the presence of objective and well-assessed outcome criteria (blind).

In Table 4.1 the main unselected population-based cohorts in studies on prognosis of adult Crohn's disease patients, used for this chapter, were summarized.

After the introduction of effective medical therapy (steroids, immunosuppressors, and biologics), it is incorrect to use the term natural history, whereas this term can be applied, for the short-term course, to the placebo arm of controlled clinical trials and, for long-term course, to the studies performed before the introduction of these therapies. The "new therapies," introduced in the last two decades, are very effective in keeping down CD activity, but their real effect on the course of disease is mostly unknown. The main events during the course of disease are activity, remission, relapse, obstruction, fistulizing,

© Springer International Publishing Switzerland 2016
G. Lo Re, M. Midiri (eds.), *Crohn's Disease: Radiological Features and Clinical-Surgical Correlations*,
DOI 10.1007/978-3-319-23066-5_4

Table 4.1 Unselected inception cohort in studies on prognosis of adult Crohn's disease patients

Region	N° CD patients	Follow-up	Inception period	Reference
Olmsted County, USA	278	Retrospective	1940–1993	[4, 21, 29]
Stockholm, Sweden	1251	Retrospective	1955–1984	[9]
Uppsala, Sweden	1469	Retrospective	1965–1983	[10]
Leicester, UK	610	Retrospective	1972–1989	[63]
Florence, Italy	231	Retrospective	1978–1992	[5, 14]
Cardiff, UK	341	Retrospective	1986–2003	[30, 64]
Copenhagen, Denmark	373	Prospective	1962–1987	[2, 3, 22]
IBSEN, Norway	232	Prospective	1990–1993	[23]
UK	5640	Prospective	1989–2010	[13]
Copenhagen, Denmark	231	Prospective	2003–2004	[32]
Veszprem, Hungary	506	Retrospective-prospective	1977–2008	[8, 19]
SIBDCS, Switzerland	1137	Retrospective-prospective	2006–onward	[48]

surgical resection, recurrence after surgery, cancer, and death.

4.1 Activity and Remission

In observational studies of chronic course diseases, the calculation of activity indices is not easy. There is not a well-established activity classification system. In a study from Olmsted County, remission was assumed in absence of symptoms without treatment; mild disease was assumed in absence of symptoms under treatment with 5-aminosalicylates (5-ASA), antibiotic, or topical therapy; severe disease was reserved to the responsive forms to oral corticosteroids (CS) or immunosuppressive medications (IM); patients under oral (CS) or IM therapy lasting more than 6 months were considered drug-dependent or drug-refractory, in absence of documented improvement within 2 months for corticosteroids or within 3 months for immunosuppressive medication [21]. In a study from the Copenhagen cohort, low activity was defined as a number of bowel movements not exceeding four, without blood and systemic symptoms; high activity was assumed in presence of systemic symptoms; moderate activity was attributed to the other cases. In the same reports by the Copenhagen group, the disease course is classified as inactive in absence of bowel symptoms during 1 year, intermittent in all cases of occur-

rence of at least 1 month symptom-free without therapy, and continuous for symptomatic disease without intervals during 1 year [22].

In another tertiary clinical French database, a panel of IBD experts was interviewed to establish the most relevant criteria for discriminating a severe from a mild-to-moderate CD course. The following criteria were proposed: (1) number of years with active disease, (2) chronic, disabling extraintestinal manifestations, (3) number of intestinal surgeries, (4) disabling perianal disease, (5) number of perianal surgical procedures, (6) requirement for a temporary or permanent stoma, and (7) death related to CD or complications of CD or complications of CD treatment [7].

This heterogeneity is the reason of the objective difficulty to perform comparative studies of course of CD.

Despite all these limits, a more benign course of CD seems to emerge from data produced using inception cohort. As shown by Munkholm et al. in a Copenhagen cohort of 373 patients, after 7 years, about 55 % of patients were in remission, whereas 15 % had low activity and 30 % had high activity, indicating that mostly the course of disease is favorable (Fig. 4.1); the probability of a continuously active course was 5 % after 5 years, while considering a period of 5 years only a quarter of patients were active, about 20 % were conversely inactive, and the remaining patients experience fluctuating symptoms, often influenced by medical treatments (Fig. 4.2).

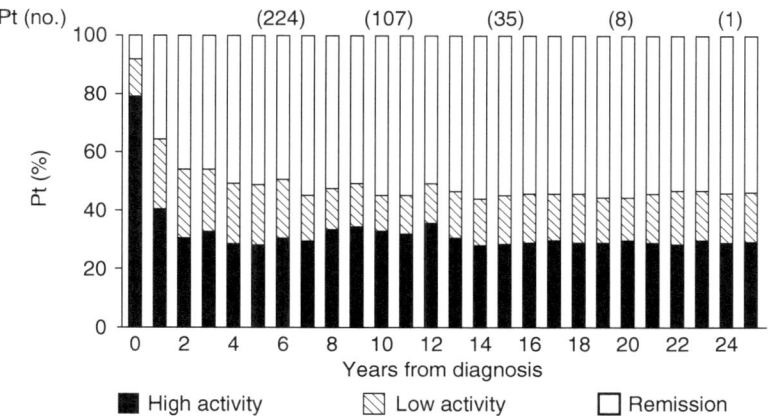

Fig. 4.1 Distribution according to disease activity after diagnosis. Reprinted from Munkholm et al. [22]

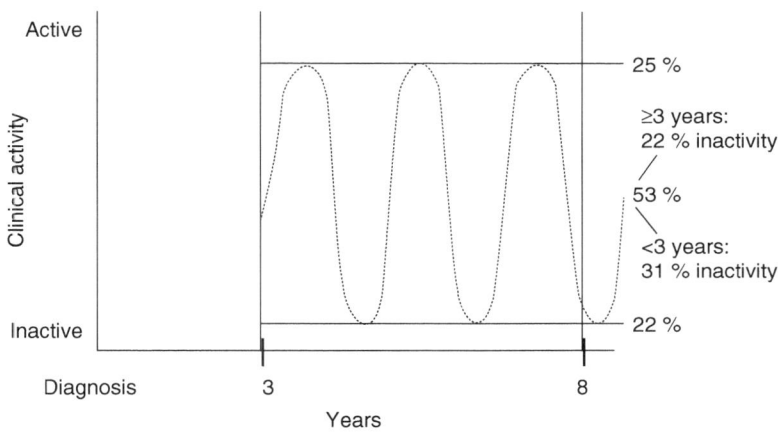

Fig. 4.2 Distribution according to disease activity over time. Reprinted from Munkholm et al. [22]

This observation is confirmed in almost all the studies based on unselected inception cohort.

Data from Olmsted County had shown that, using the Markov model [15], a presumed patient spent most time in remission or mild disease (53 %) and only 8 % of the time in severe disease or surgery (Fig. 4.3).

In the IBSEN cohort more than 60 % of patients were in clinical remission after 10 years of follow-up [23].

This trend is also confirmed in some referral cohort. Recently in a study from a cohort of 600 patients from Paris, the percentage of patient-years with inactive disease was significantly higher than that of patient-years with hospitalization and even more than that of patient-years with abdominal surgery [7].

4.2 Early Crohn's Disease

Early CD needs a dedicated discussion, because of its relevance in clinical practice and in research. Studies of referral centers and population-based studies have shown that about one-fifth of patients already have evidence of a stricturing or penetrating intestinal complication at diagnosis. From one of the most extensive clinical course studies in children with CD [24], based on an IBD registry in northwestern France (404 children with median follow-up time of 84 months), it emerges that childhood-onset CD is characterized by widespread extent, frequent evolution toward more complicated forms, and early prescription of corticosteroids (CS); furthermore the cumulative risk for the

Fig. 4.3 Identification of the main disease states and probability of each of them over time (Markov model analysis). Reprinted from Silverstein et al. [21]

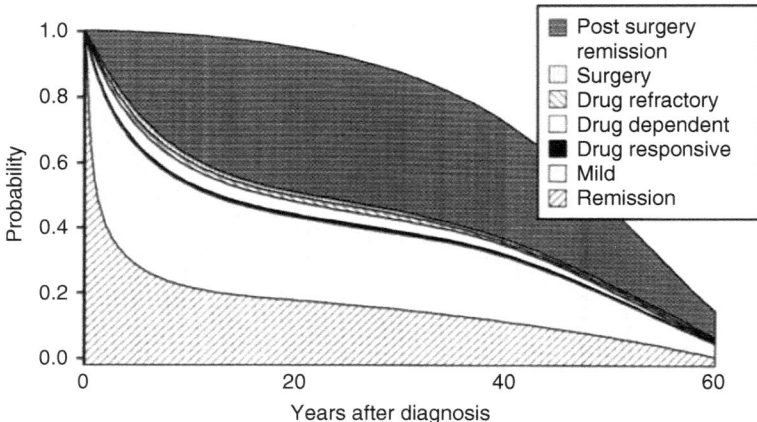

first intestinal resection is approximately 34 % at 5 years from diagnosis.

Our efforts are directed at early detection of disease to perform effective intervention before the onset of bowel damage (stricture, fistula, abscess). Also in clinical research settings, the development of new therapeutic strategies to implement the early treatment of CD patients is now a relevant target.

According to Laurent Peyrin-Biroulet et al. [16], an early CD meets the following criteria:

1. Crohn's disease activity index (CDAI) >220
2. C-reactive protein >10 mg/l or significant endoscopic (large coalescent and deep ulcerations covering more than 10 % of the mucosal area of at least one segment of the colorectum) or radiological evidence (computed tomography [CT] or magnetic resonance imaging [MRI] bowel enhancement) of disease activity or positive fecal markers
3. No limit of age (both pediatric and adult patients can be included)
4. No previous or current use of immunomodulators (azathioprine, 6-mercaptopurine, methotrexate), biologics, and corticosteroids (previously steroid-dependent with oral steroids or any treatment with intravenous steroids)
5. No fistula (including perianal fistulas), abscess, and stricture (wall thickening and luminal narrowing with prestenotic dilatation defined as a diameter greater than the normal diameter of the small bowel or colon) on CT or MRI

6. No history of CD-related surgery (minor or major surgical procedures, no history of endoscopic balloon dilation of a stricture)
7. No impaired GI functioning: normal fecal continence, no previous or current use of oral or parenteral substitution (vitamins, minerals), and no enteral or parenteral nutrition since diagnosis
8. Disease duration less than 2 years

If early treatment has an impact on the course of the disease, it is not fully understood, because of the general lack of long-term data. From the D'Haens trial [25] and from the subgroup analysis of the placebo-controlled CHARM trial [26], early treated patients were less likely to have mucosal ulceration after 2 years of treatment, and increased remission rates were observed in those patients with disease duration <2 years. Data collected by Abraham et al., from a cohort of veterans with CD, suggest that early treatment could prevent the fibrosis development with a reduction of the rate of surgery [27]. However only prospective population-based studies comparing early vs. late treatment could give an answer to this question. Of course these studies are difficult to carry out.

4.3 Surgery

In the course of CD, surgery could be necessary if some complications occur, such as strictures, fistulas, and intra-abdominal abscesses. Over the disease course the majority of patients undergo surgery. In the Swedish and Danish cohort, the cumulative rates of surgery after 10 years were 83 % and 61 %, respectively; in the Copenhagen cohort 35 % of patients were operated in the first year.

Now in the era of rapidly evolving treatments, it is important to evaluate the surgical risk trend. In a recent systematic review of 30 population-based studies, diagnosed from 1955 to 2011, the authors concluded that the risk of surgery had decreased over time at 1, 5, and 10 years after diagnosis [28].

These data are consistent with the majority of evidences produced in recent studies in which a reduction in surgical rates was observed, even if contrary data were also not lacking. For example, the cumulative probability of first major abdominal surgery from time of diagnosis remained stable over time, without any evidence of treatment benefit in Olmsted County [29].

The most debated question is the role of the introduction of immunomodulators in reducing the risk of surgery, since the reduction of surgical rates has coincided with the increased and earlier use of IM and biologics.

In the Cardiff [30] and West Hungary cohorts [8], the increased and earlier use of thiopurine was an independent factor influencing the likelihood of surgery. In a prospective UK population-based cohort [13], patients treated with 6 months of IM therapy had a 44 % reduction in the risk of surgery (hazards ratio (HR): 0.56; 95 % confidence interval (CI): 0.37–0.85), and those receiving 12 months of thiopurine therapy had a 69 % reduction in the risk of surgery (HR: 0.31; 95 % CI: 0.22–0.44). Early treatment showed no additional benefit in reducing risk of surgery. Recently data were published from a Danish nationwide cohort study [19]. In this inception cohort of adult with IBD, 13,185 patients with CD, diagnosed during 1979-2011, were selected. Four cohorts were created according to the era of diagnosis. The authors found an increasing use of azathioprine (AZA) and tumor necrosis factor-alpha blockers (anti-TNF-α) in the more recent cohorts, together with a decreased use of 5-ASA and oral CS. The use of biologic agents and IM in the first 4 years from diagnosis was significantly higher, whereas the use of oral CS was lower.

Likewise the cumulative probability of undergoing first major surgery was lowest in the most recent cohorts within the first year and 5th and 9th years after diagnosis, and the same significant decrease in surgery over time was observed for minor surgery (intra-abdominal fistulas or perianal complication).

In a tertiary unit-referred patient cohort from France [17], the percentage of patients who were operated on during the first 3 months remained less than 5 %. After the first 3 months, the operative rate (number of operations performed per year) fluctuated within a narrow range (3.3–7.5 %), without any significant change over 26 years. In a Spanish study, a comparison between two referred cohorts, one selected before and another after the introduction of infliximab (IFX), did not show a reduction of surgical requirements [31].

How much the introduction of immunomodulators and anti-TNF-α has changed the course of disease still remains debated, despite all the economic and scientific efforts that have been made over the years in clinical and basic research. In the Paris referral cohort, abovementioned, an increased trend of use of anti-TNF-α and IM was observed in mild-to-moderate diseases and in severe diseases, together with an increased proportion of untreated patients over time, mostly in the more recent years and in the mild-to-moderate forms. The authors concluded that despite the proportion of patients under immunosuppressants (comprising steroids and anti-TNF) that had not changed over the years, the percentage of patients with active disease was decreased both in mild-to-moderate forms and in severe forms. This led the authors to conclude that the decrease in disease activity, especially in moderate CD, observed over time, was not related to the treatment regimen.

In a prospective inception cohort from Copenhagen [32] (inception period between 2003 and 2004), it was not possible to infer that biologics have reduced significantly the risk of surgery. This study is very relevant because, differently from the other upper mentioned, it is the only one in which the use of biologics was possible from the beginning of enrollment. The authors found a 7-year cumulative risk of anti-TNF- α treatment of 23.3 %.

Historically a high rate of response to placebo has been shown in randomized controlled trials (RCT) on IBD, with a significant heterogeneity among the studies, ranging between rates near zero and thirty percent [33]. This observation might suggest that the course of the disease is not always influenced by therapies, whereas it could spontaneously switch between periods of activity and inactivity. However in most of the trials there was a lack of disease activity-based eligibility criteria. This omission had led to the inclusion of patients with minimal disease activity, in whom it is difficult to assess the benefit of treatment. Moreover primary end points for induction trials were often clinical response or improvement, and a wide variety of non-validated instruments to assess disease activity were used.

Summarizing according to the advances in treatment, there is a lower use of aminosalicylates and topical treatment, the time to exposure to steroids tends to be reduced, and concurrently the use of thiopurines and anti-TNF has grown. However, no convincing surgery-sparing effect of newer medications can be definitively assessed. Other factors might affect the risk of surgery over time: new therapies, change in diagnostic approach (availability of CT and MRI), advance in surgery techniques, increasing use of endoscopy, and the reduction of exposure to harmful substances (smoking, etc.). An interesting issue is the rapid evolution of surgical techniques, for example, laparoscopic surgery. Limited resections were more widely used than in the past, with an increased use of this surgical technique, in more selected patients. This approach has contributed to maintain stable the rates of surgery over time.

Only long-term data from prospective unselected inception cohort could give more definite answers.

4.4   Relapse and Recurrence After Surgery

After a complete resection there is a high rate of endoscopic recurrence. In a meta-analysis of placebo arm of studies on prevention therapy of endoscopic recurrence [18], the pooled data of severe endoscopic recurrence was 50 %, meaning, according to the Rutgeerts' study [34], that this population will be affected by clinical symptoms within a short time. A recent multicenter study by Orlando et al. [35] has shown that even after 6 months there is a 62 % rate of severe endoscopic recurrence. Many variables have been associated with risk of recurrence: smoking, site, extent and pattern of disease, type of anastomosis, disease duration, and extraintestinal manifestation, but with discordant results among the studies.

Many drugs have been evaluated for prevention of endoscopic recurrence. Mesalazine and metronidazole seem to have a marginal role [36, 37], whereas it seems that biologics therapy influences significantly the rate of recurrence [38, 39].

4.5   Predictors

The classification of CD in different phenotypes is useful to predict the clinical course. According to the Vienna classification system [40], CD could be classified, based on:

- Location: L1 (terminal ileum), L2 (colon), L3 (ileocolon), and L4 (upper gastrointestinal)
- Behavior: B1 (non-stricturing, non-penetrating), B2 (stricturing), and B3 (penetrating)
- Age at diagnosis: A1 (below 40 years) and A2 (above 40 years)

The Montreal statement provided the addiction of the perianal disease as a modifier [41].

Disease location at diagnosis is relatively homogeneous and quite stable, with the exception of the reported variance in the frequency of upper gastrointestinal location, comparing pediatric- and adult-onset populations. Data from the population-based cohorts suggest that 20–30 % of patients have an L1, the percentages of L2 and L3 range between 30 and 45 % and 20 and 35 %, respectively, and 2 % have an L4, correlated with a worsened prognosis. The extent of disease is also a negative predictor.

The clinical features of CD change over time with a decreasing frequency of inflammatory disease behavior and an increasing frequency of stricturing and/or penetrating disease behavior. In the Veszprem cohort [19] at 7 years, the risk of progression to more complicated forms was 25 %. In a Mayo Clinic study, 81.4 % had non-stricturing, non-penetrating disease, 4.6 % had stricturing disease, and 14.0 % had penetrating disease at diagnosis. The cumulative risk of developing either complication in the Mayo cohort was 18.6 % at 90 days, 22.0 % at 1 year, 33.7 % at 5 years, and 50.8 % at 20 years after diagnosis [42]. In a noteworthy study by Cosnes et al., up to 70 % of CD patients developed either penetrating or stricturing disease during the course of the disease (Fig. 4.4). During the first 10 years, 27 % of patients had a change in disease behavior from non-stricturing, non-penetrating to structuring disease, while 30 % developed penetrating phenotypes [44].

Pediatric onset has been associated with a more complicated course: high prevalence of upper forms, high cumulative risk of use of immunosuppressors, and increased frequency of active periods, but it is not definitively clear if there is also a higher risk of surgery over time [25, 43, 45, 46].

In a landmark study by Beaugerie et al. [47], factors predictive of disabling CD course during a 5-year period following the diagnosis were analyzed in a prospective-retrospective referral cohort. Among 1123 patients the rate of disabling disease was 85.2 %. At the multivariate analysis independent factors present at diagnosis, significantly associated with subsequent 5-year disabling course, were the initial requirement for steroid use, an age below 40 years, and the presence of perianal disease.

This study is particularly relevant because the early identification of patients at increased risk of developing a severe disease could help clinicians to identify patients that would benefit more from an aggressive treatment, limiting the side effects of therapies.

Furthermore the length of diagnostic delay is another negative predictor. Data reported from the IBD Swiss cohort [48] showed that the length of diagnostic delay was positively correlated with the occurrence of bowel stenosis and intestinal surgery in a cohort of about 1000 CD patients, stratified into four groups according to the quartiles of diagnostic delay.

The younger age at diagnosis is a predictor of worsened prognosis, whereas the older age at diagnosis seems to be a predictor of favorable course of disease [49], even if older IBD patients might have a higher morbidity and mortality than younger if they underwent hospitalization. In a Wisconsin cross-sectional study, patients older than 65 years with an IBD-related hospitalization in 2004, even after adjusting for comorbidity, had

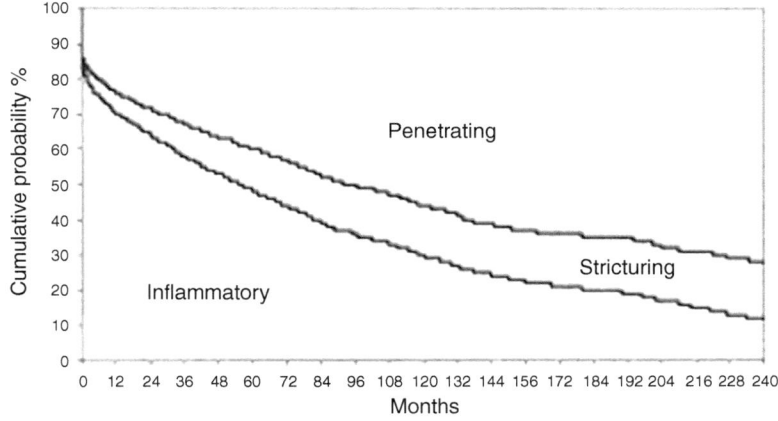

Fig. 4.4 Long-term evolution of disease behavior in CD [43]

higher in-hospital mortality. Older patients with fistulizing disease are more likely to undergo surgery. Among IBD patients who underwent surgery, older patients also had a longer postoperative stay [20].

Another well-known negative prognostic factor is smoking. Smokers are at risk of having a disease with more exacerbations. In a French study of 622 consecutive inpatients, the number of flare-ups was significantly higher in smoking patients than nonsmoking; the former smokers had the same risk of nonsmokers [50]. In an Italian series of 182 patients who underwent surgery for CD, smoking was independently associated with the risk of clinical, endoscopic, and surgical recurrence; the presence of extraintestinal manifestations and the extent of disease were other independent factors [51].

A great number of genetic factors have been associated as possible predictors of different courses of disease, but despite a high number of genes, associated with CD, that were identified [52], none of these have emerged as a real predictor of worse course [53].

4.6   Risk of Malignancies

The real risk of intestinal malignancies in CD is also debated. Although in the past IBD were considered at higher risk of developing cancer [54, 55], some authors have suggested that the higher prevalence of intestinal cancer reported in the various studies on CD might depend mainly on a selection bias in the referral cohorts. In a landmark work by Jess et al. [56], a meta-analysis of six population-based cohort studies was carried out to evaluate the risk of colorectal cancer (CRC) and the risk of small bowel cancer. The study revealed an overall increased risk of both CRC and small bowel cancer among patients with CD; the risk of CRC in two of the six included studies was greater in patients with CD involving the colon than in patients with pure ileal CD.

The risk of cancer in patients using immunosuppressants is another debated issue, since in the posttransplant settings immunosuppressants are associated with a higher risk of cancer and recurrence of cancer in patients with a positive story [57]. Furthermore thiopurines have been shown to promote EBV-related lymphomas and nonmelanoma skin cancers in patients with IBD [58, 59].

Recently a noteworthy study by Beaugerie et al. has shown an increased risk of malignancies in IBD patients [60]. In this study 19,500 patients were enrolled in a prospective referral cohort (CESAME), 400 of which had history of cancer. Authors found that patients with IBD with previous cancer had a doubled risk of new or recurrent cancer, compared with the risk of an incident first cancer in patients without history of malignancy, whereas the exposure to immunosuppressors was not associated with new or recurrent cancer. In another study on the same population [61], the risk of lymphoproliferative disorders in IBD patients receiving thiopurines was five times higher in patients exposed to thiopurines than in those never exposed to these drugs. Other independent factors associated with risk of incident lymphoproliferative disorder were old age, male sex, and longer duration of inflammatory bowel disease.

Even if it is less common, hepatosplenic T-cell lymphoma is not less important. It has been associated with use of combination therapies (anti-TNF-α + IM), especially in young males [62].

4.7   Mortality

Data on mortality in CD range between a wideness of values. The standardized mortality ratios (SMR) for Crohn's disease vary from 0.72 to more than 2.0 [63, 64]. Generally the excess risk of dying in CD as compared with the general population is different in referral cohorts and in population-based studies, because of the referral filter bias. In unselected cohorts an overall increased risk of dying is not always detectable; a very large sample size is needed to detect small differences. In Tables 4.2 and 4.3 SMR of population-based and referral cohorts were summarized. Standardized mortality ratios are calculated as the ratio of deaths observed in a cohort to those expected in a group of the same size from

Table 4.2 CD-related mortality from selected population-based cohorts was reported as standardized mortality ratios

Author	Site	N° of patients	SMR (95 % CI)
Jess [4]	Olmsted County, USA	314	1.2 (0.9–1.6)
Persson [9]	Stockholm, Sweden	1251	1.5 (1.3–1.7)
Jess [3]	Copenhagen, Denmark	374	1.3 (1.0–1.6)
Sjoberg [10]	Uppsala, Sweden	1469	1.6 (1.4–1.9)
Masala [14]	Florence, Italy	231	1.5 (1.1–2.1)
Card [65]	GPRD, UK	5960	1.7 (1.5–2.0)
Wolters [66]	Europe	371	1.9 (1.3–2.5)

Table 4.3 CD-related mortality from hospital-based cohorts was reported as standardized mortality ratios

Author	Site	N° of patients	SMR (95 % CI)
Prior [67]	Birmingham, UK	513	2 (1.8–2.19)
Weterman [68]	Leiden, Netherlands	659	2.23 (1.75–2.85)
Cottone [69]	Palermo, Italy	531	0.97 (0.4–1.8)
Farrokhyar [70]	Southern England, UK	196	0.94 (0.59–1.4)
Uno [12]	Kyushu and Fukuoka, Japan	544	1.43 (0.53–3.12)

the general population in the same area and standardized for age and sex of the individuals in the study cohort.

In a recent meta-analysis, including 13 studies that were conducted within general and specialist health care settings and results from different countries, the risk of dying for patients with CD is over 50 % higher than would be expected for someone in the general population of the same age and sex [11]. Specialist centers had the highest combined SMR and community-based studies the lowest.

A significant decrease in SMR of 1.9 % per year from 1955 to 1985 has been showed. The introduction of AZA (1970 in Europe), along with corticosteroids, coincides with the reduction seen in SMR. This meta-analysis has not shown a significant impact on SMR of anti-TNF-α. The use of biologics agents has spread recently, so it is not definitively possible to assess their real long-term impact.

Interestingly authors noted no significant increase in mortality with duration of disease, while an increased mortality risk was assessed for patients within 5 years from diagnosis. The major cause of death was surgical complications. Mortality was finally highest in patients diagnosed under 20 years old and women diagnosed before the age of 50 years. Smoking was associated with an excess mortality in the Florence cohort [14].

Conclusions

- Studies evaluating the course of the disease have produced different results according to the adopted methodology. Unselected inception cohort studies the best ones on which we rely in order to avoid the selection bias from referral centers.
- The main events during the course of the disease are activity, remission, relapse, obstruction, fistulizing, surgical resection, cancer, and death.
- A more benign course of CD than expected seems to emerge from data produced using inception cohort. In the studies from the most important unselected population-based cohorts, more than 50 % of patients were in remission after several years of disease, and only a few of the patients had high activity.
- The true impact of early treatment with immunomodulators on the course of the disease is not fully understood, because of the general lack of long-term data.
- Data from inception cohorts have shown a high risk of surgery, increasing over time (more than 60 % at 10 years), but in the last decades this trend has been being reduced. It is not definitively established if this reduction of surgical rates over time is correlated with an increased use of immunomodulators and biologic therapies.

- The clinical features of CD change over time with a decreasing frequency of inflammatory disease behavior and an increasing frequency of stricturing and/or penetrating disease behavior. The main predictors of disabling course are the presence of L4, the extension of disease, pediatric onset, the initial requirement for steroid use at diagnosis, an age below 40 years at diagnosis, the presence of perianal disease at diagnosis, the length of diagnostic delay, and smoking habitus. Genetic factors have not been definitively correlated with prognosis. The older age at diagnosis seems to be a positive predictor.

- An increased risk of colorectal cancer and small bowel cancer has been described in CD. Patients receiving long-term thiopurine are at higher risk of lymphoproliferative disorders (especially B-cell lymphoma) and nonmelanoma skin cancer. The less common hepatosplenic T-cell lymphoma has been associated with use of combination therapies (anti-TNF-α + IM), especially in young males.

- The risk of dying in a CD patient when compared with the general population is higher, even if in inception cohort studies the increased risk is not always detectable.

References

1. Crohn BB, Ginzburg L, Oppenheimer GD. (From the Mount Sinai Hospital New York) "Regional Ileitis" A pathologic and clinical entity. JAMA. 1932;99:1323–8.
2. Jess T, Riis L, Vind I, et al. Changes in clinical characteristics, course, and prognosis of inflammatory bowel disease during the last 5 decades: a population-based study from Copenhagen, Denmark. Inflamm Bowel Dis. 2007;13(4):481–9.
3. Jess T, Winther KV, Munkholm P, et al. Mortality and causes of death in Crohn's disease: follow-up of a population-based cohort in Copenhagen County, Denmark. Gastroenterology. 2002;122(7):1808–14.
4. Jess T, Loftus Jr EV, Harmsen WS, et al. Survival and cause specific mortality in patients with inflammatory bowel disease: a long term outcome study in Olmsted County, Minnesota, 1940–2004. Gut. 2006;55(9):1248–54.
5. Palli D, Trallori G, Masala G. General and cancer specific mortality of a population based cohort of patients with inflammatory bowel disease: the Florence Study. Gut. 1998;42(2):175–9.
6. Sackett DL, Hayness RB, Guyatt G, Tugwell P. Clinical epidemiology. A basic science for clinical medicine. 2nd ed. London: Little, Brown and Company; 1991.
7. Cosnes J, Bourrier A, Nion-Larmurier I, et al. Factors affecting outcomes in Crohn's disease over 15 years. Gut. 2012;61:1140–5.
8. Lakatos PL, Golovics PA, David G, et al. Has there been a change in the natural history of Crohn's disease? Surgical rates and medical management in a population-based inception cohort from Western Hungary between 1977–2009. Am J Gastroenterol. 2012;107:579–88.
9. Persson PG, Bernell O, Leijonmarck CE, et al. Survival and cause-specific mortality in inflammatory bowel disease: a population-based cohort study. Gastroenterology. 1996;110(5):1339–45.
10. Sjöberg D, Holmström T, Larsson M, et al. Incidence and clinical course of Crohn's disease during the first year – results from the IBD Cohort of the Uppsala Region (ICURE) of Sweden 2005–2009. J Crohns Colitis. 2014;8(3):215–22.
11. Canavan C, Abrams KR, Mayberry JF, et al. Meta-analysis: mortality in Crohn's disease. Aliment Pharmacol Ther. 2007;25:861–70.
12. Uno H, Yao T, Matsui T, Sakurai T, et al. Mortality and cause of death in Japanese patients with Crohn's disease. Dis Colon Rectum. 2003;46(10 Suppl):S15–21.
13. Chatu S, Saxena S, Subramanian V, et al. The impact of timing and duration of thiopurine treatment on first intestinal resection in Crohn's Disease: national UK population-based study 1989–2010. Am J Gastroenterol. 2014;109:409–16.
14. Masala G, Bagnoli S, Ceroti M, et al. Divergent patterns of total and cancer mortality in ulcerative colitis and Crohn's disease patients: the Florence IBD study 1978–2001. Gut. 2004;53(9):1309–13.
15. Sonnenberg FA, Beck JR. Markov models in medical decision making: a practical guide. Med Decis Making. 1993;13(4):322–38.
16. Peyrin-Biroulet L, Loftus Jr EV, Colombel J-F, et al. Early Crohn disease: a proposed definition for use in disease-modification trials. Gut. 2010;59:141–7.
17. Cosnes J, Nion-Larmurier I, Beaugerie L, et al. Impact of the increasing use of immunosuppressants in Crohn's disease on the need for intestinal surgery. Gut. 2005;54:237–41.
18. Renna S, Cammà C, Modesto I, et al. Meta-analysis of the placebo rates of clinical relapse and severe endoscopic recurrence in postoperative Crohn's disease. Gastroenterology. 2008;135(5):1500–9.
19. Rungoe C, Langholz E, Andersson M, et al. Changes in medical treatment and surgery rates in inflammatory bowel disease: a nationwide cohort study 1979–2011. Gut. 2014;63:1607–16.

20. Ananthakrishnan AN, McGinley EL, et al. Inflammatory bowel disease in the elderly is associated with worse outcomes: a national study of hospitalizations. Inflamm Bowel Dis. 2009;15: 182–9.

21. Silverstein MD, Loftus EV, Sandborn WJ, et al. Clinical course and costs of care for Crohn's disease: Markov model analysis of a population-based cohort. Gastroenterology. 1999;117:49–57.

22. Munkholm P, Langholz E, Davidsen M, et al. Disease activity courses in a regional cohort of Crohn's disease patients. Scand J Gastroenterol. 1995;30:699–706.

23. Solberg IC, Vatn MH, Hoie O, et al. Clinical course in Crohn's disease: results of a Norwegian population-based ten-year follow-up study. Clin Gastroenterol Hepatol. 2007;5:1430–8.

24. Vernier-Massouille G, Balde M, Salleron J, et al. Natural history of pediatric Crohn's disease: a population-based cohort study. Gastroenterology. 2008;135:1106–13.

25. D'Haens G, Baert F, van Assche G, et al. Early combined immunosuppression or conventional management in patients with newly diagnosed Crohn's disease: an open randomised trial. Lancet. 2008;371:660.

26. Schreiber S, Reinisch W, Colombel JF, et al. Subgroup analysis of the placebocontrolled CHARM trial: increased remission rates through 3 years for adalimumab-treated patients with early Crohn's disease. J Crohn's Colitis. 2013;7:213–21.

27. Abraham NS, Richardson P, Castillo D, et al. Dual therapy with infliximab and immunomodulator reduces one-year rates of hospitalization and surgery among veterans with inflammatory bowel disease. Clin Gastroenterol Hepatol. 2013;11(10): 1281–7.

28. Frolkis AD, Dykeman J, Negrón ME, et al. Risk of surgery for inflammatory bowel diseases has decreased over time: a systematic review and meta-analysis of population-based studies. Gastroenterology. 2013;145(5):996–1006.

29. Peyrin-Biroulet L, Harmsen WS, Tremaine WJ, et al. Surgery in a population-based cohort of Crohn's disease from Olmsted County, Minnesota (1970–2004). Am J Gastroenterol. 2012;107:1693–701.

30. Ramadas AV, Gunesh S, Thomas GA, et al. Natural history of Crohn's disease in a population-based cohort from Cardiff (1986–2003): a study of changes in medical treatment and surgical resection rates. Gut. 2010;59:1200–6.

31. Domenech E, Zabana Y, Garcia-Planella E, et al. Clinical outcome of newly diagnosed Crohn's disease: a comparative, retrospective study before and after infliximab availability. Aliment Pharmacol Ther. 2010;31:233–9.

32. Vester-Andersen MK, Michelle V, et al. Disease course and surgery rates in inflammatory bowel disease: a population-based, 7-year follow-up study in the era of immunomodulating therapy. Am J Gastroenterol. 2014;109:705–14.

33. Sandborn WJ, Colombel JF, Enns R, et al. Natalizumab induction and main- tenance therapy for Crohn's disease. N Engl J Med. 2005;353:1912–25.

34. Hanauer SB, Korelitz BI, Rutgeerts P. Postoperative maintenance of Crohn's disease remission with 6-mercaptopurine, mesalamine, or placebo: a 2-year trial. Gastroenterology. 2004;127(3): 723–9.

35. Orlando A, Mocciaro F, Renna S. Early post-operative endoscopic recurrence in Crohn's disease patients: data from an Italian Group for the study of inflammatory bowel disease (IG-IBD) study on a large prospective multicenter cohort. J Crohns Colitis. 2014;8(10):1217–21.

36. Caprilli R, Cottone M, Tonelli F, et al. Two mesalazine regimens in the prevention of the post-operative recurrence of Crohn's disease: a pragmatic, double-blind, randomized controlled trial. Aliment Pharmacol Ther. 2003;17(4):517–23.

37. Cottone M, Cammà C. Mesalamine and relapse prevention in Crohn's disease. Gastroenterology. 2000;119(2):597.

38. Regueiro M, Schraut W, Baidoo L, et al. Infliximab prevents Crohn's disease recurrence after ileal resection. Gastroenterology. 2009;136(2):441–50.

39. Savarino E, Bodini G, Dulbecco P, et al. Adalimumab is more effective than azathioprine and mesalamine at preventing postoperative recurrence of Crohn's disease: a randomized controlled trial. Am J Gastroenterol. 2013;108(11):1731–42.

40. Gasche C, Scholmerich J, Brynskov J, et al. A simple classification of Crohn's disease: report of the working party of the world congresses of gastroenterology, Vienna 1998. Inflamm Bowel Dis. 2000;6: 8–15.

41. Silverberg MS, Satsangi J, Ahmad T, et al. Toward an integrated clinical, molecular and serological classification of inflammatory bowel disease: report of a Working Party of the 2005 Montreal World Congress of Gastroenterology. Can J Gastroenterol. 2005;19(Suppl A):5–36.

42. Thia KT, Sandborn WJ, Harmsen WS, et al. Risk factors associated with progression to intestinal complications of Crohn's disease in a population-based cohort. Gastroenterology. 2010;139:1147–55.

43. Gower-Rousseau C, Vasseur F, Fumery M, et al. Epidemiology of inflammatory bowel diseases: new insights from a French population-based registry (EPIMAD). Dig Liver Dis. 2013;45:89–94.

44. Cosnes J, Cattan S, Blain A, et al. Long-term evolution of disease behavior of Crohn's disease. Inflamm Bowel Dis. 2002;8:244–50.

45. De Bie CI, Paerregaard A, Kolacek S, et al. Disease phenotype at diagnosis in pediatric Crohn's disease: 5-year analyses of the EUROKIDS Registry. Inflamm Bowel Dis. 2013;19:378–85.

46. Pigneur B, Seksik P, Viola S, et al. Natural history of Crohn's disease: comparison between childhood- and adult-onset disease. Inflamm Bowel Dis. 2010;16:953–61.

47. Beaugerie L, Seksik P, Nion–Larmurier I, et al. Predictors of Crohn's disease. Gastroenterology. 2006;130:650–6.

48. Schoepfer AM, Dehlavi M-A, Fournier N, et al.; On behalf of the Swiss IBD Cohort Study Group. Diagnostic delay in Crohn's disease is associated with a complicated disease course and increased operation rate. Am J Gastroenterol. 2013;108:1744–53

49. Choi JH, Kim ES, Cho KB, et al. Old age at diagnosis is associated with favorable. Outcomes in Korean patients with inflammatory bowel disease gastrointestinal study group. Intest Res. 2015;13(1):60–7.

50. Cosnes J, Carbonnel F, Carrat F, et al. Effects of current and former cigarette smoking on the clinical course of Crohn's disease. J Aliment Pharmacol Ther. 1999;13:1403–11.

51. Cottone M, Rosselli M, Pagliaro L, et al. Smoking habits and recurrence in Crohn's disease. Gastroenterology. 1994;106(3):643–8.

52. Franke A, McGovern DP, Barrett JC, et al. Genome-wide meta-analysis increases to 71 the number of confirmed Crohn's disease susceptibility loci. Nat Genet. 2010;42(12):1118–25.

53. Maus B, Jung C, Mahachie John JM, et al. Molecular reclassification of Crohn's disease: a cautionary note on population stratification. PLoS One. 2013;17:8(10).

54. Weedon DD, Shorter RG, Ilstrup DM, et al. Crohn's disease and cancer. N Engl J Med. 1973;289:1099–103.

55. Greenstein AJ, Sachar DB, Smith H, et al. A comparison of cancer risk in Crohn's disease and ulcerative colitis. Cancer. 1981;48:2742–5.

56. Jess T, Gamborg M, Matzen P, et al. Increased risk of intestinal cancer in Crohn's disease: a meta-analysis of population-based cohort studies. Am J Gastroenterol. 2005;100:2724–9.

57. Gutierrez-Dalmau A, Campistol JM. Immunosuppressive therapy and malignancy in organ transplant recipients: a systematic review. Drugs. 2007;67:1167–98.

58. Beaugerie L, Brousse N, Bouvier AM, et al. Lymphoproliferative disorders in patients receiving thiopurines for inflammatory bowel disease: a prospective observational cohort study. Lancet. 2009;374:1617–25.

59. Peyrin-Biroulet L, Khosrotehrani K, Carrat F, et al. Increased risk for non-melanoma skin cancers in patients who receive thiopurines for inflammatory bowel disease. Gastroenterology. 2011;141:1621–8.e5.

60. Beaugerie L, Carrat F, Colombel J-F et al.; and the CESAME Study Group. Risk of new or recurrent cancer under immunosuppressive therapy in patients with IBD and previous cancer. Gut. 2014;63: 1416–23

61. Beaugerie L, Brousse N, Bouvier AM, et al.; CESAME Study Group. Lymphoproliferative disorders in patients receiving thiopurines for inflammatory bowel disease: a prospective observational cohort study. Lancet. 2009;374(9701):1617–25

62. Kotlyar DS, Osterman MT, Diamond RH, et al. A systematic review of factors that contribute to hepatosplenic T-cell lymphoma in patients with inflammatory bowel disease. Clin Gastroenterol Hepatol. 2011;9(1):36–41.

63. Probert CSJ, Jayanthi V, Wicks ACB. Mortality in Crohn's disease in Leicestershire, 1972–1989: an epidemiological community based study. Gut. 1992;33:1226–8.

64. Canavan C, Abrams KR, Hawthorne B. Long-term prognosis in Crohn's disease: an epidemiological study of patients diagnosed more than 20 years ago in Cardiff. Alim Pharmacol Therapeut. 2007;25(1):59–65.

65. van Staa TP, Card T, Logan RF, et al. 5-aminisalicylate use and colorectal cancer risk in inflammatory bowel disease: a large epidemiological study. Gut. 2005;54(11):1573–8.

66. Wolters FL, Russel MG, Sijbrandij J, et al.; European Collaborative study group on Inflammatory Bowel Disease (EC-IBD). Crohn's disease: increased mortality 10 years after diagnosis in a Europe-wide population based cohort. Gut. 2006;55(4):510–8.

67. Prior P, Gyde S, Cooke WT, Waterhouse JAH, Allen RN. Mortality in Crohn's disease. Gastroenterology. 1981;80:307–12.

68. Weterman IT, Biermond I, Pena AS. Mortality and causes of death in Crohn's disease. Review of 50 years' experience in Leiden University Hospital. Gut. 1990;31:1387–90.

69. Cottone M, Magliocco A, Rosselli M, et al. Mortality in patients with Crohn's disease. Scand J Gastroenterol. 1996;31:372–5.

70. Farrokhyar F, Swarbrik ET, Grace RH, et al. Low mortality in ulcerative colitis and Crohn's disease in three regional centres in England. Am J Gastroenterol. 2001;96(2):501–7.

Diagnostic and Therapeutic Role of Endoscopy in Crohn's Disease

Gianfranco Cocorullo, Nicola Falco,
Tommaso Fontana, Roberta Tutino,
Sebastiano Bonventre, Francesco D'Arpa,
and Gaspare Gulotta

Endoscopy plays a very important role in the management of Crohn's disease (CD).

It is an extremely important diagnostic tool in the period of symptoms onset, allowing the evaluation of the activity and of the extent of the disease; moreover, it is very useful in follow-up giving an evaluation of the response to the medical therapy, a detection of recurrences following surgery, and providing an oncological screening [1].

Several procedures like traditional colonoscopy, single- and double-balloon enteroscopy, endocapsule examination, and endoscopic ultrasound are today available.

CD can be diagnosed with endoscopy by a skilled gastroenterologist in the setting of a suggestive clinical presentation [2].

The "European Crohn's and Colitis Organization" (ECCO) guidelines recommend colonoscopy, including exploration of the last ileal loop, as the golden standard procedure to establish a diagnosis of CD since it allows performing multiple biopsies of the small bowel, as well as of each colonic tract.

However, further investigations are needed to study each part of the bowel and to show the overall extension of the disease.

The detectable endoscopic lesions are 40 % in ileum/colon, 30 % only in the ileum, 20 % only in the colon, 5 % in the duodenum, and 5 % in the rectum [3].

Bernell et al. [4] categorized CD on the basis of its localization in:

- Orojejunal (oral till the Treitz's ligament)
- Small bowel excluding terminal ileum (last 30 cm.)
- Ileocecal (last 30 cm. of ileum with or without cecal involvement)
- Continuous ileocolic (continuous ileocolic involvement)
- Discontinuous ileocolic (both small and large bowel involvement but without continuous inflammation in the ileocecal region)
- Colorectal (confined to the colon or to the rectum or both)

The correct localization of CD and the evaluation of its activity degree, obtained by the histological examination of multiple biopsies, play an indispensable role in the right orientation of treatments and for the choice of medical or surgical therapy. According to statistical data, the major role in the diagnosis of CD affords the

G. Cocorullo (✉) • N. Falco • T. Fontana • R. Tutino
S. Bonventre • F. D'Arpa • G. Gulotta
Department of surgical oncological and
stomatological sciences, University Hospital
P. Giaccone, University of Palermo, Palermo, Italy
e-mail: gianfranco.cocorullo@unipa.it

© Springer International Publishing Switzerland 2016
G. Lo Re, M. Midiri (eds.), *Cronn's Disease: Radiological Features and Clinical-Surgical Correlations*,
DOI 10.1007/978-3-319-23066-5_5

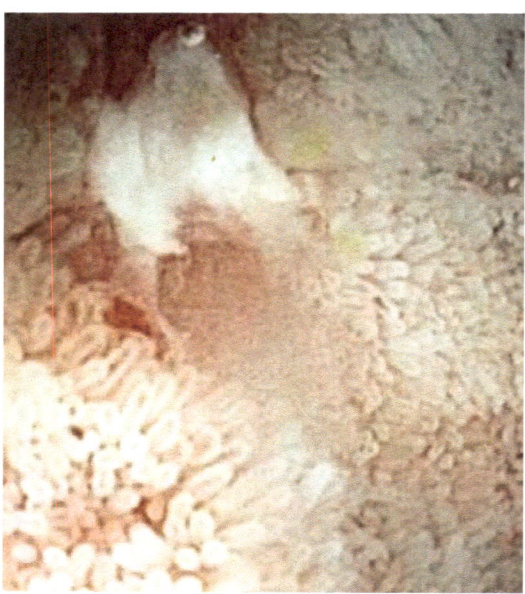

Fig. 5.1 Aphthous ulcer

Table 5.1 Score for diagnosis of CD versus UC

1	Discontinuity of mucosal involvement	+55
2	Cobblestone-like lesions	+8
3	Aphthous/serpiginous/linear ulcers	+4
4	Large/deep ulcers	+4
5	Sparing of the rectum	+5
6	Anal lesions	+15
7	Continuous mucosal involvement	−2
8	Granularity	−3
9	Not visible vascular frame	−2
10	Erosions or micro-ulcers	−7
11	Rectal involvement	−2

Table 5.2 Rutgeerts' score for ileal involvement

Grade	
0	No lesions in terminal ileum
1	Less than five aphthous lesions
2	More than five aphthous lesions and normal mucosa between them or skip areas of larger lesions or lesions limited to the ileocolonic anastomosis
3	Diffuse aphthous ileitis with diffusely inflamed mucosa
4	Diffuse inflammation with larger ulcers, nodules, and/or narrowing

retrograde ileoscopy that has got an overall importance [5, 6].

Colonoscopy can highlight areas involved by disease separated by normal colonic mucosa. The colonic disease is more present in the cecum-right colon, usually with rectal sparing. On the contrary, anal lesions can often occur.

Characteristic lesions are small aphthous ulcers (Fig. 5.1) that can form star ulcers and large linear or deep serpiginous ulcers; these can develop the cobblestone-like colonic mucosa aspect with deep ulcers interposed between areas of edematous mucosa [7].

Endoscopic examination is also essential in the differential diagnosis of inflammatory bowel disease (IBD) from other causes of colitis including infectious and noninfectious conditions such as ischemic colitis, diverticulitis, solitary ulcer of the rectum, drug-induced colitis, and others. Moreover, it consents to distinguish between CD and the others IBD such as ulcerative colitis, indeterminate colitis, collagenase colitis, and lymphocytic colitis.

In ulcerative colitis (UC), the distribution of lesions is continuous, in contrast to CD where it is discontinuous and segmental; both show a fra-gility of the mucosa; however, this is much more common in the UC in conjunction with proctocolitis, too [8, 9]. Conversely, the involvement of the terminal ileum is almost present in CD while is absent in UC. Another endoscopic sign of the CD is the characteristic cobblestone-like aspect, absent in UC.

An endoscopic score system was developed which has a sensitivity of 92 % in differential diagnosis between CD and UC. A score >4 is suggestive for CD, while a score <4 is suggestive for the second one [8, 9]. Criteria are showed in Table 5.1.

Moreover, Rutgeerts proposed an endoscopic score system to assess ileal lesions in patients with diagnosis of CD. The score plays a very important role also with regard to the postsurgical recurrence detection, and it is used for the relapses classification (Table 5.2) [10, 11].

Endoscopic indexes were developed, also, to evaluate the ileocolonic CD activity; these are the "Crohn's disease endoscopic index of severity"

Table 5.3 Scoring system for Crohn's disease endoscopic index of severity (CDEIS)

	Rectum	Sigmoid and left colon	Transverse colon	Right colon	Ileum	Total
Deep ulcerations (12 if present)						Total 1
Superficial ulcerations (12 if present)						Total 2
Surface involved by disease (cm)						Total 3
Surface involved by ulcerations (cm)						Total 4

Total 1 + Total 2 + Total 3 + Total 4 = Total A
Number of segments totally or partially explored = n
Total A/n = Total B
If an ulcerated stenosis is present anywhere, add 3 = C
If a nonulcerated stenosis is present anywhere, add 3 = D
Total B + C + D = CDEIS

Table 5.4 Definitions of the simple endoscopic score for Crohn's disease (SES-CD) variables

	0	1	2	3
Presence of ulcers	None	Aphthous ulcers (0.1–0.5 cm)	Large ulcers (0.5–2 cm)	Very large ulcers (>2 cm)
Ulcerated surface	None	<10 %	10–30 %	>30 %
Affected surface	Unaffected segment	<50 %	50–75 %	>75 %
Presence of narrowings	None	Single, can be passed	Multiple, can be passed	Cannot be passed

Values are given to each variable for every examined bowel segment
SES-CD sum of all variables for the five bowel segments

(CDEIS) (Table 5.3) and the "simple endoscopic score for Crohn's disease" (SES-CD) (Table 5.4).

In these indexes, bowel is divided into five segments that are evaluated individually and then collected.

SES-CD provides a numerical score (0–3) for four endoscopic parameters in each segment; these are size of ulcers, degree of ulcerated surface, degree of affected surface, and presence of narrowing in the colon. The sum constitutes the SES-CD score.

However, the evaluation of bowel endoscopic lesions does not reflect the systemic manifestation of symptomatic inflammatory process.

Thus, endoscopic recurrences of CD, following colectomy or ileocolectomy, occur in 73–93 % of patients within 1 year, while clinical recurrences affect only 20 % of these patients.

Unfortunately, Rutgeerts score 3–4 is predictive of early recurrences of symptoms and development of complications in the next course of CD [2].

For patients with a high suspicion of CD despite the negativity of the ileoscopy and/or of

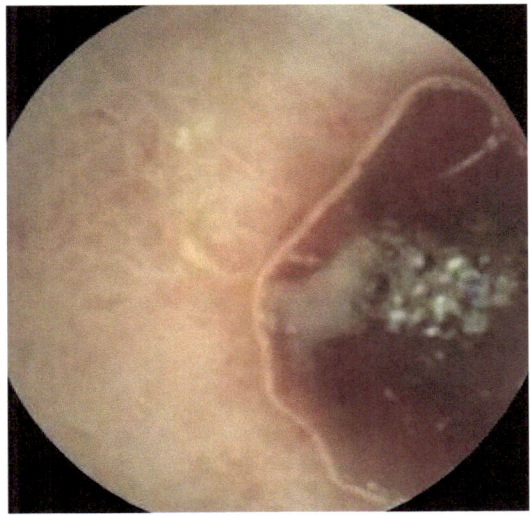

Fig. 5.2 VCE in CD

radiological examinations (CT or MR), the ECCO proposes, in the statement 2 I, the use of video-capsule endoscopy (VCE) for the study of the entire small bowel (Fig. 5.2) [12]. Of course, this

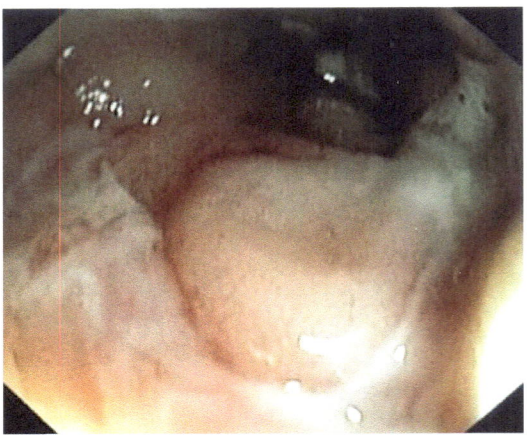

Fig. 5.3 Ileal stricture

is not the first-line modality to assess the initial diagnosis of CD. This exam that is superior to the CT or RM in the diagnosis of bowel lesions needs the integration with radiological exams to evaluate the presence of even severe extra-luminal lesion [13]. VCE is indeed useful to determine the extent, severity, and recurrence following surgery and to evaluate the response to medical therapy of the disease; it has a high negative predictive level but a lower specificity. The exam is contraindicated in patients with suspected gastrointestinal obstruction, strictures, or fistulas and is relatively contraindicated when dysphagia, Zenker's diverticulum, colonic diverticulosis, extensive Crohn's enteritis, and prior pelvic or abdominal surgery occur [13].

Double-balloon enteroscopy allows examining the entire small bowel mucosa. The exam is indicated for endoscopic examination and therapy following VCE findings; it should be reserved to patients in whom the biopsy specimens from suspicious areas are important for the diagnosis, the technique is useful in cases needing a small bowel stricture dilatation too (Fig. 5.3) [12].

In this regard, the ECCO guidelines propose endoscopic dilatation, as a therapeutic tool, in the conservative treatment of brief, mild to moderate strictures, as alternative to strictureplasty [14]. Some authors suggest that endoscopic dilatation has to be preferred to strictureplasty in short strictures and in anastomotic stenosis [13]. Patients that have short (<8 cm) and localized strictures without active inflammation at the site of stricture

are the most suitable for endoscopic treatment. Endoscopic dilatation permits a deferral of surgery of at least 3 years in cases of regular course of the procedure; however, some authors report a rate of perforation following endoscopic dilatation up to 11 % needing emergency surgery [15]. So, dilatation should be performed only in presence of an available surgical team [13].

Endoscopy plays a role, also, in the detection of the origin and in the treatment of acute gastrointestinal bleedings. Bleedings are often caused by an ulcer, mainly located in the left colon; these can be endoscopically treated with laser coagulation or bipolar coagulation when medical therapy fails [2].

The treatment of perianal abscesses and fistulas takes advantages by transrectal endoscopic ultrasound (EUS) in association to MR. EUS with hydrogen peroxide as contrast medium and MRI with contrast medium have a diagnostic accuracy of 100 % in the evaluation of perianal abscesses and fistulas [16], allowing to localize lesions that are not identified and so probably untreated during surgical evaluation, guarantying so better outcomes.

Since it was found that inflammatory bowel diseases have an increased risk (2–3 times higher than the general population) of developing neoplasms, endoscopy finds an important role in their detection, too [17]. The ASGE (American Society of Gastrointestinal Endoscopy) international guidelines recommended biopsies as four-quadrant biopsies every 10 cm, with a minimum of 32 samples, during each colonoscopy.

Endoscopic surveillance should be done every 3 years after 8–10 years of disease, every 2 years after 20 years of disease, and every year after 30 years of disease [18].

Any histological diagnoses of high-grade dysplasia or multifocal low-grade dysplasia find a surgical indication [19].

References

1. Ueno F, Matsui T, Matsumoto T, et al. On Behalf of the Guidelines Project Group of the Research Group of Intractable Inflammatory Bowel Disease subsidized by the Ministry of Health, Labour and

Welfare of Japan and the Guidelines Committee of the Japanese Society of Gastroenterology. Evidence-based clinical practice guidelines for Crohn's disease, integrated with formal consensus of experts in Japan. J Gastroenterol. 2012;48:31–72.

2. Blonski W, Kotlyar D, Lichtenstein G. Endoscopy of inflammatory Bowel Disease. In: Classen M, Tytgat GNJ, Lightdale CJ. Gastroenterological Endoscopy. 2nd edition, Stuttgart. New York: Thieme; 2010. p. 617–640.

3. van der Woude CJ, Ardizzone S, Bengtson MB, et al. ECCO Guidelines/Consensus Paper ECCO Guidelines/Consensus Paper. The second European evidenced-based consensus on reproduction and pregnancy in inflammatory bowel disease for the European Crohn's and Colitis Organization (ECCO). J Crohns Colitis. 2015;1–18. doi:10.1093/ecco-jcc/jju006.

4. Bwernell O, Lapidus A, Hellers G. Risk factors for surgery and post-operative recurrence in Crohn's disease. Ann Surg. 2000;231:38.

5. Geboes K, Ectors N, D'Haens G, Rutgeerts P. Is ileoscopy with biopsy worthwhile in patients presenting with symptoms of inflammatory bowel disease? Am J Gastroenterol. 1998;93(2):201–6.

6. Cherian S, Singh P. Is routine ileoscopy useful? An observational study of procedure times, diagnostic yield, and learning curve. Am J Gastroenterol. 2004;99(12):2324–9.

7. Nahon S, Bouhnik Y, Lavergne-Slove A, et al. Colonoscopy accurately predicts the anatomical severity of colonic Crohn's disease attacks: correlation with findings from colectomy specimens. Am J Gastroenterol. 2002;97(12):3102–7.

8. Pera A, Bellando P, Caldera D, et al. Colonoscopy in inflammatory bowel disease. Diagnostic accuracy and proposal of an endoscopic score. Gastroenterology. 1987;92(1):181–5.

9. Mary JY, Modigliani R. Development and validation of an endoscopic index of the severity for Crohn's disease: a prospective multicentre study. Gut. 1989;30:983–9.

10. Sandborn WJ, Feagan BG, Hanauer SB, et al. A review of activity indices and efficacy endpoints for clinical trials of medical therapy in adults with Crohn's disease. Gastroenterology. 2002;122:512–30.

11. Rutgeerts P, Geboes K, Vantrappen G, et al. Predictability of the postoperative course of Crohn's disease. Gastroenterology. 1990;99:956–63.

12. O'Connor M, Bager P, Duncan J, et al. N-ECCO Consensus statements on the European nursing roles in caring for patients with Crohn's disease or ulcerative colitis. J Crohns Colitis. 2013;7:744–64.

13. Aratari A, Botti F, Carrara A, et al. Linee Guida della Malattia of Crohn ACOI - (In collaborazione con SICCR) www.acoi.it/pratica-clinica-e-pubblication/linee-Guida

14. Thomas-Gibson S, Brooker JC, Hayward CM, et al. Colonoscopic balloon dilation of Crohn's strictures: a review of long-term outcomes. Eur J Gastroenterol Hepatol. 2003;15:485–8.

15. Scimeca D, Mocciaro F, Cottone M, et al. Efficacy and safety of endoscopic balloon dilation of symptomatic intestinal Crohn's disease strictures. Dig Liver Dis. 2011;43:121–5.

16. Orsoni P, Barthet M, Portie F, et al. Prospective comparison of endosonography, magnetic resonance imaging and surgical findings in anorectal fistula and abscess complicating Crohn's disease. Br J Surg. 1999;86:360–4.

17. Laukoetter MG, Mennigen R, MareikeHannig C, et al. Intestinal cancer risk in Crohn's disease: a meta-analysis. J Gastrointest Surg. 2011;15:576–83.

18. ASGE guideline: endoscopy in the diagnosis and treatment of inflammatory bowel disease. GIE. 2006;63(4):558–65.

19. Mitchell PJ, Salmo E, Haboubi NY. Inflammatory bowel disease: the problems of dysplasia and surveillance. Tech Coloproctol. 2007;11:299–309.

Medical Treatment of Perianal Crohn's Disease

6

Ambrogio Orlando, Sara Renna, Gaspare Solina, and Mario Cottone

6.1 Epidemiology and Clinical Course of Perianal Crohn's Disease

Crohn's disease (CD) is characterised by a transmural inflammation of the bowel, which can lead to the development of fistulas in 17–43 % of the cases [1, 2].

It is possible to recognise four types of fistulas: enterocutaneous, enteroenteric or enterocolic, enterovaginal and enterovesicular. The cumulative risk for developing fistulas is 33 % after 10 years and 50 % after 20 years from the diagnosis of CD [3]. Of these fistulas, 54 % involve the perianal region [4]. Various classifications of perianal fistulas have been proposed,

where the anal sphincters are the reference point. From the surgical point of view, Parks' classification [5] is more descriptive, but it is too complicated to use in routine practice. More empiric and easier classifications in simple and complex fistulas have been proposed [6, 7].

The presence of perianal disease is considered an independent factor predicting a disabling course of CD, and it has a negative impact on the quality of life [8]. Since these fistulas often involve the anal sphincters, they can be a source of significant morbidity, with an increased risk for incontinence in case of complex fistulas, which may require an aggressive surgical intervention.

Based on a recent consensus [9], the best management of complex perianal CD fistulas requires a multidisciplinary approach. Surgical drainage of sepsis is the first-line therapy followed by medical treatment. Anti-TNFα is indicated as the first-line medical treatment. Definitive surgical repair of fistulas is only of consideration in the absence of luminal inflammation. Proctectomy with permanent stoma is the last resort for severe, therapy refractory disease.

However, the management of the complex perianal Crohn's fistulas is challenging, and despite intensive medical and surgical treatment, a significant percentage of patients will continue to have debilitating perianal symptoms. Furthermore, fistulas frequently recur after discontinuation of treatment [10, 11].

A. Orlando, MD, PhD (✉) • S. Renna, MD
M. Cottone, MD, PhD
UOC Internal Medicine,
"V. Cervello" Hospital, Azienda Ospedaliera
"Ospedali Riuniti Villa Sofia-Cervello",
Palermo, Italy
e-mail: ambrogiorlando@gmail.com;
cottonedickens@gmail.com

G. Solina, MD, PhD
UOC General Surgery,
"V. Cervello" Hospital, Azienda Ospedaliera
"Ospedali Riuniti Villa Sofia-Cervello",
Palermo, Italy

© Springer International Publishing Switzerland 2016
G. Lo Re, M. Midiri (eds.), *Crohn's Disease: Radiological Features and Clinical-Surgical Correlations*,
DOI 10.1007/978-3-319-23066-5_6

In the presence of perianal disease, the choice of medical treatment, surgical treatment or both is determined by the severity of symptoms, the disease activity, the presence of proctitis and the type of fistula. Patients with complex perianal disease must be treated with a multidisciplinary approach, involving the cooperation among dedicated gastroenterologists and colorectal surgeons. The drainage of any local sepsis has to be considered the initial step before medical treatment, because persisting fistula tracts after premature skin closure are predisposed to sepsis worsening [12, 13]. Furthermore, combining the placement of non-cutting seton drainage with the subsequent medical treatment seems to achieve a better treatment response, reducing fistula recurrence [14, 15]. Many studies evaluated the efficacy of medical treatments, alone or in combination with surgical procedures, to improve the outcomes in this subgroup of CD patients. However, most of these studies are small, open label and considered the efficacy on perianal CD as a second outcome or as the result of a post hoc analysis from controlled clinical trials [16].

Few randomised controlled trials (RCTs) are available on treatments of perianal CD Table 6.1, and in all of them, the efficacy outcomes were evaluated by the Fistula Drainage Assessment. A fistula was considered opened if the investigator can express purulent material from the fistula with the application of gentle pressure. Fistula response was defined as closure of at least 50 % of fistulas for at least 4 weeks. Complete fistula closure was defined as closure of all fistulas for at least 4 weeks. Recently, it was observed that inflamed fistula tracts often persist, despite the apparent closure of external orifices, causing recurrent fistulas and pelvic abscesses. Based on this observation, radiological outcomes, especially using MRI examination, have been considered with promising results. In presence of perianal disease, the choice of medical, surgical or a combination of both medical and surgical treatment is determined by the type of fistula and the degree of rectal inflammation.

Recently, the Italian guidelines [17] on the use of antitumour necrosis factor-α treatment (TNFα), in the case of complex perianal fistulas

anti-TNFα, should be considered as the first choice of medical therapy, in combination with a preliminary surgical therapy. Surgical procedures should include a "cone-like" fistulectomy of each fistula tract with sparing of sphincteric structures and loose seton placement, which will be removed according with the subsequent therapy. Antibiotics and/or immunosuppressants should be used as a second-line medical treatment. These recommendations are quite different from those reported in the ECCO guidelines in which anti-TNFα agents are considered to be second-line options after antibiotics and immunosuppressants. However, in the new ECCO guidelines that will be published soon, this statement should be revised [18].

In this chapter, we analysed the literature evidence in which the efficacy of medical therapy and of the different drugs (antibiotics, immunosuppressants, tacrolimus and anti-TNF alpha) has been evaluated.

6.2 Medical Therapy

6.2.1 Antibiotics

Antibiotics have been used for the treatment of fistulising CD for both their antiseptic and anti-inflammatory properties. The most common used antibiotics are metronidazole, at the dosage of 750–1000 mg daily, and ciprofloxacin, at the dosage of 1000–1500 mg daily. Many studies, most of which open-label case series involving few patients, have been performed with only modest results [19–21].

A RCT was presented comparing the efficacy of ciprofloxacin and metronidazole on perianal fistulas [22]. Twenty-five patients were randomised to receive ciprofloxacin (500 mg), metronidazole (500 mg) or placebo twice daily for 10 weeks. The primary outcome was considered the closure of all open actively draining fistulas. The closure of a fistula was defined as the absence of drainage, both spontaneous and on gentle compression. The closure of all fistulas at week 10 occurred in 3 patients (30 %) treated with ciprofloxacin, no patients (0 %) treated with

Table 6.1 Results of the trials on fistulising CD

Study	Drug	N° Patients	Follow-up	Rate of remission treated (%)	Rate of remission placebo (%)	Outcome definition
West 2004[a] [23]	Ciprofloxacin + infliximab	24	18	73	39	No drainage despite finger compression
Thia 2009 [22]	Ciprofloxacin/ metronidazole	25	10	30/0	12.5	Absence of drainage, both spontaneous and on gentle compression
Sandborn 2003 [26]	Tacrolimus	42	10	10	8	Absence of either spontaneous drainage or the ability to express drainage with gentle compression
Hart 2007 [27]	Topical tacrolimus	19	12	0	0	Drainage cessation of all fistulas, maintained until the end of the treatment period or for 2 consecutive visits
Present 1999 [28]	Infliximab	94	2–6	55	13	No drainage despite gentle finger compression
Sands 2004 [12]	Infliximab	306	54	36	19	Drainage cessation of all fistulas, maintained until the end of the treatment period or for 2 consecutive visits
Colombel 2007[b] [36]	Adalimumab	117	56	33	13	No drainage despite gentle finger compression
Dewint 2014[c] [38]	Adalimumab ± ciprofloxacin	76	24	71	47	At least 50 % reduction of number of draining fistulas from baseline to week 12
Schreiber 2011[d] [39]	Certolizumab pegol	58	26	36	17	Absence of drainage on gentle compression at any two consecutive visits

[a]Only response rate was considered
[b]Subgroup analysis of CHARM study
[c]After adalimumab induction therapy (160/80 mg week 0, 2), patients received 40 mg every other week together with ciprofloxacin 500 mg or placebo twice daily for 12 weeks
[d]Subgroup analysis of PRECISE 2 study

metronidazole, and 1 patient (12.5 %) treated with placebo ($p=0.41$). This small study suggested that remission occurred more often in patients treated with ciprofloxacin, but the differences were not significant.

Another RCT [23] was also conducted to evaluate the effect of combined ciprofloxacin and infliximab treatment in perianal CD. Twenty-four patients, treated with infliximab (5 mg/kg) at weeks 6, 8 and 12, were randomly assigned to receive ciprofloxacin (500 mg) twice daily or placebo for 12 weeks. The closure of perianal fistula was defined as no drainage despite firm finger compression. At week 18, the response rate was 73 % in the ciprofloxacin group and 39 % in the placebo group ($p=0.12$). Using logistic regression analysis, patients treated with cipro-floxacin tended to respond better (OR = 2.37, $p = 0.07$). The use of logistic regression analysis in this type of study is methodologically questionable.

A limit of the antibiotic treatment is the adverse events commonly associated with the long-term therapy. They can include glossitis, nausea, sensory neuropathy, headache, diarrhoea and rash.

To avoid the systemic side effects of antibiotic treatment, the potential efficacy of metronidazole 10 % ointment has been evaluated in a RCT [24]. Seventy-four patients with perianal fistulas were randomised to metronidazole ointment, applied perianally three times daily, or placebo ointment. At the end of the study, more subjects in the met-ronidazole group showed a reduction in perianal discharge and in perianal pain, but a significant difference with placebo was not showed. The authors concluded that topical treatment with metronidazole is well tolerated, with minimal adverse effects, and could be useful for the treat-ment of the pain and discharge associated with perianal CD.

6.2.2 Immunosuppressants

There are no controlled trials where the efficacy of immunosuppressants in fistulising CD was considered as a primary endpoint. The efficacy of azathioprine (AZA) and 6-mercaptopurine (6MP) in this setting was analysed in several trials where the treatment of perianal disease was considered as a secondary endpoint. Because of the small sample size of these studies, a meta-analysis was conducted to have a more reliable result on the efficacy of immunosuppressants in the treatment of perianal CD.

The meta-analysis of these trials [25] found that 54 % of patients with perianal disease who received AZA/6MP responded versus 21 % of patients who received placebo (odds ratio 4.44 [CI, 1.50–13.20]). The limits of these studies were the small number of analysed patients and being not designed primarily to look at the

effect of the treatment on perianal fistulas but on active inflammatory disease. The relatively low reported remission rates, with high recurrence rates, represent probably the reason for the lack of new trials focused on these drugs in favour of much more evidences on other new treatments like biologics.

6.2.3 Tacrolimus

The efficacy of tacrolimus in the treatment of perianal CD has been studied in few studies. In a RCT by Sandborn [26], patients with perianal fis-tulas were treated with tacrolimus (0.2 mg/kg daily) or placebo for 10 weeks. The fistula clo-sure was defined as the absence of either sponta-neous drainage or the ability to express drainage with gentle compression. In the tacrolimus group, 43 % of the patients reached the closure of at least 50 % of fistulas for longer than 4 weeks, compared with 8 % of the patients treated with placebo ($p = 0.004$). Complete fistula closure, however, was only achieved in 10 % of the patients who received tacrolimus. The authors observed that fistula closure was not affected by the concomitant immunosuppressive therapy with AZA/6MP (38 % closure with therapy vs 50 % without).

Despite the encouraging results, a limit of the treatment with tacrolimus is represented by the high rate of adverse events, including headache, insomnia, elevated creatinine, paraesthesia and tremor.

To avoid these systemic adverse events, the efficacy of a treatment with topical tacrolimus was investigated in a RCT [27]. Nineteen patients were stratified according to whether they had ulcerating (7 patients) or fistulising (12 patients) disease and randomised to topical tacrolimus (1 g ointment twice a day) or placebo for 12 weeks. In the sub-group of patients with fistulising CD, the complete response was defined as clinically evaluated ces-sation of drainage of all fistulas, maintained until the end of the treatment period or for 2 consecutive visits. At the end of the study, 3 of the 4 patients treated with topical tacrolimus for ulcerating disease improved, compared with none of the 3 patients in the placebo group, but a complete healing was not achieved. In fistulising disease, topical tacrolimus resulted to be not effective.

Adverse events were infrequent and mild. The results of this study suggest that topical tacrolimus could be effective and safe in the treatment of perianal ulcerating CD, but not of fistulising CD.

6.2.4   Anti-TNF Alpha

6.2.4.1 Infliximab

Infliximab has been proven to be efficacious in the treatment of fistulas in patients with CD. The first evidence on its efficacy comes from a trial published in 1999 [28]. In this study, 94 patients with fistulising CD (85 of whom with perianal fistulas) were randomly assigned to receive infliximab or placebo at weeks 0, 2 and 6. A fistula was considered to be closed when it no longer drained despite gentle finger compression. At the end of the study, 55 % of the patients assigned to 5 mg/kg of infliximab had a closure of all fistulas, compared with 13 % of the patients assigned to placebo.

Some years later, a controlled trial (ACCENT II) [12] demonstrated the superiority of infliximab (36 %) compared with placebo (19 %) in maintaining a long-term healing of fistulas. In this study, the response was defined as a reduction of at least 50 % from baseline in the number of draining fistulas at consecutive visits four or more weeks apart. A complete response was defined as the absence of draining fistulas.

It is important to underline that in these two large trials, 11 and 15 % of the treated patients developed abscesses related to their fistulas during the study, probably because of an early closure of the cutaneous opening of the fistula tract. To minimise this complication, a combined surgical and medical treatment was proposed. Some small studies [13, 29–32] reported a better response (from 47 to 100 %), a lower recurrence and a longer time to recurrence rates in patients who had placed a seton prior to infliximab infusions compared with patients receiving

infliximab alone. The more recent trials focused on the efficacy of this combined treatment.

Data from an Italian multicentric open study including 573 patients with luminal refractory CD (312 patients) or with fistulising disease (190 patients) or both of them (71 patients) treated with infliximab, the global response of perianal fistulas was 76 % (143 out of 188), whereas abdominal and rectovaginal fistulae showed a global response to infliximab in 63 % of the patients (44 out of 70); no variable was related to response [33].

Recently, another prospective Italian study [34] was conducted to compare the outcomes of the management of perianal fistulas in CD between infliximab, surgery or a combination of surgery and infliximab. Thirty-four patients with complex perianal fistulas were included into 1 of the following 3 treatment groups: infliximab (11 patients), surgery (10 patients) or a combination of surgery and postoperative infliximab (14 patients). Patients who received surgery and infliximab experienced a shorter time to healing of fistulas and a longer mean time to relapse compared to those who received infliximab or surgery alone. This is the only RCT in which the combination therapy (medical + surgical) was compared with the classic approach (medical or surgical).

A recent retrospective study [35] evaluated 156 patients treated with infliximab for fistulising perianal CD. Of these patients, 128 had a complex fistula, but only 98 of them (76 %) were treated with seton placement. The final results showed that about 65 % of patients reached fistula closure at 2 years, but the number of patients healed from a complex perianal disease was not reported.

Although the initial response to infliximab resulted to be very good, the median duration of fistula closure is approximately 3 months, and repeated IV infusions are often required. However, it is known that after discontinuation of infliximab therapy, most fistulas recurred. Which is the best maintaining treatment for fistulising CD after infliximab and what is the best time to stop the treatment is up to now a question. New trials focused on these topics are warranted.

6.2.4.2 Adalimumab

The first data on the efficacy of adalimumab in the treatment of perianal CD come from a subgroup analysis of a large trial [36] in which 117 patients with perianal disease were treated with adalimumab at the induction dosage of 80/40 mg at weeks 0/2 and then randomised to placebo, adalimumab every other week or adalimumab every week. The closure of fistulas was assessed draining upon gentle compression. Complete fistula closure was achieved in a greater percentage of adalimumab treated patients versus those receiving placebo at both week 26 (30 and 13 % for combined adalimumab groups and placebo group, respectively) and week 56 (33 and 13 % for combined adalimumab and placebo group, respectively). Of patients with complete fistula, closure at week 26, 100 % continued to have a complete fistula closure at week 56.

To evaluate the long-term efficacy of adalimumab in the healing of draining fistulas, the patients completing week 56 were then enrolled in an open-label extension [37]. Of all patients with healed fistulas at week 56, 90 % maintained healing after 1 year of open-label adalimumab therapy. The authors concluded that adalimumab therapy is not only effective for inducing fistula healing, but a complete fistula healing is sustained for up to 2 years by most patients.

In the recent RCT (ADAFI) [38] planned on patients with perianal disease treated with biologics (± ciprofloxacin), the fistula closure rate at 24 weeks was 33 % (12 out of 36) in those treated with adalimumab and 53 % (18 out of 34) in those treated with adalimumab plus ciprofloxacin, but this difference was not significant ($p = 0.098$). Similarly, nonsignificant differences between the two groups were observed at week 24 considering both 50 and 100 % reduction of the number of draining fistulas. The primary outcome of the study was the "at least 50 % reduction of number of draining fistulas from baseline to week 12." Both response and remission rates resulted significantly higher in the adalimumab plus ciprofloxacin group in respect of the adalimumab group with the following p values: $p = 0.047$ in the intention to treat analysis (71 % vs 47 %) and $p = 0.0498$ in the per-protocol analysis (75 % vs 51.5 %), considering the response to treatment, and $p = 0.009$ in the intention to treat analysis (65 % vs 33 %) and $p = 0.009$ in the per-protocol analysis (69 % vs 36 %), considering the overall remission. In this trial, the number of patients with complex perianal disease was not reported; about 20 % of patients were treated with seton placement presuming that the number of patients with complex perianal disease was low.

The available data on the efficacy of adalimumab in fistulising CD are still insufficient because they come from post hoc analyses of RCTs, and in the ADAFI trial, the patients with complex perianal disease was not specified, and at 24 weeks no difference in clinical between the two treatment group was observed ($p = 0.02$). New RCTs where closure of fistulas will be the major endpoint are warranted.

6.2.4.3 Certolizumab Pegol

Certolizumab pegol was approved for the treatment of CD in America and in Switzerland, but not in the other European countries. Data on its efficacy in the treatment of perianal CD come from subgroup analysis of large trials. Studies focused on the efficacy of this drug in perianal CD are not available. In a subgroup analysis of the PRECISE 2 trial [39], the efficacy of maintaining treatment with certolizumab pegol in fistulising CD was evaluated. In the PRECISE 2 trial, patients with draining fistulas had received an open-label induction with certolizumab pegol 400 mg at weeks 0, 2 and 4. At week 6, responders with draining fistulas had been randomised to certolizumab pegol 400 mg or placebo every 4 weeks. Fistula closure was defined as the absence of drainage on gentle compression at any two consecutive visits. At week 26, 36 % of patients in the certolizumab pegol group had 100 % of fistula closure compared with 17 % of patients in the placebo group ($p = 0.038$).

A prospective phase IV study [40] evaluating the efficacy and safety of certolizumab pegol in a multicentre cohort of CD patients was recently published. Sixty patients were included, 53 % of whom had stricturing or penetrating disease. In the subgroup of patients with perianal disease, a complete fistula closure was observed in 36 % of patients at week 6 and in 55 % of patients at week 26. These results are promising but not still sufficient to consider certolizumab pegol a good treatment for perianal CD. New RCTs are warranted.

The results of RCTs are reported in Table 6.1.

6.3   Miscellaneous

In some small open-label studies, the efficacy of other drugs has been analysed. For example, patients treated with thalidomide demonstrated a significant improvement on their perianal disease in short-term follow-up, but the long-term treatment is limited by its toxicity [41–43]. A few evidences, from small case series, are also available to support the use of methotrexate, alone [44] or in combination with infliximab [45]. Based on the results of uncontrolled small studies, an improvement in fistula drainage was observed in 3/4 of patients treated with ev cyclosporine (4 mg/kg), but most patients relapsed after transition to oral therapy or discontinuation of the drug [46–48]. It has recently been suggested the potential benefit of local injection of infliximab and adalimumab, associated with surgical procedure in patients who have an intolerance to systemic treatment. Also the data on this type of treatment come from small studies [49–51].

An alternative treatment with stem cell local injection was proposed for the treatment of perianal fistulas. In a recent study [52], the efficacy and safety of intrafistular injections of autologous bone marrow-derived mesenchymal stromal cells were analysed, and complete closure of fistula tracts was reported in 70 % of patients without any adverse effects. These preliminary results are encouraging, but RCTs are warranted to assess the real efficacy of cellular therapy in CD complicated by perianal fistulas.

A more recent, open-label, single-arm clinical trial was conducted at six Spanish hospitals [53]. Twenty-four patients were administered intralesionally with 20 million expanded adipose-derived allogeneic mesenchymal stem cells (eASCs) in one draining fistula tract. A subsequent administration of 40 million eASCs was

performed if fistula closure was incomplete at week 12. Subjects were followed until week 24 after the initial administration. Treatment-related adverse events did not indicate any clinical safety concerns after 6 months follow-up. The full analysis of efficacy data at week 24 showed 69.2 % of the patients with a reduction in the number of draining fistulas, 56.3 % of the patients achieved complete closure of the treated fistula achieved, and 30 % of the cases presented complete closure of all existing fistula tracts. Of note, closure was strictly defined as absence of suppuration through the external orifice and complete re-epithelisation, plus absence of collections measured by magnetic resonance image scan (MRI). Furthermore, MRI Score of Severity showed statistically significant differences at week 12 with a marked reduction at week 24. The authors concluded that locally injected eASCs appear to be a simple, safe and beneficial therapy for perianal fistula in Crohn's disease patients, but additional studies are needed to further confirm the efficacy of the eASCs.

The efficacy of oral spherical adsorptive carbon (AST-120) was also evaluated in recent years. In a RCT [54], 57 patients with CD and active anal fistula were assigned to receive oral spherical adsorptive carbon or placebo for 8 weeks. The reported remission rates were 29.6 % in the oral spherical adsorptive carbon group and 6.7 % in the placebo group ($p = 0.035$), but in a recent largest phase 3 placebo RCT [55] to date to evaluate the impact of a therapeutic agent on perianal fistulae in CD, the efficacy of AST-120 could not be confirmed. An inverse relationship was observed between both inflammatory and clinical disease activity and fistula response.

Conclusion

The treatment of complex perianal CD is difficult and the chance of complete fistula healing remains no more than 50 %. It is now clear that the best management of this condition is a combining medical and surgical therapy. Up to now the most strongly evaluated medical treatments for perianal CD are the anti-TNF alpha antibodies. Regarding the other medical treatments, antibiotics and immunomodulators have not been demonstrated to result in sustained closure of fistulas in CD. The use of tacrolimus is limited by its side effects, and the efficacy of topical treatment seems to be confined to perianal ulcerating CD.

Up to now some questions remain unanswered: how to treat patients who do not respond to biologic treatments, which is the best strategy from long-term maintenance therapy in responders and which is the best evaluation instrument in future RCTs on perianal CD, considering the limits of the old used Fistula Drainage Assessment?

Regarding the medical treatments, we expect further RCTs to improve the management of these CD patients. Regarding the evaluation instrument, as therapy outcome resulted to be worse among patients with persisting fistulas in the MRI evaluation, despite a good Fistula Drainage Assessment, we think that MRI examination could be considered as a more reliable evaluation instrument to use in future RCTs on perianal CD.

References

1. Sands BE. Crohn's disease. In: Feldman M, Friedman LS, Sleisenger MH, editors. Sleisenger & Fordtran's gastrointestinal and liver disease: pathophysiology/diagnosis/management, vol. 2. 7th ed. Philadelphia: Saunders; 2002. p. 2005–38.
2. Schwartz DA, Pemberton JH, Sandborn WJ. Diagnosis and treatment of perianal fistulas in Crohn disease. Ann Intern Med. 2001;135:906–18.
3. Schwartz DA, Loftus Jr EV, Tremaine WJ, et al. The natural history of fistulizing Crohn's disease in Olmsted County, Minnesota. Gastroenterology. 2002;122:875–80.
4. Tang LY, Rawsthorne P, Bernstein CN. Are perineal and luminal fistulas associated in Crohn's disease? A population- based study. Clin Gastroenterol Hepatol. 2006;4:1130–4.
5. Parks AG, Gordon PH, Hardcastle J. A classification of fistula- in-ano. Br J Surg. 1976;63:1–12.
6. Bell SJ, Williams AB, Wiesel P, et al. The clinical course of fistulating Crohn's disease. Aliment Pharmacol Ther. 2003;17:1145–51.
7. Sandborn WJ, Fazio VW, Feagan BG, et al. Gastroenterological Association Clinical Practice Committee. AGA technical review on perianal Crohn's disease. Gastroenterology. 2003;125:1508–30.
8. Beaugerie L, Seksik P, Nion-Larmurier I, et al. Predictors of Crohn's disease. Gastroenterology. 2006;130:650–6.
9. Gecse KB, Bemelman W, Kamm MA, et al. A global consensus on the classification, diagnosis and multidisciplinary treatment of perianal fistulising Crohn's disease. Gut. 2014;63:1381–92.
10. Nordgren S, Fasth S, Hulten L. Anal fistulas in Crohn's disease: incidence and outcome of surgical treatment. Int J Colorectal Dis. 1992;7:214–8.
11. Williams JG, Rothenberger DA, Nemer FD, et al. Fistula-in-ano in Crohn's disease. Results of aggressive surgical treatment. Dis Colon Rectum. 1991;34:378–84.
12. Sands BE, Anderson FH, Bernstein CN, et al. Infliximab maintenance therapy for fistulizing Crohn's disease. N Engl J Med. 2004;350:876–85.
13. Regueiro M, Mardini H. Treatment of perianal fistulizing Crohn's disease with infliximab alone or as an adjunct to exam under anesthesia with seton placement. Inflamm Bowel Dis. 2003;9:98–103.
14. Taxonera C, Schwartz DA, Garcia-Olmo D. Emerging treatments for complex perianal fistula in Crohn's disease. World J Gastroenterol. 2009;15:4263–72.
15. Duff S, Sagar PM, Rao M, et al. Infliximab and surgical treatment of complex anal Crohn's disease. Colorectal Dis. 2011;14:972–6.
16. Renna S, Orlando A, Cottone M. Randomized controlled trials in perianal Crohn's disease. Rev Recent Clin Trials. 2012;7:297–302.
17. Orlando A, Armuzzi A, Papi C, et al. The Italian Society of Gastroenterology (SIGE) and the Italian Group for the study of Inflammatory Bowel Disease (IG-IBD) Clinical Practice Guidelines: The use of tumor necrosis factor-alpha antagonist therapy in Inflammatory Bowel Disease. Dig Liver Dis. 2011;43(1):1–20.
18. Dignass A, Van Assche G, Lindsay JO et al.; European Crohn's and Colitis Organisation (ECCO). The second European evidence-based Consensus on the diagnosis and management of Crohn's disease: current management. J Crohns Colitis. 2010;4:28–62.
19. Brandt LJ, Bernstein LH, Boley SJ, et al. Metronidazole therapy for perineal Crohn's disease: a follow-up study. Gastroenterology. 1982;83:383–7.
20. Present DH, Korelitz BI, Wisch N, et al. Treatment of Crohn's disease with 6-mercaptopurine. A long-term, randomized, double blind study. N Engl J Med. 1980;302:981–7.
21. Bernstein LH, Frank MS, Brandt LJ, et al. Healing of perineal Crohn's disease with metronidazole. Gastroenterology. 1980;79:599.
22. Thia KT, Mahadevan U, Feagan BG, et al. Ciprofloxacin or metronidazole for the treatment of perianal fistulas in patients with Crohn's disease: a randomized, double-blind, placebo-controlled pilot study. Inflamm Bowel Dis. 2009;15:17–24.

23. West RL, Van der Woude CJ, Hansen BE, et al. Clinical and endosonographic effect of ciprofloxacin on the treatment of perianal fistulae in Crohn's disease with infliximab: a double-blind-placebocontrolled study. Aliment Pharmacol Ther. 2004;20:1329–36.
24. Maeda Y, Ng SC, Durdey P, Torkington J, et al. Randomized clinical trial of metronidazole ointment versus placebo in perianal Crohn's disease. Br J Surg. 2010;97:1340–7.
25. Pearson DC, May GR, Fick GH, et al. Azathioprine and 6- mercaptopurine in Crohn disease. A meta-analysis. Ann Intern Med. 1995;123:132–42.
26. Sandborn WJ, Present DH, Isaacs KL, et al. Tacrolimus for the treatment of fistulas in patients with Crohn's disease: a randomized, placebo-controlled trial. Gastroenterology. 2003;125:380–8.
27. Hart AL, Plamondon S, Kamm MA. Topical tacrolimus in the treatment of perianal Crohn's disease: exploratory randomized controlled trial. Inflamm Bowel Dis. 2007;13:245–53.
28. Present DH, Rutgeerts P, Targan S, et al. Infliximab for the treatment of fistulas in patients with Crohn's disease. N Engl J Med. 1999;340:1398–405.
29. Topstad DR, Panaccione R, Heine JA, et al. Combined seton placement, infliximab infusion, and maintenance immunosuppressives improve healing rate in fistulising anorectal Crohn's disease: a single center experience. Dis Colon Rectum. 2003;46:577–83.
30. Van der Hagen SJ, Baeten CG, Soeters PB, et al. Anti-TNF-alpha (infliximab) used as induction treatment in case of active proctitis in a multistep strategy followed by definitive surgery of complex anal fistulas in Crohn's disease: a preliminary report. Dis Colon Rectum. 2005;48:758–67.
31. Talbot C, Sagar PM, Johnston MJ, et al. Infliximab in the surgical management of complex fistulating anal Crohn's disease. Colorectal Dis. 2005;7:164–8.
32. Hyder SA, Travis SP, Jewell DP, et al. Fistulating anal Crohn's disease: results of combined surgical and infliximab treatment. Dis Colon Rectum. 2006;49:1837–41.
33. Orlando A, Colombo E, Kohn A, et al. Infliximab in the treatment of Crohn's disease: predictor of response in an Italian multicentric open study. Dig Liver Dis. 2005;37:577–83.
34. Sciaudone G, Di Stazio C, Limongelli P, et al. Treatment of complex perianal fistulas in Crohn disease: infliximab, surgery or combined approach. Can J Surg. 2010;53:299–304.
35. Bouguen G, Siproudhis L, Gizard E, et al. Long-term outcome of perianal fistulizing Crohn's disease treated with infliximab. Clin Gastroenterol Hepatol. 2013;11:975–81.
36. Colombel JF, Sandborn WJ, Rutgeerts P, et al. Adalimumab for maintenance of clinical response and remission in patients with Crohn's disease: the CHARM trial. Gastroenterology. 2007;132:52–65.
37. Colombel JF, Schwartz DA, Sandborn WJ, et al. Adalimumab for the treatment of fistulas in patients with Crohn's disease. Gut. 2009;58:940–8.
38. Dewint P, Hansen BE, Verhey E, et al. Adalimumab combined with ciprofloxacin is superior to adalimumab monotherapy in perianal fistula closure in Crohn's disease: a randomised, double-blind, placebo controlled trial (ADAFI). Gut. 2014;63:292–9.
39. Schreiber S, Lawrance IC, Thomsen OØ, et al. Randomised clinical trial: certolizumab pegol for fistulas in Crohn's disease subgroup results from a placebo-controlled study. Aliment Pharmacol Ther. 2011;33:185–93.
40. Vavricka SR, Schoepfer AM, Bansky G, et al. Efficacy and safety of certolizumab pegol in an unselected Crohn's disease population: 26-week data of the FACTS II survey. Inflamm Bowel Dis. 2011;17:1530–9.
41. Vasiliauskas EA, Kam LY, Abreu-Martin MT, et al. An open-label pilot study of low-dose thalidomide in chronically active, steroid dependent Crohn's disease. Gastroenterology. 1999;117:1278–87.
42. Ehrenpreis ED, Kane SV, Cohen LB, et al. Thalidomide therapy for patients with refractory Crohn's disease: an open-label trial. Gastroenterology. 1999;117:1271–7.
43. Plamondon S, Ng SC, Kamm MA. Thalidomide in luminal and fistulizing Crohn's disease resistant to standard therapies. Aliment Pharmacol Ther. 2007;25:557–67.
44. Mahadevan U, Marion JF, Present DH. Fistula response to methotrexate in Crohn's disease: a case series. Aliment Pharmacol Ther. 2003;18:1003–8.
45. Schroder O, Blumenstein I, Schulte-Bockholt A, et al. Combining infliximab and methotrexate in fistulizing Crohn's disease resistant or intolerant to azathioprine. Aliment Pharmacol Ther. 2004;19:295–301.
46. Fukushima T, Sugita A, Masuzawa S, et al. Effects of cyclosporin A on active Crohn's disease. Gastroenterol Jpn. 1989;24:12–5.
47. Lichtiger S. Cyclosporine therapy in inflammatory bowel disease: open-label experience. Mt Sinai J Med. 1990;57:315–9.
48. Hanauer SB, Smith MB. Rapid closure of Crohn's disease fistulas with continuous intravenous cyclosporin A. Am J Gastroenterol. 1993;88:646–9.
49. Poggioli G, Laureti S, Pierangeli F, et al. Local injection of Infliximab for the treatment of perianal Crohn's disease. Dis Colon Rectum. 2005;48:768–74.
50. Asteria CR, Ficari F, Bagnoli S, et al. Treatment of perianal fistulas in Crohn's disease by local injection of antibody to TNF-alpha accounts for a favourable clinical response in selected cases: a pilot study. Scand J Gastroenterol. 2006;41:1064–72.
51. Poggioli G, Laureti S, Pierangeli F, et al. Local injection of adalimumab for perianal Crohn's disease: better than infliximab? Inflamm Bowel Dis. 2010;16:1631.

52. Ciccocioppo R, Bernardo ME, Sgarella A, et al. Autologous bone marrow-derived mesenchymal stromal cells in the treatment of fistulising Crohn's disease. Gut. 2011;60:788–98.

53. La Portilla F, Alba F, García-Olmo D, et al. Expanded allogeneic adipose-derived stem cells (eASCs) for the treatment of complex perianal fistula in Crohn's disease: results from a multicenter phase I/IIa clinical trial. Int J Colorectal Dis. 2013;28(3):313–23.

54. Fukuda Y, Takazoe M, Sugita A, et al. Oral spherical adsorptive carbon for the treatment of intractable anal fistulas in Crohn's disease: a multicenter, randomized, double-blind, placebo-controlled trial. Am J Gastroenterol. 2008;103:1721–9.

55. Reinisch W, Travis S, Hanauer S, et al. AST-120 (spherical carbon adsorbent) in the treatment of perianal fistulae in mild-to-moderate Crohn's disease: FHAST-1, a phase 3, multicenter, placebo-controlled study. Inflamm Bowel Dis. 2014;20(5):872–81.

Standard Therapeutic Approach and New Therapies

Marco Mendolaro, Anna Viola,
and Maria Cappello

7.1 Introduction

7.1.1 Therapeutic Strategies and Goals

The traditional approach to therapy of Crohn's disease has been the step-up approach usually represented as a pyramid (Fig. 7.1) where, progressing from mild to severe disease, therapeutic choices proceed step by step from less potent drugs at the basement of the pyramid to more potent but also more toxic drugs at the top. The advent of biological therapies and the wider use of immunomodulators, together with the opportunity to achieve ambitious treatment goals and possibly to modify the course of disease, have led to other approaches such as the accelerated step-up or the top-down approach. This means that immunomodulators and biologics can be used earlier and de-escalated when disease is in deep remission. This could allow prolonged remission.

Treatment goals in the era of biologics are induction and maintenance of remission of course, but also mucosal healing, deep remission, improvement of quality of life, reduction in hospitalization and surgery, and finally prevention of disability.

The appropriate choice of treatment is influenced by the balance between potency and potential side effects of drugs, previous response to therapy (especially when considering treatment of a relapse, or for steroid-dependent or refractory disease), and the presence of extraintestinal manifestations or complications. Different types of drugs are currently available (from mesalazine to biologics) and best treatment choice is tailored to the individual patient.

Recommendations for clinicians approaching to treatment of CD have been developed and are constantly updated by the ECCO (European Crohn's and Colitis Organization) [2–4].

Guidelines can be downloaded free of charge from the ECCO website.

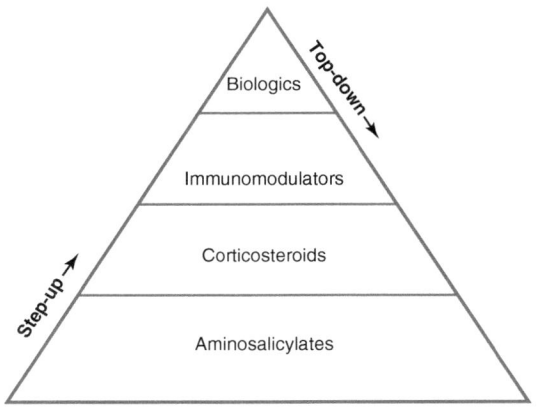

Fig. 7.1 Therapeutic pyramid. Step-up ant top-down approach (D'Haens et al. [1])

M. Mendolaro • A. Viola • M. Cappello (✉)
Gastroenterology Section,
DiBiMis, University of Palermo, Palermo, Italy
e-mail: cmarica@tin.it

© Springer International Publishing Switzerland 2016
G. Lo Re, M. Midiri (eds.), *Crohn's Disease: Radiological Features and Clinical-Surgical Correlations*,
DOI 10.1007/978-3-319-23066-5_7

Assessment of response to therapy can be made on the basis of clinical symptoms and signs, but a more objective way would include clinical and endoscopic scores, laboratory tests, and radiological findings.

At present, a number of clinical activity indices are available: the most used are Crohn's Disease Activity Index (CDAI), Harvey-Bradshaw Index (HBI), and the Inflammatory Bowel Disease Questionnaire (IBDQ), the last specifically evaluating quality of life.

CDAI, developed by Best et al., is the most widely used of the multiple-component CD indices and is used on a large scale in clinical trials. CDAI score varies between 0 and 600 points. A score of 150 is used as a cutoff between remission and active disease [5]. A score of 150-220 defines mild to moderate active disease, while a score above 220 is related to severe disease. The CDAI is a complex index and is difficult to calculate in daily clinical practice. A more suitable index is HBI that incorporated fewer clinical variables, all of which could be measured easily with five variables opposed to eight. An HBI score above 5 corresponds to a CDAI score above 150 and indicates active CD [6] (see chapter on Clinical Presentation). Both indices are mainly based on subjective findings, and their role in evaluating inflammatory activity and their specificity for CD inflammation have recently been questioned.

Quality of life is assessed by IBDQ [7], a 32-item questionnaire that includes four domains: bowel function, emotional status, systemic symptoms, and social function. High IBDQ scores indicate a better quality of life, an endpoint meeting increasing interest in clinical trials.

Laboratory tests are also used for monitoring response to therapy. They include white blood cell count, platelet count, hemoglobin, hematocrit, C-reactive protein (CRP), and erythrocyte sedimentation rate (ESR). The latter two inflammatory markers, in particular, correlate with disease activity. CRP is an acute-phase protein and can be used as a very accurate marker of disease activity and also as an independent predictor of short- and medium-term clinical relapse in patients with high levels at diagnosis [8].

Fecal biomarkers, such as the neutrophil-derived calprotectin and lactoferrin, are also useful for managing CD patients and correlate with endoscopic and histological scores of CD activity in ileocolonic or colonic disease [9, 10].

A complete blood cell count is also an important indicator of disease activity.

Mucosal healing in the era of biologics has become a fundamental treatment goal since it is related to better long-term outcomes. Endoscopy is a crucial step in assessing CD activity, and endoscopic scoring systems have been developed to classify and assess disease activity. Endoscopic scoring systems currently used are the Crohn's Disease Endoscopic Index of Severity (CDEIS), the Simple Endoscopic Score for Crohn's Disease (SES-CD), and the Rutgeerts endoscopic grading scale, the last applying to the setting of postsurgical recurrence [11–13]. The CDEIS assesses five bowel segments (terminal ileum, right colon, transverse, left colon and sigmoid, and rectum), considering specific mucosal lesions (ulcers and stenosis), extent of disease, and ranges from 0 to 44, but is complicated to use routinely. SES-CD is easier and includes four variables, each considered in five segments of the bowel: ulcer size, the extent of ulcerated surface, the extent of affected surface, and stenosis. Scores range from 0 t o 60. Ferrante et al. showed in a subanalysis of data from the SONIC trial a reduction of at least 50 % in the SES-CD or CDEIS score after 26 weeks of treatment to be predictive of corticosteroid-free clinical remission at week 50 [14].

Although endoscopy remains the gold standard for assessing CD activity, cross-sectional imaging techniques play an important complementary role. The most used are ultrasound (US), computed tomography enterography (CTE), and magnetic resonance enterography (MRE). US is particularly useful for examining the terminal ileum and colon to evaluate bowel wall thickness, strictures, loss of stratification, wall stiffness with a reduced peristalsis in the small bowel, and loss of haustra coli in the colon [15, 16]. CTE and MRE involve the use of intraluminal oral and intravenous contrast agents to evaluate the small bowel, identifying the complications of CD with greater accuracy. CT is valid for examining luminal and extraluminal structures and is widely available and standardized in its use [17]. MRI assesses mural and mucosal characteristics as presence of ulcerations, wall thickness, mural T2 signal intensity, and T1 contrast enhancement. There are also extramural features of inflammation, such as a comb sign, lymph node enlargement, and fat wrapping [18]. MRI is used to monitor treatment response, transmural healing, as well as mucosal healing, which has been correlated with a better CD course, fewer hospital admissions, less surgery, and higher steroid-free remission rates [19–21].

7.1.2 Therapeutic Armamentarium in Crohn's Disease: Conventional Therapies

7.1.2.1 Aminosalicylates

The mechanism of action of 5-ASA is still not completely known, but it has been hypothesized that the activity of 5-ASA is related to the elimination of free radicals, inhibition of T-cell proliferation and decreased production of IL1 and TNF-alpha, antigen presentation and antibody synthesis, and macrophage function. 5-ASA has been shown to downregulate nuclear factor kappa-light-chain-enhancer of activated B-cell (NF-κB) levels [22–24].

5-ASA is the active component of sulfasalazine (SASP), which is composed of a sulphapyridine molecule and the 5-ASA active moiety linked by an azo bond. The release of the 5-ASA molecule depends on azoreductase activity of the colonic flora, which breaks the azo bond. The beneficial effects of 5-ASA are due on its topical delivery to affected mucosa. Most side effects related to SASP depend on the sulphapyridine component; aminosalicylates are better tolerated. Various formulations of 5-ASA-containing compounds have been developed, including pH-dependent and time-based release systems with peculiar pharmacokinetic properties. Ph-dependent preparations are delivered in the colon, while time-release preparations are delivered throughout the whole bowel. In addition to oral 5-ASA, topical formulations (suppositories, gel, foams, and enemas), which provide the drug to the rectum and left colon, have been developed.

Older published trials showed oral aminosalicylates to be an effective treatment for active ileal, ileocolic, or colonic CD. Asacol 3.2 g/day was effective in ileocolic or colonic disease [25], and Pentasa 4 g/day was reported to be effective for ileitis, ileocolitis, and colitis [26].

However, more recent studies using different preparation sand meta-analyses have failed to demonstrate the efficacy of 5-ASA in the induction and maintenance of remission in CD. At the present time, the role of mesalazine in CD should be considered marginal and limited to mild to moderate CD [3, 27]. Mesalamine has still a role in the prevention of postsurgical relapse especially in low-risk patients (first resection, absence of prognostic factors for bad prognosis) and in those with a negative postsurgical follow-up endoscopy (absence of early relapse) [4, 27–29]. Opinion still varies about the value of topical mesalazine, which can be considered as adjunctive therapy in distal colonic CD.

Side effects of aminosalicylates are both idiosyncratic and dose dependent and occur in 10–45 % of patients. Most common dose-related side effects are headache, nausea, epigastric pain, and diarrhea. Other rare and less common adverse events are idiosyncratic reactions such as skin rashes or the rare Stevens-Johnson syndrome, pancreatitis, or agranulocytosis [30]. Aminosalicylates can induce reversible renal insufficiency, in patients with preexisting renal impairment, concomitant use of nephrotoxic drugs, or comorbid disease, and annual monitoring of renal function is recommended.

7.1.2.2 Corticosteroids

Glucocorticoids are the mainstay in the treatment of active CD for inducing remission. They have immunosuppressive activity by acting both on the inflammation cascade and on the immune system, interfering with the clonal proliferation of helper T lymphocytes and reducing transcription of genes coding for pro-inflammatory cytokines such as TNF-alpha and IFN-gamma.

The efficacy of glucocorticoids in inducing remission has been demonstrated in two large randomized controlled trials carried out in the 1980s, the NCCDS and the ECCDS.

In the National Cooperative Crohn's Disease Study (NCCDS), 60 % of patients obtained remission when treated with prednisone 0.5–0.75 mg/kg/day and tapering over 17 weeks, as compared to 30 % of the placebo group [31]. In the comparable 18-week European Cooperative Crohn's Disease Study (ECCDS), 83 % of patients achieved remission with 6-methylprednisolone 1 mg/kg/day compared with 38 % of the placebo group [32].

In view of the high prevalence of adverse events related to systemic glucocorticoid therapy, recently new topically active low-availability steroids have been developed. Budesonide is a synthetic corticosteroid derivative taken orally, which is delivered locally, and it is released in a time-dependent manner in the terminal ileum and proximal colon. Upon absorption into the portal system, the drug is highly metabolized into significantly less active metabolites in the liver, which reduces systemic exposure, potentially decreasing corticosteroid-related side effects.

In a systematic review, 9 mg/day of this preparation are superior to placebo and mesalamine in achieving remission with fewer side effects but also less efficacy of conventional steroid such as prednisolone [33]. Pushing the dose higher results in better efficacy but at the expense of increasing side effects.

Budesonide is to be preferred to prednisone in mild to moderate active terminal ileal or ileocecal disease, and a standard tapering strategy is recommended. Though better tolerated, budesonide is not effective in maintaining remission as demonstrated in clinical trials and meta-analyses, and a budesonide dependence should be approached as systemic steroid dependence [34].

Steroids should never be used for periods longer than 3 months [35] because of significant long-term side effects. Early effects due to the doses used to induce remission include cosmetics (acne, moon face, edema, and skin striae), sleep, and mood disturbs. A prolonged use of steroids leads to posterior subcapsular cataracts, osteoporosis, osteonecrosis of the femoral head, and

myopathy. Steroids increase also the risk of serious infections if associated with other immunosuppressive agents [36, 37].

Effects on withdrawal include acute adrenal insufficiency in case of sudden cessation (slow tapering is thus advised), a syndrome of pseudorheumatism with myalgia, malaise and arthralgia, and raised intracranial pressure.

If the duration of therapy is likely to be more than 12 weeks, supplements of calcium and vitamin D are recommended [38, 39].

A significant number of patients fail to respond adequately to glucocorticoids and are either steroid resistant or steroid dependent.

Steroid-dependent patients experience a relapse of symptoms as the steroid dose is tapered wile steroid-unresponsive patients do not improve even with prolonged high doses of steroids. For these patients, other therapeutic strategies with the use of thiopurines or methotrexate or biologics for maintenance are recommended.

As recommended in ECCO guidelines, "patients who are dependent on corticosteroids should be treated with thiopurines or methotrexate with or without anti-TNF therapy [EL1a, RG A for thiopurines and methotrexate], [EL1a, RG B for infliximab and adalimumab], although surgical options should also be considered and discussed" (ECCO Statement 6D) (2).

As recommended in ECCO guidelines, "patients with objective evidence of active disease refractory to corticosteroids should be treated with anti-TNF therapy, with or without thiopurines or methotrexate [EL1a, RG B for infliximab], although surgical options should also be considered and discussed at an early stage" (ECCO Statement 5H) (2).

7.1.2.3 Antibiotics

Antibiotics are coadjuvant drugs; they are considered appropriate in CD in treating CD-related complications: intra-abdominal abscesses, inflammatory masses, perianal diseases (fistulas and perirectal abscesses), bacterial overgrowth in the small bowel secondary to partial small bowel obstruction, secondary infections with organisms such as *Clostridium difficile*, and postoperative complications.

The antibiotics most frequently used are metronidazole and ciprofloxacin [40, 41].

Both drugs are more beneficial in CD of the colon than in disease restricted to the ileum probably for their action on the anaerobic flora.

They historically were considered to be first-line treatment for the management of fistulizing disease [42]. They have been a mainstay of therapy for simple fistulizing disease, while complex fistulizing disease is typically treated with a combination of approaches including immunomodulators, biologics, and surgical therapies (seton placement, drainage of abscesses). After cessation of therapy, fistula tends to recur, but long-term therapy is limited by side effect.

The largest reported experience has been with metronidazole. Beside treatment of fistulizing disease, another indication is the prevention of postsurgical recurrence in which high-dose metronidazole (20 mg/kg/day for 3 months) has been shown effective in preventing endoscopic and clinical recurrence at 1 year [43].

Metronidazole is generally well tolerated and incidence of side effects is dose dependent and time related. Most common side effects are gastrointestinal discomfort, nausea, and dysgeusia. After several months of treatment, a peripheral neuropathy can occur, and in rare occasions, this is not reversible after withdrawal of the drug.

The other antibiotic widely used is ciprofloxacin, a quinolone derivative with a selective suppressive effect on intestinal flora. Ciprofloxacin has similar efficacy to metronidazole and with fewer side effects.

Ciprofloxacin and metronidazole are often used to induce remission in mild to moderate CD, but comparison studies with corticosteroids have not clearly identified any additional benefits to induce remission [44, 45].

Another antibiotic used is rifaximin, a nonsystemic antibiotic approved for the treatment of traveler's diarrhea and also used in irritable bowel syndrome. It is not completely absorbed in the blood stream, minimizing systemic exposure and reducing the risk of side effects. Rifaximin is associated with clinical improvement in patients with mild Crohn's disease and can play an adjunctive role for inducing and maintaining remission [46].

In conclusion, although controlled studies with antibiotics used for treatment of CD are limited and inconclusive, these drugs are widely used in clinical practice. At present, metronidazole and ciprofloxacin, used alone or in association, are considered appropriate for septic complications, symptoms attributable to bacterial overgrowth, or perianal disease.

7.1.2.4 Thiopurines

Thiopurines, azathioprine (AZA) and its metabolite 6-mercaptopurine (6-MP) are widely used in the management of CD and exert their effect via inhibition of purine synthesis. In order to get activated, they must undergo a very complex metabolism. Both are prodrugs; AZA is converted to mercaptopurine, which is metabolized to the active 6-thioguanine nucleotide (6-TG). 6-TG then functions as a purine analog, inhibiting DNA synthesis, and also appears to trigger T-cell apoptosis [47, 48]. AZA and 6-MP, alone or in combination with other drugs, are effective in induction and maintaining remission in active CD and are steroid-sparing drugs in steroid-dependent or steroid-refractory patients [49, 50].

Two Cochrane meta-analyses have synthesized the existing data regarding the efficacy of AZA and 6MP in the induction and maintenance of remission in CD in patients treated with AZA/6MP versus placebo. Prefontaine et al. assessed eight RCTs of AZA/6MP for induction of remission in 425 patients with active CD.17 Overall response in the pooled treatment group was 54 versus 33 % in the placebo arm (odds ratio [OR], 2.43; 95 % CI, 1.623.64). Induction of remission in active CD by using AZA requires a long period of time (from 3 to 6 months), since the response rate increases after 17 weeks. Thiopurines were more effective than placebo for maintaining remission in CD. With respect to maintenance of remission, a recent systematic review assessing seven trials with AZA and one with 6MP demonstrated, among 550 patients, an OR of 2.32 (95 % CI, 1.553.49) for AZA and 3.32 (95 % CI, 1.407.87) for 6MP [51].

AZA and MP also showed to be more effective than placebo or mesalazine in preventing both clinical and endoscopic postoperative recurrence in CD [52].

The optimal dose of AZA is typically 2–3 mg/kg/day, whereas the dose for 6MP is half (1–1.5 mg/kg/day). To obtain a full pharmacological effect, a long-term treatment is required and frequent side effects occur. The high rate of adverse reactions reduces their use as an early therapeutic option. Adverse events due to thiopurines are classified as dose independent or dose dependent. Dose-independent or "allergic" adverse reactions include fever, malaise, nausea, abdominal pain, diarrhea, arthralgia, and pancreatitis and occur early (days or weeks). Dose-related or "nonallergic" AEs are myelotoxicity and liver toxicity and usually develop later (months or years) [53–56].

During treatment, a careful laboratory monitoring is recommended, particularly when first initiating the drug. Given the potential for significant bone marrow suppression, frequent blood cell count monitoring is recommended, particularly when initiating therapy or optimizing dosing. Liver function tests should also be monitored periodically. However, the absolute risk of developing these remains low. Pretreatment assessment of TPMT phenotype or genotype could be useful but is not widely used and recommended by ECCO guidelines. Thiopurines' use is safe during pregnancy and lactation.

Treatment with thiopurines leads to a form of chronic immunosuppression and to an increased risk of infection. The use of thiopurines has also been associated with an increased risk of lymphoma and an increase of nonmelanoma skin cancer [57–61].

Screening for opportunistic infection before immunosuppressive treatment should be performed, and vaccination history should be documented [62].

As far as concerns the duration of maintenance immunosuppressive therapy with thiopurines, an expert consensus recommends to continue immunomodulators for at least 4 years in view of the low risk of relapse after this time interval and to minimize the risk of cancer [63].

7.1.2.5 Methotrexate

Methotrexate (MTX) is a folate antagonist with cytotoxical immunosuppressive activity. Mechanism of action includes inhibition of dihydrofolate reductase, inhibiting purine and pyrimidine synthesis, resulting in decreased cellular proliferation and modulation of cytokine production. MTX has the same indications of thiopurines, but is generally reserved for treatment of active or relapsing Crohn's disease in patients with refractoriness or intolerance to thiopurines or anti-TNF agents [64] and may be preferable in patients with CD-related arthropathy. Methotrexate is effective for inducing remission and preventing relapse in CD. In a controlled study, patients treated with intramuscular MTX (25 mg/week) and a concomitant dose of prednisolone (20 mg at initiation) were able to withdraw steroids and enter remission compared with placebo. MTX also is effective in maintaining remission; in patients treated with 15 mg/week of intramuscular MTX, a significant number remained in remission at 40 weeks compared with placebo group [65]. The standard induction dose is 25 mg administered intramuscularly (IM) or subcutaneously via weekly injections. A switch to oral administration may be attempted for maintenance while carefully monitoring the clinical response.

As with thiopurines, there are significant potential side effects. Most common complications of MTX are due to its mechanism of action and include folate deficiency. Therefore, in patients taking MTX administration of folate, supplementation for 2 or 3 days a week is advisable.

Other early common side effects are fatigue, nausea, vomiting, diarrhea, and alopecia [63].

Though less common than with thiopurines, mild leukopenia can also occur. Hepatic fibrosis is the most severe idiosyncratic side effect of long-term therapy, and liver function test monitoring is recommended, though transaminase levels may not correlate with degree of fibrosis [66]. Also transient fibroelastography annually is advisable. Measurement of full blood count and liver function tests is advisable before and within 4 weeks of starting therapy, then monthly. Patients on long-term MTX should also be monitored carefully for pneumonitis, a rare but possible side effect. Methotrexate is teratogenic and is contraindicated during pregnancy and lactation [67].

7.1.3   New Approach: Biological Therapy

The introduction of biological therapy has revolutionized therapeutic strategies in CD allowing the achievement of new goals: not only response and remission and maintenance of remission but also mucosal healing, deep remission, improvement of quality of life, and reducing hospitalizations and surgery. Biological therapy could have the potential to change disease course and to prevent disability.

7.1.4   Biological Agents: Anti-TNF-Alpha

Tumor necrosis factor-alpha blockers (infliximab, adalimumab, and certolizumab) are monoclonal antibodies that block the pro-inflammatory cascade that triggers the activation and proliferation of T lymphocytes in the intestine.

TNF-α is a cytokine especially produced by activated macrophages and lymphocytes and has been shown to be elevated in the lamina propria of patients with CD. Anti-TNF agents act by binding soluble TNF-α and also by inducing apoptosis in activated T cells within the lamina propria of patients with CD. These agents have demonstrated the ability to induce apoptosis in activated monocytes, as well [68, 69].

According to ECCO guidelines, "anti-TNF therapy should be considered as an alternative to thiopurines for patients with moderately active localized ileocaecal CD who have previously been steroid-refractory, steroid-dependent, or steroid-intolerant. For those patients with severely active localized ileocaecal Crohn's disease and objective evidence of active disease who have relapsed, anti-TNF therapy with or without an immunomodulator is an appropriate option. Infliximab or adalimumab, in combination with surgical therapy, should be used, for complex perianal Crohn's disease, as a second line medical treatment after antibiotics and thiopurines" [3]. More recently, guidelines from the IG-IBD, the Italian Group for the Study of IBD, have been issued, which, while confirming indications to anti-TNF in most clinical scenarios according to ECCO, recommend anti-TNF as first clinical option in the field of perianal disease [70].

As far as concerns the duration of therapy of anti-TNF agents, according to ECCO guidelines, "Anti-TNF agents are effective for maintenance of remission up to 1 year in patients with clinical response to induction therapy. No recommendation can be given for the duration of treatment, although prolonged use of these medications may be considered if needed. Potential risks and benefits should be discussed on an individual basis."

There is evidence that long-term infliximab treatment has a good overall safety profile in cohort studies [71] and that adalimumab is able to maintain remission for up to 2 years in patients who responded to induction therapy [72].

In the STORI trial (infliximab discontinuation in Crohn's disease patients in stable remission on combined therapy with immunosuppressors), 115 patients receiving both infliximab and an immunosuppressor in stable steroid-free remission for at least 6 months discontinued infliximab therapy [73]. After a median follow-up time of 12 months, 43.9 % of patients had a relapse. Multivariate analysis showed that endoscopic activity, CRP level, and hemoglobin and infliximab trough levels predicted increasing risk of relapse. These data suggest that if discontinuation of treatment is desired, stratification of relapse risk according to predictive factors should be carefully evaluated and treatment withdrawal should be reserved to those patients at low risk of relapse.

Loss of response to anti-TNF therapy occurs at a rate of 10–20 %/year; when patients on anti-TNF loose response, an assessment of disease activity with the exclusion of complications and adherence problems is mandatory. Optimization of therapy by either dose intensification (reduction of the interval between doses) or dose escalation is appropriate strategy before switching to another agent. Switching is an effective strategy, but reduces future therapeutic options. For intolerance, especially if severe, switching to an alternative anti-TNF agent is appropriate.

Primary lack of response can occur: by definition, this usually happens within 12 weeks; current strategy suggests the use of an alternative anti-TNF agent or switch to another class of drugs [62].

Therapy with biological agents should be strictly monitored for the risk of adverse advents and opportunistic infection [37, 74]. Patients with fever, cough, systemic symptoms, or with a suspected pyogenic complication of Crohn's disease should be evaluated for opportunistic infections and treatment with antibiotics before starting or continuing biological therapy.

Whether this risk can be attributed to anti-TNF agents or concomitant use of other immunomodulators remains controversial. Recent analysis of pooled data from several clinical trials suggests that these risks may not be more elevated with anti-TNF agents when used alone, but appear to be increased when receiving both anti-TNF drugs and immunomodulators [75].

Before starting anti-TNFs, screening is mandatory. Tuberculosis screening includes a full medical history, physical examination, TST or IGRA, and a chest X-ray. Patients should be tested also for HBV (HbsAg, anti-HbcAb,), anti-HCV, and anti-HIV using antibody testing.

Furthermore, anti-TNF therapy has been associated with drug-induced lupus, demyelinating reactions, peripheral neuropathy, psoriasis, and heart failure.

A meta-analysis of all randomized controlled trials comparing all anti-TNF strategies with placebo did not show an increased risk of malignancy in patients receiving anti-TNF [76]. These figures are in contrast with the results from a previous meta-analysis including patients with rheumatoid arthritis receiving infliximab or adalimumab which reported an increased risk of malignancy [77].

The risk of lymphoma in patients on anti-TNFs seems low, but hepatosplenic T-cell lymphoma (HSTCL) has been described in patients with Crohn's disease who have been treated with anti-TNF agents in combination with immunomodulators or with immunomodulators alone (6-MP and azathioprine). This nearly fatal form of NHL predominantly affects young men, but the absolute rate of these events is low. This, in addition to the uncertain of benefit of combination therapy, has led to an emphasis on previous or concomitant treatment with conventional immunomodulators, particularly in young male patients [78, 79].

Recently, nested-case control studies have demonstrated in patients treated with anti-TNF an increased risk of melanoma [59].

7.1.4.1 Infliximab

Infliximab, administered intravenously, is a chimeric IgG 1 monoclonal antibody with a murine variable region and human immunoglobulin constant region. It neutralizes the biologic activity of TNF-alpha by inhibiting binding to its receptors.

The infliximab therapeutic schedule includes an induction phase at 0, 2, and 6 weeks and a maintenance treatment every 8 weeks.

Infliximab was the first biological response modifier that has been shown to be effective in Crohn's disease. A randomized, controlled trial (ACCENT I) provided strong confirmation of the initial impression of efficacy found in pivotal studies. Patients with moderate to severe Crohn's disease were randomized to an initial infusion of placebo or 5, 10, or 20 mg/kg infliximab. Recruited patients had moderate to severe Crohn's disease (CDAI, 220–400) despite treatment with aminosalicylates and oral glucocorticoids (59 %), or 6-MP, or azathioprine (37 %). The primary endpoint was clinical response, defined as a decrease in the CDAI of 70 or more points at week four. All treatment groups had results significantly better than those with placebo (placebo response rate of 17 %). The highest rate of response was seen at 4 weeks in the 5 mg/kg group (81 %) [80]. A smaller but still significant fraction of patients had a clinical response by week 12 (48 % for 5 mg/kg vs. 12 % for placebo). The fraction of patients in clinical remission (CDAI less than 150 and a decrease in CDAI of 70 or more points) at week four also was significantly higher among the 5 mg/kg group (33 %) compared with the placebo group (4 %). Clinical improvement was accompanied by improvement in health-related quality of life and decreases in serum C-reactive protein levels. However, the inclusion criteria have been heterogeneous including both patients with active disease naive to steroids and with steroid-refractory or steroid-dependent disease.

No trial has been designed on the maintenance of corticosteroid-dependent patients. The data of efficacy on this population can be extrapolated from the results of ACCENT I trial in which 51 % of patients received corticosteroids at the time of randomization. Twenty-four percent of those maintained on infliximab every 8 weeks at 5 mg/kg and 32 % of those receiving 10 mg/kg were in corticosteroid-free clinical remission at week 54. Only 9 % of patients receiving placebo maintained corticosteroid-free remission ($p=0.004$ for infliximab groups vs. placebo) [81].

The ACCENT II study evaluated the effectiveness of maintenance therapy with infliximab in sustaining fistula closure in patients suffering from one or more fistulas for at least 3 months immediately preceding screening and who responded to induction therapy. The primary efficacy endpoint was defined as the time from randomization until loss of response. According to researchers, results show that at week 54, 36 % of patients taking infliximab had complete absence of draining fistulas vs. 19 % of patients receiving placebo ($p=0.009$). Time to loss of response was significantly longer for patients who received maintenance therapy with infliximab (greater than 40 weeks vs. 14 weeks for placebo, $p<0.001$) [82].

The value of the concomitant use of immunomodulators (6-MP, azathioprine, or methotrexate) to improve the anti-TNF initial response and maintenance effect is controversial. In the SONIC trial, patients with moderate to severe Crohn's disease were randomized to the TNF-a inhibitor infliximab plus placebo, azathioprine plus placebo, or the combination of infliximab plus azathioprine. At the end of 26 weeks, corticosteroid-free remission was achieved in 57 % of patients on the combination, 44.4 % of those on infliximab, and 30.6 % of those on azathioprine.

The advantage for both infliximab ($p=0.009$) and the combination ($p<0.001$) over azathioprine monotherapy was highly statistically significant. The study suggested that moving immediately to infliximab should be more effective than stepping up to the immunomodulator azathioprine. A widespread early use of biologics in all CD patients cannot be recommended, but in selected patient subgroups with a predictable disabling severe course (extensive disease, severe rectal disease, young age, severe perianal diseases at diagnosis, steroid need at diagnosis), the early introduction of biologics can be empirically considered on an individual basis [83].

Treatment with the anti-TNF agents usually is well tolerated. In the largest and longer-term clinical trials, between 4 and 16 % of patients withdrew from the study due to an adverse event [84]. Injection site and infusion reactions occurred at variable rates. Severe acute infusion reactions consist of chest tightness, dyspnea, rash, and hypotension. Infusion reactions with infliximab typically are associated with antibodies to infliximab (ATIs), also referred to as HACAs (human antichimeric antibodies). ATIs developed in 13 % of infliximab-treated patients with Crohn's disease. ATIs are less likely to develop in patients treated concomitantly with glucocorticoids or immune modulators, providing a justification for continuing methotrexate, azathioprine, or 6-MP, even when these treatments have failed.

Delayed hypersensitivity reactions, manifesting as severe polyarthralgia, myalgia, facial edema, urticaria, or rash, are unusual complications that can occur two to 14 days after an infusion [85].

7.1.4.2 Adalimumab

Adalimumab, another TNF-blocking drug, is a subcutaneously administered, recombinant, fully human, IgG1 monoclonal antibody that binds to TNF-alpha. By neutralizing it, adalimumab inhibits a number of TNF-alpha events including the release of IL-6, acute-phase reactants of inflammation, and molecules enabling leukocyte migration. Furthermore, via the activation of intracellular caspases, TNF-expressing mononuclear cells undergo apoptosis [86].

The usual adult induction dose is 160 mg followed by an 80 mg dose 2 weeks later. For ongoing treatment, the usual dose is then 40 mg every other week.

Similar to infliximab, adalimumab has been evaluated for its effect in inducing and maintaining remission, its steroid-sparing effect, and its impact on hospitalizations and surgeries.

The CLASSIC I trial included a total of 299 patients with moderate to severe active Crohn's disease naive to TNF-alpha inhibitor therapy who were randomized to receive adalimumab (40/20 mg, 80/40 mg, or 160/80 mg) or placebo at weeks 0 and 2. They were randomly assigned to adalimumab at three different doses, or placebo, at zero and 2 weeks [87]. The highest dose of 160/80 mg demonstrated significantly higher rates of remission at week 4 compared with placebo (36 vs. 12 %, $p = 0.001$). Similarly, a response (CDAI decrease of 100 points) at 4 weeks was achieved significantly more often in patients who received the highest dose compared with placebo (50 % vs. 25 %, $p = 0.007$). Adverse events occurred at similar frequencies in all four treatment groups except injection site reactions, which were more common in adalimumab-treated patients.

There were 275 patients from CLASSIC I who were entered into the CLASSIC II trial. Patients who were in remission at both week 0 (week four of the CLASSIC I trial) and week 4 were re-randomized to 40 mg every other week (eow), weekly, or placebo for 56 weeks. In this re-randomized cohort of 55 patients, 79 % who received adalimumab 40 mg eow and 83 % who received 40 mg weekly maintained remission through week 56 (primary endpoint) compared with 44 % for placebo (p 0.05 for both adalimumab groups vs. placebo). The patients from CLASSIC I who were not in remission at both weeks zero and four received open-label adalimumab 40 mg every other week (dosages could be increased to 40 mg weekly if there was a nonresponse or flare). Of the 204 who entered the open-label arm, 46 % were in clinical remission and 65 % were considered responders at week 56 [88]. Thus, CLASSIC I and II showed that adalimumab induced and maintained clinical remission in patients with moderate to severe CD naive to TNF inhibitor treatment.

The results of the CHARM trial, which had the largest sample size for a maintenance trial with adalimumab in CD, confirm that this drug is more effective than placebo for long-term (56 weeks) maintenance of remission. Patients who had been exposed to infliximab in the past and either lost response or had become intolerant to infliximab were eligible for this trial [89].

In CHARM, approximately 40 % of the 499 patients with moderate to severe CD who responded to adalimumab maintained remission at 26 and 52 weeks, thus confirming long-term efficacy. ADA demonstrated steroid-sparing properties, beneficial effects in patients with perianal fistulas, and decreases rates of hospitalization and surgery. IFX-naive patients had higher response rates than those with prior IFX exposure.

7.1.4.3 Certolizumab

Certolizumab pegol is a humanized monoclonal antibody composed of a PEGylated Fab'fragment that binds to TNF-alpha. The PEGylated Fab'fragment does not interfere with the antibody's ability to neutralize TNF-alpha [90].

Certolizumab pegol is approved in the United States for treatment and maintenance of response in adults with moderate to severe Crohn's disease who had an inadequate response to conventional therapy. Approval for Crohn's disease was based upon two placebo-controlled trials [91, 92]. The drug is also available in Canada and some European Union countries where, however, approved indications are limited to rheumatoid arthritis, psoriatic arthritis, and axial spondyloarthritis. Its use in Crohn's disease in Europe has not been approved.

7.1.4.4 Alpha-4 Integrin Blocker

In the last 2 years, new molecules directed against integrins and integrin receptors have been developed and investigated in clinical trials, showing that anti-α4integrin agents can be effective and safe for the induction and maintenance of remission in active CD. Adhesion molecules, mainly integrins (α4β7, α4β1), located at the surface of endothelial cells, are responsible for cell migration to sites of inflammation and play a key role in the pathogenetic mechanisms of IBD. Drugs targeting alpha-4 integrin (natalizumab, vedolizumab) can limit the severity of inflammation inhibiting the recruitment of lymphocytes in the affected sites.

7.1.4.5 Natalizumab

Natalizumab is an IgG4 humanized monoclonal antibody that specifically antagonizes α4 integrin. Natalizumab was first developed in IBD showing efficacy for induction and maintenance of clinical remission in CD. However, cases of progressive multifocal leukoencephalopathy (PML) due to JC virus reactivation in natalizumab-treated patients have pull up the further development of the drug [93].

7.1.4.6 Vedolizumab

Vedolizumab is a humanized monoclonal antibody that binds to the α4β7integrin, blocking its interaction with mucosal addressin cell adhesion molecule-1 (MAdCAM-1). This interaction facilitates lymphocyte homing to the gut and is an important contributor to inflammation that is a hallmark of CD [94]. Because MAdCAM-1 is preferentially expressed on blood vessels in the intestinal tract, vedolizumab is theoretically more gut specific and therefore a more targeted form of immunosuppression. Concern about safety profile has been caused by previous experience with the first anti-integrin, natalizumab, available in the United States but never approved in Europe because of the risk of PML (progressive multifocal polyencephalopathy), due to JC virus reactivation. The overall rate of PML cases among patients treated with natalizumab is about 1.16 per 1000 patients. Nearly 3000 patients have been treated with vedolizumab in phase III clinical trials with no reported cases of PML.

Vedolizumab was developed as a treatment for patients with moderate to severe IBD who have failed at least one conventional therapy, including TNF antagonists. In GEMINI II (a randomized, placebo-controlled, trial) vedolizumab-treated patients with active Crohn's disease, nonresponder to immunosuppressive agents or TNF antagonists, were more likely to achieve remission but not a Crohn's Disease Activity Index-100 response at week six and more likely to be in remission at week 52 compared with patients receiving placebo. Adverse events, including nasopharyngitis, were more common than in placebo-treated patients, but usually mild [95].

Vedolizumab has been approved in Europe and is currently under evaluation of regulatory authorities in Italy.

7.1.5 Biosimilars

Biosimilars are biologic medicines that enter the market when the patent of the original reference product has expired. The approval procedures for biosimilars require a thorough demonstration of the comparability of the biosimilar to the original biologic. To secure regulatory approval, there must be no clinically significant difference, in terms of safety, purity, and potency, between the biosimilar and the originator, already-approved biologic.

Infliximab is the first anti-TNF-alpha agent that has lost its patent, and some infliximab biosimilars have already been authorized for use in the European Union. Available data from the literature have demonstrated efficacy and safety of infliximab biosimilars in rheumatoid arthritis and ankylosing spondylitis. No RCT has been performed in IBD raising some concerns in gastroenterologists about the transferability of efficacy rates from the originator to biosimilars in these diseases; reassurance however comes from observational post-marketing reports from countries in which regulatory approval is already available.

7.1.6 Future Trends

There is a rich pipeline of novel therapeutic agents [96]. Treatment strategies that appear particularly appealing include selective anti-integrin therapy with anti-interleukin 12/23p40 therapy with ustekinumab [97] and Janus kinase 1, 2, and 3 inhibition with tofacitinib [98].

Another approach was proposed by Monteleone et al. In a phase 2 study, a *SMAD7*

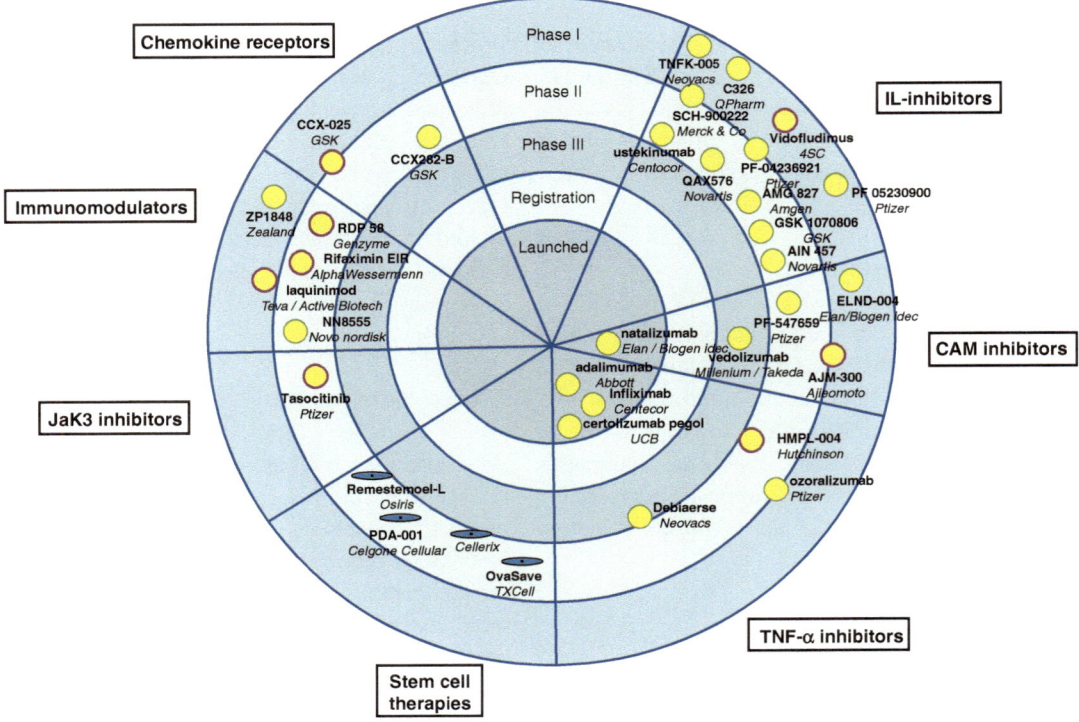

Fig. 7.2 Crohn's disease new biologics pipeline (From Danese et al. [96])

antisense oligonucleotide, called mongersen, targets SMAD7 proteins in the ileum and colon to increase TGF-β1, which is an immunosuppressive cytokine that can attenuate Crohn's disease-related inflammation. Patients who received mongersen had significantly higher rates of remission and clinical response than those who received placebo [99].

With the availability of more biologics, therapeutic strategies will probably undergo more radical changes: patients' profiling according to prognostic factors and previous therapeutic history will be increasingly relevant to target therapeutical approach (Fig. 7.2).

References

1. D'Haens G, Baert F, van Assche G, et al., for the Belgian Inflammatory Bowel Disease Research Group; North-Holland Gut Club. Early combined immunosuppression or conventional management in patients with newly diagnosed Crohn's disease: an open randomised trial. Lancet. 2008;371:660–7.

2. Gert Van Assche, Axel Dignass, Julian Panes, Laurent Beaugerie et al. for the European Crohn's and Colitis Organisation (ECCO). The second European evidence-based consensus on the diagnosis and management of Crohn's disease: definitions and diagnosis. J Crohns Colitis. 2010;4:7–27.

3. Dignass A, Van Assche G, Lindsay JO, Lémann M, et al. for the European Crohn's and Colitis Organisation (ECCO). The second European evidence-based consensus on the diagnosis and management of Crohn's disease: Current management. J Crohns Colitis. 2010;4: 28–62.

4. Gert Van Assche, Axel Dignass, Walter Reinisch, et al. for the European Crohn's and Colitis Organisation (ECCO). The second European evidence-based Consensus on the diagnosis and management of Crohn's disease: special situations. J Crohns Colitis. 2010;4:63–101.

5. Best WR, Becktel JM, Singleton JW, Kern Jr F. Development of a Crohn's disease activity index. National Cooperative Crohn's Disease Study. Gastroenterology. 1976;70:439–44.

6. Harvey FR, Bradshaw JM. A simple index of Crohn's disease activity. Lancet. 1980;1:514.

7. Irvine EJ, Feagan B, Rochon J, et al. Quality of life: a valid and reliable measure of therapeutic efficacy in the treatment of inflammatory bowel disease. Canadian Crohn's Relapse Prevention Trial Study Group. Gastroenterology. 1994;106:287–96.

8. Kiss LS, Papp M, Lovasz BD, et al. High-sensitivity C-reactive protein for identification of disease phenotype, active disease, and clinical relapses in Crohn's disease: a marker for patient classification? Inflamm Bowel Dis. 2012;18(9):1647–54.

9. Sipponen T, Karkkainen P, Savilahti E, et al. Correlation of faecal calprotectin and lactoferrin with an endoscopic score for Crohn's disease and histological findings. Aliment Pharmacol Ther. 2008;28(10):1221–9.

10. Sipponen T, Savilahti E, Kohlo KL, Nuutinen H, Turunen U, Farkkila M. Crohn's disease activity assessed by fecal calprotectin and lactoferrin: correlation with Crohn's disease activity index and endoscopic findings. Inflamm Bowel Dis. 2008;14(1):40–6.

11. Mary JY, Modigliani R. Development and validation of an endoscopic index of the severity for Crohn's disease: a prospective multicentre study. Grouped'EtudesTherapeutiques des Affections Inflammatoires du Tube Digestif (GETAID). Gut. 1989;30(7):983–9.

12. Daperno M, D'Haens G, Van Assche G, et al. Development and validation of a new, simplified endoscopic activity score for Crohn's disease: the SES-CD. Gastrointest Endosc. 2004;60(4):505–12.

13. Rutgeerts P, Geboes K, Vantrappen G, Beyls J, Kerremans R, Hiele M. Predictability of the postoperative course of Crohn's disease. Gastroenterology. 1990;99(4):956–63.

14. Ferrante M, Colombel JF, Sandborn WJ, et al. International Organization for the Study of Inflammatory Bowel Diseases. Validation of endoscopic activity scores in patients with Crohn's disease based on a post hoc analysis of data from SONIC. Gastroenterology. 2013;145(5):978–86.

15. Maconi G, Radice E, Greco S, Bianchi Porro G. Bowel ultrasound in Crohn's disease. Best Pract Res Clin Gastroenterol. 2006;20(1):93–112.

16. Di Mizio R, Maconi G, Romano S, D'Amario F, Bianchi Porro G, Grassi R. Small bowel Crohn disease: sonographic features. Abdom Imaging. 2004;29(1):23–35.

17. Panes J, Bouhnik Y, Reinisch W, et al. Imaging techniques for assessment of inflammatory bowel disease: joint ECCO and ESGAR evidence-based consensus guidelines. J Crohns Colitis. 2013;7(7):556–85.

18. Makanyanga JC, Taylor SA. Current and future role of MR enterography in the management of Crohn disease. AJR Am J Roentgenol. 2013;201(1):56–64.

19. Hommes D, Colombel JF, Emery P, Greco M, Sandborn WJ. Changing Crohn's disease management: need for new goals and indices to prevent disability and improve quality of life. J Crohns Colitis. 2012;6 Suppl 2:S224–34.

20. Schnitzler F, Fidder H, Ferrante M, et al. Mucosal healing predicts long-term outcome of maintenance therapy with infliximab in Crohn's disease. Inflamm Bowel Dis. 2009;15(9):1295–301.

21. Baert F, Moortgat L, Van Assche G, et al. Belgian Inflammatory Bowel Disease Research Group. North-Holland Gut Club Mucosal healing predicts sustained clinical remission in patients with early-stage Crohn's disease. Gastroenterology. 2010;138(2):463–8.

22. Bantel H, Berg C, Vieth M, Stolte M, Kruis W, Schulze-Osthoff K. Mesalazine inhibits activation of transcription factor NF-kappaB in inflamed mucosa of patients with ulcerative colitis. Am J Gastroenterol. 2000;95(12):3452–7.

23. Haskó G, Szabó C, Németh ZH, Deitch EA. Sulphasalazine inhibits macrophage activation: inhibitory effects on inducible nitric oxide synthase expression, interleukin-12 production and major histocompatibility complex II expression. Immunology. 2001;103(4):473–8.

24. Kaiser GC, Yan F, Polk DB. Mesalamine blocks tumor necrosis factor growth inhibition and nuclear factor kappaB activation in mouse colonocytes. Gastroenterology. 1999;116(3):602–9.

25. Tremaine WJ, Schroeder KW, Harrison JM, Zinsmeister AR. A randomized, double-blind, placebo-controlled trial of the oral mesalamine (5-ASA) preparation, Asacol, in the treatment of symptomatic Crohn's colitis and ileocolitis. J Clin Gastroenterol. 1994;19:278–82.

26. Singleton JW, Hanauer SB, Gitnick GL, et al. Mesalamine capsules for the treatment of active Crohn's disease: results of a 16-week trial. Gastroenterology. 1993;104:1293–301.

27. Ford AC, Khan KJ, Talley NJ, Moayyedi P. 5-aminosalicylates prevent relapse of Crohn's disease after surgically induced remission: systematic review and meta-analysis. Am J Gastroenterol. 2011;106(3):413–20.

28. Cammá C, Giunta M, Roselli M, et al. Mesalamine in the maintenance treatment of Crohn's disease: a meta-analysis adjusted for confounding variables. Gastroenterology. 1997;113:1465–73.

29. Feagan BG. Editorial: 5-ASA therapy for active Crohn's disease: old friends, old data and a new conclusion. Clin Gastroenterol Hepatol. 2004;2:376–8.

30. Ransford RAJ, Langman MJS. Sulphasalazine and mesalazine: serious adverse reactions re-evaluated on the basis of suspected adverse reaction reports to the Committee on Safety of Medicines. Gut. 2002;51:536–9.

31. Summers RW, Switz DM, Sessions JT, et al. National cooperative Crohn's disease study group: results of drug treatment. Gastroenterology. 1979;77:847–69.

32. Malchow H, Ewe K, Brandes JW, et al. European cooperative Crohn's disease study (ECCDS): results of drug treatment. Gastroenterology. 1984;86:249–66.

33. Otley A, Steinhart AH. Budesonide for induction of remission in Crohn's disease. Cochrane Database Syst Rev. 2005;(4):CD000296. Review.

34. Benchimol EI, Seow CH, Otley AR, Steinhart AH. Budesonide for maintenance of remission in Crohn's disease. Cochrane Database Syst Rev. 2009;(1):CD002913.

35. Steinhart AH, Ewe K, Griffiths AM, Modigliani R, Thomsen OO. Corticosteroids for maintaining remission of Crohn's disease. Cochrane Database Syst Rev. 2003;(4):CD000301.

36. Lichtenstein GR, Feagan BG, Cohen RD, Salzberg BA, Diamond RH, Chen DM, et al. Serious infections and mortality in association with therapies for Crohn's disease: TREAT registry. Clin Gastroenterol Hepatol. 2006;4:621–30.

37. Toruner M, Loftus EV, Harmsen WS, et al. Risk factors for opportunistic infections in patients with inflammatory bowel disease. Gastroenterology. 2008;134:929–36.

38. British Society of Gastroenterology. Guidelines for osteoporosis in celiac disease and inflammatory bowel disease. Gut. 2000;46(Suppl1):i1–8.

39. Compston J. Osteoporosis in inflammatory bowel disease. Gut. 2003;52:63–4.

40. Arnold GL, Beaves MR, Pryjdun VO, Mook WJ. Preliminary study of ciprofloxacin in active Crohn's disease. Inflamm Bowel Dis. 2002;8:10–5.

41. Sutherland L, Singleton J, Sessions J, Hanauer S, Krawitt E, Rankin G, Summers R, et al. Double blind, placebo-controlled trial of metronidazole in Crohn's disease. Gut. 1991;32:1071–5.

42. Thia KT, Mahadevan U, Feagan BG, et al. Ciprofloxacin or metronidazole for the treatment of perianal fistulas in patients with Crohn's disease: a randomized, double-blind, placebo controlled pilot study. Inflamm Bowel Dis. 2009;15(1):17–24.

43. Rutgeerts P, Hiele M, Geboes K, Peeters M, Penninckx F, Aerts R, Kerremans R. Controlled trial of metronidazole treatment for prevention of Crohn's recurrence after ileal resection. Gastroenterology. 1995;108:1617–21.

44. Prantera C, Zannoni F, Scribano ML, et al. An antibiotic regimen for the treatment of active Crohn's disease: a randomized, controlled clinical trial of metronidazole plus ciprofloxacin. Am J Gastroenterol. 1996;91:328–32.

45. Borgaonkar MR, MacIntosh DG, Fardy JM. A meta-analysis of anti-mycobacterial therapy for Crohn's disease. Am J Gastroenterol. 2000;95:725–9.

46. Shafran I, Burgunder P. Adjunctive antibiotic therapy with rifaximin may help reduce Crohn's disease activity. Dig Dis Sci. 2010;4:1079–84.

47. Maltzman JS, Koretzky GA. Azathioprine: old drug, new actions. J Clin Invest. 2003;111(8):1122–4.

48. Tiede I, Fritz G, Strand S, et al. CD28-dependent Rac1 activation is the molecular target of azathioprine in primary human CD4þ T lymphocytes. J Clin Invest. 2003;111(8):1133–45.

49. Sandborn WJ, Sutherland L, Pearson D, May G, Modigliani R, Prantera C. Azathioprine or 6-mercaptopurine for inducing remission of Crohn's disease. Cochrane Database Syst Rev. 2000;(2):CD000545.

50. Pearson DC, May GR, Fick G, Sutherland LR. Azathioprine for maintaining remission of Crohn's disease. Cochrane Database Syst Rev. 2000;(2):CD000067.

51. Prefontaine E, Sutherland LR, Macdonald JK, Cepoiu M. Azathioprineor 6-mercaptopurine for maintenance of remission in Crohn's disease. Cochrane Database Syst Rev. 2009;(1):CD000067.

52. Reinisch W, Angelberger S, Petritsch W, Shonova O, Lukas M, Bar-Meir S, et al. Azathioprine versus mesalazine for prevention of postoperative clinical recurrence in patients with Crohn's disease with endoscopic recurrence: efficacy and safety results of a randomised, double-blind, double-dummy, multicentre trial. Gut. 2010;59:752–9.

53. Fraser AG, Orchard TR, Jewell DP. The efficacy of azathioprine for the treatment of inflammatory bowel disease: a 30 years review. Gut. 2002;50:485–9.

54. Nielsen OH, Vainer B, Rask-Madsen J. Review article: the treatment of inflammatory bowel disease with 6-mercaptopurine or azathioprine. Aliment Pharmacol Ther. 2001;15:1699–708.

55. Al Hadithy AFY, de Boer NKH, Derijks LJJ, Escher JC, Mulder CJ, Brouwers JR. Thiopurines in inflammatory bowel disease: pharmacogenetics, therapeutic drug monitoring and clinical recommendations. Dig Liver Dis. 2005;37:282–97.

56. Connel WR, Kamm MA, Ritchie JK, Lennard-Jones JE. Bone marrow toxicity caused by azathioprine in inflammatory bowel disease: 27 years of experience. Gut. 1993;34:1081–5.

57. Beaugerie L, Brousse N, Bouvier AM, CESAME Study Group, et al. Lymphoproliferative disorders in patients receiving thiopurines for inflammatory bowel disease: a prospective observational cohort study. Lancet. 2009;374(9701):1617–25.

58. Peyrin-Biroulet L, Khosrotehrani K, Carrat F, Cesame Study Group, et al. Increased risk for nonmelanoma skin cancers in patients who receive thiopurines for inflammatory bowel disease. Gastroenterology. 2011;141(5):1621–8. e1–e5.

59. Long MD, Martin CF, Pipkin CA, Herfarth HH, Sandler RS, Kappelman MD. Risk of melanoma and non melanoma skin cancer among patients with inflammatory bowel disease. Gastroenterology. 2012;143(2):390–9.

60. Singh H, Nugent Z, Demers AA, Bernstein CN. Increased risk of non-melanoma skin cancers among individuals with inflammatory bowel disease. Gastroenterology. 2011;141(5):1612–20.

61. Long MD, Herfarth HH, Pipkin CA, Porter CQ, Sandler RS, Kappelman MD. Increased risk for non-melanoma skin cancer in patients with inflammatory bowel disease. Clin Gastroenterol Hepatol. 2010;8(3):268–74.

62. Rahier aF, Magrob cd, Abreue C, ArmuzziA, f Ben-Horing S, Chowers Y, h M. et al. on behalf of the European Crohn's and Colitis Organisation (ECCO). Second European evidence-based consensus on the prevention, diagnosis and management of opportunistic infections in inflammatory bowel disease J.F. J Crohns Colitis. 2014;8:443–68.

63. Pittet V, Froehlich F, Maillard MH, EPACT-II Update Panelists. When do we dare to stop biological or immunomodulator therapy for Crohn's disease? Results of a multidisciplinary European expert panel. J Crohns Colitis. 2013;7:820–926.

64. Fraser AG. Methotrexate: first or second-line immunomodulator? Eur J Gastroenterol Hepatol. 2003;15:225–31.

65. Feagan BG, Fedorak RN, Irvine EJ, et al; North American Crohn's Study Group Investigators. A comparison of methotrexate with placebo for the maintenance of remission in Crohn's disease. N Engl J Med. 2000;342(22):1627–32.

66. Te HS, Schiano TD, Kuan SF, et al. Hepatic effects of long-term methotrexate use in the treatment of inflammatory bowel disease. Am J Gastroenterol. 2000;95:3150–6.

67. van der Woude CJ, Ardizzone S, Bengtson MB, Fiorino G, Fraser G, Katsamos K, Kolacek S, Juillerat P, Mulders AGMJ, Pedersen N, Selinger C, Sebastian S, Sturm A, Zelinova Z, Magro F, for the European Crohn's and Colitis Organization (ECCO). The second European evidence- based consensus on reproduction and pregnancy in inflammatory bowel disease. J Crohns Colitis. 2015;9:107–24.1–18.

68. Van den Brande JM, Braat H, van den Brink GR, et al. Infliximab but not etanercept induces apoptosis in lamina propria T-lymphocytes from patients with Crohn's disease. Gastroenterology. 2003;124(7):1774–85.

69. Hove T, van Montfrans C, Peppelenbosch MP, van Deventer SJ. Infliximab treatment induces apoptosis of lamina propria T lymphocytes in Crohn's disease. Gut. 2002;50(2):206–11.

70. Orlando A, et al. The Italian Society of Gastroenterology (SIGE) and the Italian Group for the study of Inflammatory Bowel Disease (IG-IBD) Clinical Practice Guidelines: The use of tumor necrosis factor-alpha antagonist therapy in inflammatory bowel disease. Dig Liver Dis. 2010;43:1–20.

71. Fidder H, Schnitzler F, Ferrante M, et al. Long-term safety of infliximab for the treatment of inflammatory bowel disease: a single-centre cohort study. Gut. 2009;58:501–8.

72. Panaccione R, Colombel JF, Sandborn WJ, et al. Adalimumab sustains clini- cal remission and overall clinical benefit after 2 years of therapy for Crohn's disease. Aliment Pharmacol Ther. 2010;31:1296–309.

73. Louis E, Vernier-Massouille G, Grimaud JC, et al. Infliximab discontinuation in Crohn's disease patients in stable remission on combined therapy with immunosuppressors: interim analysis of a prospective cohort study. Gut. 2008;57(Supp 2):A66.

74. Lichtenstein GR, Rutgeerts P, Sandborn WJ, et al. A pooled analysis of infections, malignancy, and mortality in infliximab and immunomodulator-treated adult patients with inflammatory bowel disease. Am J Gastroenterol. 2012;107(7):1051–63.

75. Sandborn W, Rutgeerts P, Reinisch W, et al. Study of biologic and immunomodulator naive patients in Crohn's disease (SONIC). Presented at the annual scientific meeting of the American College of Gastroenterology, Orlando; 7 Oct 2008.

76. Peyrin-Biroulet L, Deltenre P, de Suray N, et al. Efficacy and safety of tumor necrosis factor antagonists in Crohn's disease: meta-analysis of placebo- controlled trials. Clin Gastroenterol Hepatol. 2008;6:644–53.

77. Bongartz T, Sutton AJ, Sweeting MJ, et al. Anti-TNF antibody therapy in rheumatoid arthritis and the risk of serious infections and malignancies: systematic review and meta-analysis of rare harmful effects in randomized controlled trials. JAMA. 2006;295:2275–85.

78. Shale M, Kanfer E, Panaccione R, et al. Hepatosplenic T cell lymphoma in inflammatory bowel disease. Gut. 2008;57:1639–41.

79. Ochenrider MG, Patterson DJ, Aboulafia DM. Hepatosplenic T-cell lymphoma in a young man with Crohn's disease: casa report and literature review. Clin Lymphoma Myeloma Leuk. 2010;10(2):144–8.

80. Targan SR, Hanauer SB, van Deventer SJ, et al. A short-term study of chimeric monoclonal antibody cA2 to tumor necrosis factor alpha for Crohn's disease. Crohn's Disease cA2 Study Group. N Engl J Med. 1997;337:1029–35.

81. Hanauer SB, Feagan BG, Lichtenstein GR, et al; ACCENT I Study Group. Maintenance infliximab for Crohn's disease: the ACCENT I randomised trial. Lancet. 2002;359(9317):1541–9.

82. Sands BE, Blank MA, Patel K, van Deventer SJ, ACCENT II Study. Long-term treatment of rectovaginal fistulas in Crohn's disease: response to infliximab in the ACCENT II Study. Clin Gastroenterol Hepatol. 2004;2(10):912–20.

83. Colombel JF, Sandborn WJ, Reinisch W, SONIC Study Group, et al. Infliximab, azathioprine, or combination therapy for Crohn's disease. N Engl J Med. 2010;362(15):1383–95.

84. Sands BE, Anderson FH, Bernstein CN, et al. Infliximab maintenance therapy for fistulizing Crohn's disease. N Engl J Med. 2004;350:876–85.

85. Hanauer SB, Rutgeerts PJ, D'Haens G, et al. Delayed hypersensitivity to infliximab (Remicade) re-infusion after 2–4 year interval without treatment. Gastroenterology. 1999;116:A731.

86. Cvetkovic R, Scott L. Adalimumab: a review of its use in adult patients with rheumatoid arthritis. BioDrugs. 2006;20:293–311.

87. Hanauer SB, Sandborn WJ, Rutgeerts P, et al. Human anti-tumor necrosis factor monoclonal antibody (adalimumab) in Crohn's disease: the CLASSIC-I trial. Gastroenterology. 2006;130(2):323–33. quiz 591.

88. Sandborn WJ, Hanauer SB, Rutgeerts P, et al. Adalimumab for maintenance treatment of Crohn's disease: results of the CLASSIC II trial. Gut. 2007;56(9):1232–9.

89. Colombel JF, Sandborn WJ, Rutgeerts P, et al. Adalimumab for maintenance of clinical response and remission in patients with Crohn's disease: the CHARM trial. Gastroenterology. 2007;132(1):52–65.

90. Nesbitt A, Fossati G, Bergin M, et al. Mechanism of action of certolizumab pegol (CDP870): in vitro comparison with other anti-tumor necrosis factor alpha agents. Inflamm Bowel Dis. 2007;13:1323–32.

91. Sandborn W, Feagan B, Stoinov S, et al. Certolizumab pegol for the treatment of Crohn's disease. N Engl J Med. 2007;357:228–38.

92. Schreiber S, Khaliq-Kareemi M, Lawrance IC, et al. Maintenance therapy with certolizumab pegol for Crohn's disease. N Engl J Med. 2007;357:239–50.

93. Clifford D, De Luca A, Simpson D, et al. Natalizumab-associated progressive multifocal leukoencephalopathy in patients with multiple sclerosis: lessons from 28 cases. Lancet Neurol. 2010;9:438–46.

94. Soler D, Chapman T, Yang LL, Wyant T, Egan R, Fedyk ER. The binding specificity and selective antagonism of vedolizumab, an anti-alpha4beta7 integrin therapeutic antibody in development for inflammatory bowel diseases. J Pharmacol Exp Ther. 2009;330:864–75.

95. Sandborn WJ, et al. Vedolizumab as induction and maintenance therapy for Crohn's disease. N Engl J Med. 2013;369:711.

96. Danese S. New therapies for inflammatory bowel disease: from the bench to the bedside. Gut. 2012;61:918e932.

97. Sandborn WJ, Gasink C, et al. Ustekinumab induction and maintenance therapy in refractory Crohn's disease. N Engl J Med. 2012;367:1519–28.

98. Sandborn WJ, Ghosh S, Panes J, et al. A phase 2 study of tofacitinib, an oral Janus kinase inhibitor, in patients with Crohn's disease. Clin Gastroenterol Hepatol. 2014;12(9):1485–93.

99. Monteleone G, Neurath MF, Ardizzone S, et al. Mongersen, an oral SMAD7 antisense oligonucleotide, and Crohn's disease. N Engl J Med. 2015;372(12):1104–13.

Current Status of Imaging in Small and Large Bowel Diseases

Gian Andrea Rollandi and Luca Cevasco

Over the years, radiological examinations for small and large bowel are radically changed: milestones were the introduction of barium meals in the 1950s, of enteroclysis in the 1980s, and of cross-sectional techniques in the 1990s.

Until the 1980s, gold standard examinations were the *small bowel follow-through (SBFT)* [1] and the *single-contrast colon enema* [2]. In the 1980s, Sellink JL [3], Herlinger H [4], and Maglinte DD [5] developed *single- and double-contrast small bowel enteroclysis*, while Welin S [6], Altaras J [7], and Cittadini G [8] encoded the method of *the double-contrast barium enema of the colon*. These examinations provide an extraordinary evaluation of the mucosal layer with a reported sensitivity and a specificity respectively of 85–95 % and 89–94 % in the detection of the typical Crohn's disease lesions, when performed by expert radiologists [9]. Unfortunately, they give only indirect information on transmural and extraintestinal involvement, with difficulties in the assessment of single bowel loops, even if displayed in transparency [10].

Since the second half of the 1990s, already known cross-sectional techniques, mainly CT and MRI, have been specifically developed for the assessment of gastrointestinal pathology [11], with excellent results. These examinations allow a simultaneous evaluation of mucosal, mural, and extraintestinal pathologies without any possible superposition of bowel loops.

Conventional techniques have so largely lost their role in the everyday clinical practice, being less and less used in the last years. Only plain abdominal film still plays a role as the first-line examination in the acute abdomen, being able to identify signs of obstruction and perforation (Fig. 8.1).

Each cross-sectional imaging technique is characterized by peculiar advantages and limitations (diagnostic accuracy, availability, cost, X-ray dose, spatial and contrast resolution). In some circumstances, different modalities can be used to complement each other [12].

8.1 Technical Principles of Cross-Sectional Techniques

The most used cross-sectional techniques for the evaluation of small and large bowel are ultrasound, CT, and MRI. They share some essential technical common points that must be satisfied:

- Intestinal cleansing
- Bowel distension
- Bowel wall enhancement

G.A. Rollandi (✉) • L. Cevasco
Radiodiagnostic Unit, E.O. Ospedali Galliera,
Mura della Cappuccine 14, Genoa 16128, Italy
e-mail: gianandrea.rollandi@galliera.it

© Springer International Publishing Switzerland 2016
G. Lo Re, M. Midiri (eds.), *Crohn's Disease: Radiological Features and Clinical-Surgical Correlations*,
DOI 10.1007/978-3-319-23066-5_8

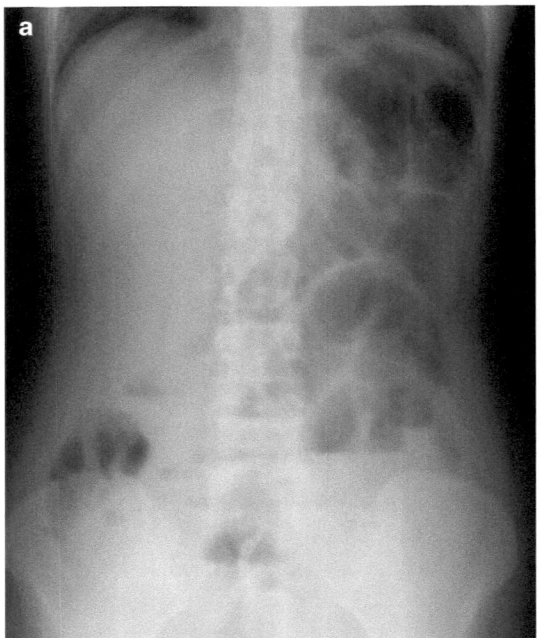 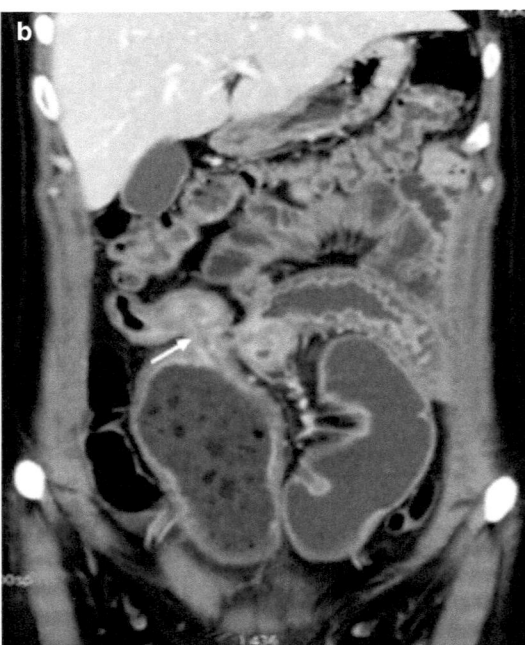

Fig. 8.1 Acute ileal obstruction. Plain abdominal film (**a**) shows signs of acute obstruction (small bowel loop distension with multiple air-fluid levels). Contrast-enhanced CT (**b**) detects a Crohn's stenotic lesion of the last ileal loop (*arrow* in **b**)

8.1.1 Intestinal Cleansing

The aim of a complete cleansing is to remove residual stool, which obviously may mimic pathologic findings; it also allows an easier anterograde and retrograde bowel filling.

8.1.2 Bowel Distension

An optimal distention allows a correct and complete evaluation of the bowel, since collapsed intestinal loops can hide small lesions or mimic diseases, so leading to false-positive or false-negative results.

In the past, it was widely debated about the most performing route of administration of enteral contrast media, and if positive contrast agents (baritated or iodinated), neutral (water solutions), or negative ones (air or carbon dioxide) were to be preferred. Enteral contrast agent can be orally administrated, infused through a nasojejunal tube or retrograde introduced by an enema [13].

8.1.3 Bowel Wall Enhancement

The injection of intravenous contrast media ensures bowel wall enhancement, improving contrast resolution and allowing to distinguish between different mural layers. In this way, it is possible to combine anatomical and functional information. In fact a functional analysis of bowel wall microcirculation allows to get the right differential diagnosis between different inflammatory diseases or between inflammations and tumors. Intravenous contrast media injection also provides an overall enhancement of the entire abdomen, improving the detection of extraintestinal findings, related to Crohn's disease or unexpected.

8.2   Small Bowel

Due to its anatomical location, the small bowel remains beyond the reach of conventional upper and lower endoscopy techniques, and a radiological evaluation of luminal and extraluminal findings is still quite a challenge.

8.2.1   Ultrasound

In the last decade, interesting results were reported about the use of *ultrasound (US)* in many common intestinal diseases, such as appendicitis, diverticulitis, bowel obstructions, and Crohn's disease [14]. Right iliac fossa and its structures, as cecum and last ileal loop, could be properly evaluated by ultrasound. So Crohn's lesions of the last ileal loop can be detected, while early ileal lesions localized elsewhere are still challenging findings, due to the lack of sure anatomical landmarks. For these reasons, a fully comprehensive examination of all ileal loops is rarely achievable, leading to a possible false-negative examination. Ultrasound can also detect and characterize bowel mural thickening and strictures that are Crohn's typical pathologic findings. It has been reported that the cause of small bowel obstructions can be sonographically detected up to 76 % of the patients [14]. Also the presence of mesenteric nodes, phlegmon, and abscesses can be quite easily identified, even if with less accuracy than CT.

An improvement in small bowel evaluation with ultrasound is the use of SICUS (small intestine contrast ultrasonography with oral administration of enteral contrast medium) or CEUS (contrast-enhanced ultrasonography) [9]. However, the timing and costs of these US techniques are similar to CT ones but with less accuracy and less panoramic view.

Ultrasound strengths remain its wide availability and relatively low cost (except for CEUS).

Furthermore, ultrasound allows a continuous and direct contact with the patient during the examinations, with the possibility to use the probe as "a hand" to visit the patient.

Since Crohn's disease is a chronic pathology needing multiple follow-ups and affecting also pediatric or very young patients, US can be safely implied, thanks to the lack of radiation exposure.

Ultrasound should be so considered as a valid first-line examination in symptomatic patients with suspected Crohn's disease and a useful tool for the follow-up of already known lesions, especially when located in the last ileal loop. US however is unsuitable for lesion's staging because it lacks of panoramic view.

The use of ultrasound in Crohn's disease has however several limitations, and high dependence on the skillness of the operator remains the main one. The experience in the use of US for bowel disease evaluation is in fact still quite limited [11, 15].

8.2.2   CT

CT is an accurate and panoramic imaging technique ensuring the visualization of both the bowel and the surrounding structures.

In the past it was widely debated if positive contrast agents (baritated or iodinated) or neutral ones (water solutions) were to be preferred for bowel distension in CT examinations. Nowadays, neutral enteral agents are usually preferred. In fact they have attenuation values and signal intensity similar to water, allowing a better depiction of mesenteric wall. Positive contrast agent could be sometimes used in TC examinations in peculiar conditions, such as to better detect fistulous tracts.

Another controversial issue regards the route of administration of enteral contrast. Two main techniques have been proposed:

- *Enteroclysis*, with infusion of neutral contrast material through a nasojejunal tube
- *Enterography*, with oral administration of a nonabsorbable isotonic solution

With enteroclysis, a better luminal distension in both jejunal and ileal tracts in comparison to the one achieved with enterography, especially for jejunal loops, is achievable [16].

However, in Crohn's disease, some studies demonstrated no significant difference in the overall detection of clinically significant findings [11] (Fig. 8.2). The question is still debated, and a consensus conference has been issued by The European Society of Gastrointestinal and Abdominal Radiology (ESGAR).

Usually, enterographic studies are preferred to the enteroclysis-based ones because they are easier to perform and better tolerated by the patient [10]. Patient's discomfort due to nasojejunal catheter, along with the radiation exposure during its placing (about 0.5–1 mSv), is an important disadvantage of enteroclysis [11, 17].

According to our experience, the most performing examination is obtained with the association of a small bowel enterography to a colon water enema [18]. *CT enterography of small bowel associated with colon water enema (CTe-WE)* allows a simultaneous, combined, and constant distension of both small and large bowels, with some limitations only in the depiction of

jejunum loops. With this technique, it is so possible to obtain a whole digestive tube examination with high diagnostic accuracy, allowing to simultaneously detect pathologic findings in different gastrointestinal tracts [13] (Fig. 8.3).

Regardless of the bowel filling technique, the injection of intravenous iodinated contrast media ensures mural and mucosal enhancement, improving contrast resolution, so allowing to detect the typical trilaminar mural stratification of Crohn's disease.

Nowadays, CT is the most comprehensive, accurate, and repeatable radiological examination for Crohn's disease evaluation. CT limitations remain the use of ionizing radiations and the need of intravenous injection of iodinated contrast media, possibly leading to acute adverse reactions and to renal failure. New reduction dose techniques have overcome the problem of ionizing radiation, and this result probably will improve in the future. Cost to replace older equipment is the only present limitation to the spread of these new reduction dose techniques [11]. The other limitation due to the need of contrast media could be overcome

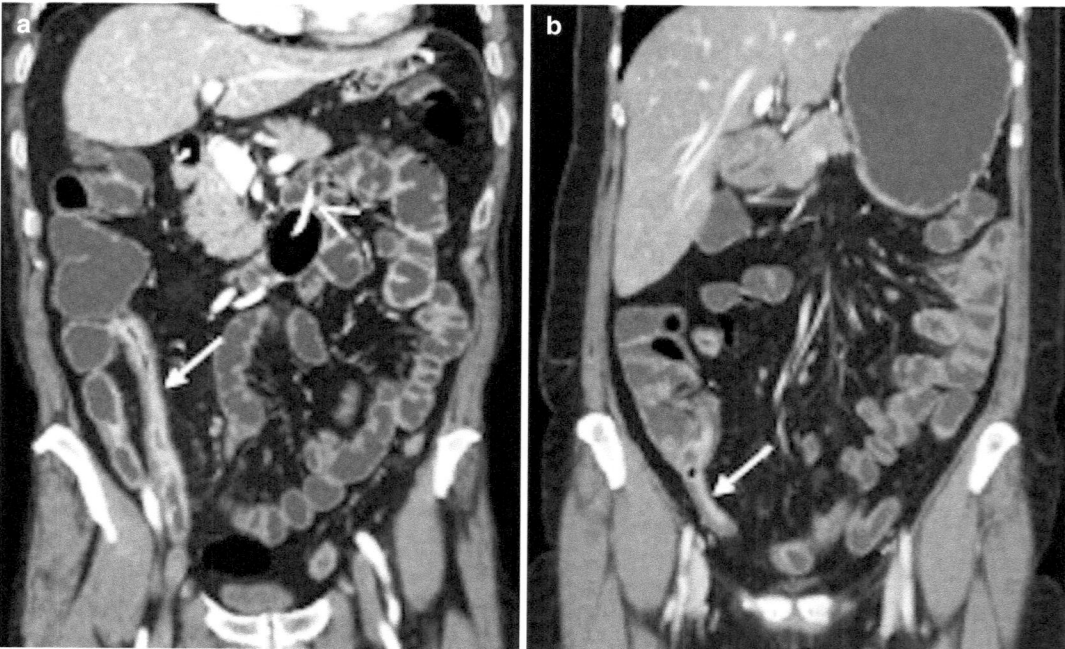

Fig. 8.2 CT enteroclysis (CTE) vs. CT enterography (CTe). Both CTE (**a**) and CTe (**b**) show adequate luminal distension of small bowel loops and a Crohn's lesion of the last ileal loop (*arrow* in **a** and **b**). Nasojejunal catheter in CTE (*arrowhead* in **a**)

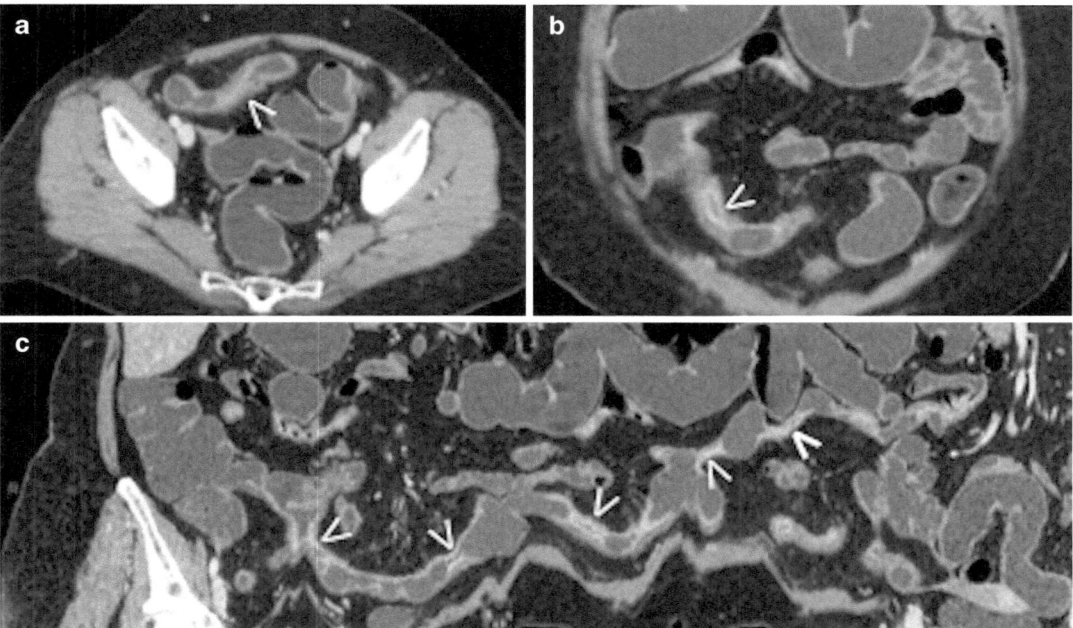

Fig. 8.3 CTe-WE. Typical trilaminar mural stratification of Crohn's disease (*arrowheads* in **a** and **b**) seen on axial (**a**) and coronal (**b**) planes. Curved reformatted image (**c**) shows multiple inflammatory skip lesions involving the terminal ileum (*arrowheads* in **c**)

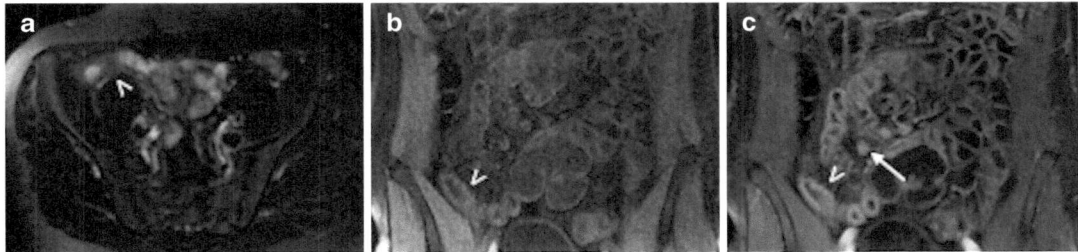

Fig. 8.4 MR enterography. (**a**) Axial T2-weighted acquisition with fat suppression. (**b**, **c**) Coronal GET1 acquisition with fat suppression. Crohn's lesion of the last ileal loop (*arrowheads*) with enlarged local nodes (*arrow* in **c**), better shown on coronal planes after paramagnetic contrast media injection (**c**)

by using new drugs, but unfortunately, iodinated ones are the only choice on the market, probably because of their low production costs. Anyway a substantial contrast media dose reduction can be achieved with new dual-energy CT scanners [19].

Nowadays, CT allows an almost infinite number of planar or curved reconstructions, thanks to volume acquisitions with isotropic and submillimeter voxel, with advanced workstation's post-processing. A multiplanar assessment is particularly useful for bowel's evaluation: according to the anatomical orientation of ileal loops, the best plane for bowel examination is in fact the coronal one.

8.2.3 MRI

Magnetic resonance imaging of small bowel is mainly based on T1-weighted images with and without paramagnetic contrast media injection, T2-weighted images with and without fat suppression technique, and diffusion-weighted images (DWI), in multiplanar scansions (Fig. 8.4).

MR enteroclysis (MREc) and MR enterography (MRE) share common technical points with CT-based enteroclysis and enterography techniques. Like CT examinations, the bowel must be adequately cleansed, distended, and enhanced. The most performing route of administration of the endoluminal contrast media is still debated [9, 20].

The spatial resolution achievable with MRI is lower than with CT [17], but MRI demonstrated higher contrast resolution. The use of intravenous contrast media, as for CT and US, could improve the detection of bowel hyperemia and edema and of inflammatory mucosal erosions and ulcers. These typical Crohn's disease signs are useful to assess the activity grade of the pathology. MRI seems to be superior also in the detection of fistulous tracts [16], a common Crohn's complication.

Another advantage of MRI is the possibility to evaluate bowel motility, with the use of fast T2-weighted SSFP or echo planar imaging sequences comprehensively called "MRI-fluoroscopy sequences" that can be visualized in a cine-like mode [17]. A chronic Crohn's fibrotic stricture is shown as aperistaltic [16], while an acute inflammatory one may present wall spasms and hyperenhancement. New studies have to be done in order to develop MR motility imaging, but interesting results about the improvement of Crohn's disease lesions detection are encouraging [21, 22]. The possibility to check bowel motility and its grade of filling is also very useful during the technical execution of MRI with the possibility to achieve better bowel distension.

Other recent MRI innovation is the analysis of Brownian motion of water among cellular structures using diffusion-weighted imaging (DWI) [23, 24]. Although it is already known that DWI signal and ADC values directly reflect tissue structure, recent studies have reported a higher sensibility of these sequences in the detection of bowel inflammatory lesions compared with contrast-enhanced MR imaging [25].

The longer time of acquisition, the lower spatial resolution, the low availability, and the higher cost of the examination suggest the use of magnetic resonance imaging only in selected patients. MRI should be preferred in pediatric or very young patients who need multiple follow-ups over a lifetime [10, 16], in patients with known chronic renal failure, or in patients allergic to iodinated contrast media.

8.2.4 Endoscopy

Small bowel loops cannot be reached easily by conventional upper and lower endoscopy. In order to overcome this limitation, new endoscopic techniques have been used, such as single-balloon endoscopy (SBE) [26] and double-balloon endoscopy (DBE) [27, 28]. The main advantages of endoscopic examinations are the availability of biopsies and the possibility to perform therapeutic procedures such as balloon dilatation of stenosis [29]. However, these endoscopic techniques have great limitations: they are not universally available and it takes quite long time to be performed. Furthermore, they highly depend on the operator experience, on the patient's conditions, and on the number and the entity of ileal stenosis.

8.2.5 Capsule

Video capsule endoscopy (VCE) [10, 29] is an alternative technique used for small and large bowel investigation. The patient swallows a capsule of less than 2 cm of length lighting the lumen and acquiring about 2 images per second during its way. All data are radiotransmitted wireless to an external recorder [11]. Capsule endoscopy should be performed mainly in case of suspected gastrointestinal bleeding with previous negative upper and lower endoscopy [30, 31]. The main limitation of capsule endoscopy is its possible retention in case of bowel strictures, quite common in Crohn's disease. To overcome this limitation, the proper VCE capsule should be administrated only after capsule patency test, implying the previous use of a dissolvable capsule.

Furthermore, capsule is able to demonstrate nonspecific mucosal ulcers only, so resulting poor in the assessment of typical Crohn's mural involvement. High costs and long time for interpretation are other limitations of this technique. The European consensus group [32] recommends the use of capsule endoscopy when standard imaging techniques and endoscopy cannot detect the pathology [11], mainly in the suspect of angiodysplastic lesions.

8.2.6 Nuclear Medicine

Nowadays, nuclear medicine has no more a main role in the diagnosis of Crohn's disease, except for differential diagnosis between Crohn's lesion and Meckel's diverticulum by means of *scintigraphy* and in case of suspected neoplastic degeneration of chronic Crohn's lesions with the use of *fluorodeoxyglucose positron emission tomography CT (18F-FDG PET-CT)*.

Generally, nuclear medicine examinations could be performed when other imaging modalities have been negative [11].

8.3 Large Bowel

8.3.1 Ultrasound

Ultrasound examinations in Crohn's disease have a role in the detection and evaluation of lesions localized in the cecum and in the differential diagnosis between inflammatory bowel diseases and acute appendicitis in acute scenarios. It can be also performed to evaluate Crohn's perianal complications, such as fistula and abscesses [33].

8.3.2 CT

Two main CT techniques have been developed to adequately analyze the large bowel:

- *CT with water enema (CT-WE)*, with introduction of tap water through a rectal enema in a previously cleansed colon, with the patient placed on the CT table. The neutral contrast agent may sometimes reflux through the ileocecal valve from the cecum into the ileum, revealing pathologic findings of the last ileal loop. An intravenous iodinated contrast media injection ensures mural and mucosal enhancement, improving contrast resolution.
- *Computed tomographic colonography (CTC) or virtual colonoscopy (VC)*, with inflation of air or carbon dioxide through a rectal catheter. The morphology of colonic surface is emphasized by reflections arising from a virtual external light source, obtaining images similar to conventional endoscopic vision.

Main advantages of CTC over CT-WE are the lower X-ray dose and the absence of iodinated contrast media injection. Nowadays, CTC is included as a colorectal cancer (CRC) screening option for asymptomatic average-risk adults aged 50 years and older [34].

However, polyps are not pathognomonic findings of Crohn's disease. Main Crohn's pathological signs are hyperemic thickening of bowel wall and perienteric fat stranding with engorged vasa recta, better depicted by CT-WE.

In the case of CTC, air or carbon dioxide is used to achieve lumen distension. The gas provides an extreme HU difference between bowel wall and the lumen. This extreme HU difference affects the bowel enhancement evaluation. In CT-WE, water is used to distend the lumen, and a better wall-lumen interface is achieved, allowing to distinguish the three-layered structure of the bowel walls and to easily detect Crohn's lesions [35]. For these reasons, CT-WE in Crohn's disease seems to be superior to CTC.

8.3.3 MRI

MR colonography (MRC) is a recent colonic imaging technique offering an alternative to CTC without the use of ionizing radiations [36]. Similar to CTC, colon distension is commonly achieved by inflation of air or carbon dioxide. Data on the accuracy of MRI colonography for the detection of inflammatory colonic lesions in IBD are still limited.

MR imaging, due to its high contrast resolution, is instead the most accurate tool to evaluate

Crohn's perianal complications: fistulous tracts, abscesses, and their anatomical relationship with pelvic floor muscles are very well depicted.

8.3.4 Colonoscopy

Conventional colonoscopy is currently considered the reference standard for the evaluation of inflammatory bowel diseases. However, technical failure of colonoscopy is not uncommon. Causes of incomplete colonoscopy are anatomic variants, patient intolerance, strictures, and severe diverticulosis. Up to 10 % of colonoscopy is technically difficult, even if performed by skilled operators [37]. Moreover, optical colonoscopy is poorly tolerated diagnostic procedure with possible complications, mainly represented by bowel perforation [9].

> **Conclusions**
> Nowadays, cross-sectional imaging techniques, mainly CT and MRI, have overtaken the conventional radiological methods for the evaluation of small and large bowel, with the possibility to detect both luminal and extraluminal pathological findings [10].
>
> The wider availability of CT equipments, the lower cost of the examination and the rapidity of image acquisition, with less motion artifacts, and a better patient's compliance represent strengths of CT over MR imaging. In fact, with a 64-slice CT equipment, it is possible to cover the entire abdomen and the pelvis in less than 10 s, while the acquisition of standard MRI sequences for a complete small bowel examination needs approximately 20 min [17].
>
> The sensitivity and specificity of CT and MRI techniques are however referred to be overall comparable [38–43], both in excess of 90 % and 80 %, respectively [11], and so the choice of the best examination has to be suited to the needs of each patient.
>
> Nowadays, CT could be the technique of choice in the detection and follow-up of inflammatory pathologies [15] especially

when occurred complications are suspected. MRI should be preferred in pediatric or very young patients who need multiple follow-ups over a lifetime [10, 16], in patients with known chronic renal failure, or in patients allergic to iodinated contrast media.

References

1. Gasche C, Schober E, Turetschek K. Small bowel barium studies in Crohn's disease. Gastroenterology. 1998;114(6):1349.
2. ROBINSON JM. Detection of small lesions of the large bowel; barium enema versus double contrast. Calif Med. 1954;81(5):321–4.
3. Sellink JL. Radiologic examination of the small intestine by duodenal intubation. Acta Radiol Diagn (Stockh). 1974;15(3):318–32.
4. Rubesin SE, Levine MS, Laufer I, Herlinger H. Double-contrast barium enema examination technique. Radiology. 2000;215(3):642–50.
5. Rubesin SE, Maglinte DD. Double-contrast barium enema technique. Radiol Clin North Am. 2003;41(2):365–76.
6. Welin S, Welin G. The double contrast examination of the colon. Experience with the Welin modification. Stuttgart: Georg Thieme Publishers; 1976. p. 110–1.
7. Altaras J. Radiologischer Atlas. Kolon und Rektum. Munchen: Urban & Schwarzenberg; 1982.
8. Cittadini G. Double contrast barium enema: the Genoa approach. Milan: Springer; 1998.
9. Paparo F, Denegri A, Revelli M, Puppo C, Garello I, Bacigalupo L, Garlaschi A, Rollandi L, Fornaro R. Crohn's disease: value of diagnostic imaging in the evaluation of anastomotic recurrence. Ann Ital Chir. 2014;85(3):271–81.
10. Algin O, Evrimler S, Arslan H. Advances in radiologic evaluation of small bowel diseases. J Comput Assist Tomogr. 2013;37(6):862–71.
11. Murphy KP, McLaughlin PD, O'Connor OJ, Maher MM. Imaging the small bowel. Curr Opin Gastroenterol. 2014;30(2):134–40.
12. Saibeni S, Rondonotti E, Iozzelli A, Spina L, Tontini GE, Cavallaro F, Ciscato C, De Franchis R, Sardanelli F, Vecchi M. Imaging of the small bowel in Crohn's disease: a review of old and new technique. World J Gastroenterol. 2007;13(24):3279–87.
13. Paparo F, Garlaschi A, Biscaldi E, Bacigalupo L, Cevasco L, Rollandi GA. Computed tomography of the bowel: a prospective comparison study between four techniques. Eur J Radiol. 2013;82(1):e1–10.
14. Gritzmann N, Hollerweger A, Macheiner P, Rettenbacher T. Transabdominal sonography of the gastrointestinal tract. Eur Radiol. 2002;12(7): 1748–61.

15. Dambha F, Tanner J, Carroll N. Diagnostic imaging in Crohn's disease: what is the new gold standard? Best Pract Res Clin Gastroenterol. 2014;28(3): 421–36.

16. Masselli G, Gualdi G. CT and MR enterography in evaluating small bowel diseases: when to use which modality? Abdom Imaging. 2013;38(2):249–59.

17. Soyer P, Boudiaf M, Fishman EK, Hoeffel C, Dray X, Manfredi R, Marteau P. Imaging of malignant neoplasms of the mesenteric small bowel: new trends and perspectives. Crit Rev Oncol Hematol. 2011;80(1):10–30.

18. Paparo F, Bacigalupo L, Garello I, et al. Crohn's disease: prevalence of intestinal and extraintestinal manifestations detected by computed tomography enterography with water enema. Abdom Imaging. 2012;37(3):326–37.

19. Mileto A, Ramirez-Giraldo JC, Marin D, Alfaro-Cordoba M, Eusemann CD, Scribano E, Blandino A, Mazziotti S, Ascenti G. Nonlinear image blending for dual-energy MDCT of the abdomen: can image quality be preserved if the contrast medium dose is reduced? AJR Am J Roentgenol. 2014;203(4):838–45.

20. Horsthuis K, Bipat S, Bennink RJ, Stoker J. Inflammation bowel disease diagnosed with US, MR, scintigraphy, and CT: Meta-analysis of prospective studies. Radiology. 2008;241(1):64–79.

21. Froehlich JM, Patak MA, von Weymarn C, Juli CF, Zollikofer CL, Wentz KU. Small bowel motility assessment with magnetic resonance imaging. J Magn Reson Imaging. 2005;21(4):370–5.

22. Froehlich JM, Waldherr C, Stoupis C, Erturk SM, Patak MA. MR motility imaging in Crohn's disease improves lesion detection compared with standard MR imaging. Eur Radiol. 2010;20(8):1945–51.

23. Maccioni F, Patak MA, Signore A, Laghi A. New frontiers of MRI in Crohn's disease: motility imaging, diffusion-weighted imaging, perfusion MRI, MR spectroscopy, molecular imaging, and hybrid imaging (PET/MRI). Abdom Imaging. 2012;37(6): 974–82.

24. Oussalah A, Laurent V, Bruot O, Bressenot A, Bigard MA, Régent D, Peyrin-Biroulet L. Diffusion-weighted magnetic resonance without bowel preparation for detecting colonic inflammation in inflammatory bowel disease. Gut. 2010;59(8):1056–65.

25. Oto A, Kayhan A, Williams JT, Fan X, Yun L, Arkani S, Rubin DT. Active Crohn's disease in the small bowel: evaluation by diffusion weighted imaging and quantitative dynamic contrast enhanced MR imaging. J Magn Reson Imaging. 2011;33(3): 615–24.

26. Boudiaf M, Soyer P, Terem C, Pelage JP, Maissiat E, Rymer R. Ct evaluation of small bowel obstruction. Radiographics. 2001;21(3):613–24.

27. Algin O, Evrimler S, Ozmen E. Metin MR, Ocakoglu G, Ersoy O, Karaoglanoglu M, Arslan H. A novel biphasic oral contrast solution for enterographic studies. J Comput Assist Tomogr. 2013;37(1):65–74.

28. Schreyer AG, Stroszczynski C. Radiological imaging of the small bowel. Dig Dis. 2011;29 Suppl 1:22–6.

29. Takenaka K, Ohtsuka K, Kitazume Y, Nagahori M, Fujii T, Saito E, Naganuma M, Araki A, Watanabe M. Comparison of magnetic resonance and balloon enteroscopic examination of the small intestine in patients with Crohn's disease. Gastroenterology. 2014;147(2):334–42.

30. Elsayes KM, Al-Hawary MM, Jagdish J, Ganesh HS, Platt JF. CT enterography: principles, trends, and interpretation of findings. Radiographics. 2010;30(7):55–70.

31. Maglinte DD. Capsule imaging and the role of radiology in the investigation of diseases of the small bowel. Radiology. 2005;236(3):763–7.

32. Van Assche G, Dignass A, Panes J, Beaugerie L, Karagiannis J, Allez M, Ochsenkühn T, Orchard T, Rogler G, Louis E, Kupcinskas L, Mantzaris G, Travis S, Stange E, European Crohn's and Colitis Organisation (ECCO). The second European evidence-based consensus on the diagnosis and management of Crohn's disease: definitions and diagnosis. J Crohns Colitis. 2010;4(1):7–27.

33. Nevler A, Beer-Gabel M, Lebedyev A, Soffer A, Gutman M, Carter D, Zbar AP. Transperineal ultrasonography in perianal Crohn's disease and recurrent cryptogenic fistula-in-ano. Colorectal Dis. 2013;15(8):1011–8.

34. Farraye FA, Adler DG, Chand B, Conway JD, Diehl DL, Kantsevoy SV, Kwon RS, Mamula P, Rodriguez SA, Shah RJ, Wong Kee Song LM, Tierney WM, ASGE Technology Committee. Update on CT colonography. Gastrointest Endosc. 2009;69(3):393–8.

35. Soyer P, Hamzi L, Sirol M, Duchat F, Dray X, Hristova L, Placé V, Pocard M, Boudiaf M. Colon cancer: comprehensive evaluation with 64-section CT colonography using water enema as intraluminal contrast agent-a pictorial review. Clin Imaging. 2012;36(2):113–25.

36. Rimola J, Ordás I. MR colonography in inflammatory bowel disease. Magn Reson Imaging Clin N Am. 2014;22(1):23–33.

37. Laghi A, Bellini D, Petrozza V, Piccazzo R, Santoro GA, Fabbri C, van der Paardt MP, Stoker J. Imaging of colorectal polyps and early rectal cancer. Colorectal Dis. 2015;17 Suppl 1:36–43.

38. Horsthuis K, Bipat S, Bennink RJ, Stoker J. Inflammatory bowel disease diagnosed with US, MR, scintigraphy, and CT: meta-analysis of prospective studies. Radiology. 2008;247(1):64–79.

39. Siddiki HA, Fidler JL, Fletcher JG, Burton SS, Huprich JE, Hough DM, Johnson CD, Bruining DH, Loftus Jr EV, Sandborn WJ, Pardi DS, Mandrekar JN. Prospective comparison of state-of-the-art MR enterography and CT enterography in small-bowel Crohn's disease. AJR Am J Roentgenol. 2009;193(1):113–21.

40. Amzallag-Bellenger E, Oudjit A, Ruiz A, Cadiot G, Soyer PA, Hoeffel CC. Effectiveness of MR enterography for the assessment of small-bowel

diseases beyond Crohn disease. Radiographics. 2012;32(5):1423–44.

41. Quencer KB, Nimkin K, Mino-Kenudson M, Gee MS. Detecting active inflammation and fibrosis in pediatric Crohn's disease: prospective evaluation of MR-E and CT-E. Abdom Imaging. 2013;38(4):705–13.

42. Grand DJ, Kampalath V, Harris A, Patel A, Resnick MB, Machan J, Beland M, Chen WT, Shah SA. MR enterography correlates highly with colonoscopy and histology for both distal ileal and colonic Crohn's disease in 310 patients. Eur J Radiol. 2012;81(5): e763–9.

43. Jensen MD, Kjeldsen J, Rafaelsen SR, Nathan T. Diagnostic accuracies of MR enterography and CT enterography in symptomatic Crohn's disease. Scand J Gastroenterol. 2011;46(12):1449–57.

Conventional Radiology in the Evaluation of the Small Bowel

9

Giuseppe Lo Re, Federica Vernuccio,
Dario Picone, Federico Midiri,
Maria Cristina Galfano, Sergio Salerno,
Roberto Lagalla, and Massimo Midiri

9.1 Introduction

For many years, the small bowel has been considered as the "black box" of the gastrointestinal system because it could not be evaluated through endoscopy. For this reason, the conventional radiological methods, such as small bowel enteroclysis (SBE) and small bowel follow-through (SBFT), have been considered the standard approach for the evaluation of the small bowel in the diagnosis and management of Crohn's disease for years [1]. However, due to technological limits, the study of small bowel through conventional radiology has been focused mainly on its function than on its anatomy. To date, the conventional examination with the study of intestinal transit is now rarely used, if not obsolete, but it has still a historical value in the diagnosis of inflammatory bowel diseases.

9.2 Techniques

9.2.1 Small Bowel Follow-Through

The SBFT is an examination that allows the visualization of the small bowel, which would not otherwise be visible on x-ray, by using barium as contrast medium. Barium is an inert substance that enters and exits the body without interacting or being metabolized, making it a very safe and effective contrast medium. However, considering the risk of granuloma formation in both lungs and the peritoneal cavity, and of abdominal adhesions or peritonitis, the use of barium is contraindicated whenever bowel perforation or predisposition for pulmonary aspiration is suspected.

The patient is asked to drink approximately 200–300 ml of barium while supine abdominal films are obtained until the terminal ileum and cecum are filled with barium [2]. The esophagus, stomach, and duodenum are easily evaluated through SBTF. This type of SBFT can take 2–3 h to complete and a detailed evaluation of the bowel lumen is not possible due to the overlapping loops of the small intestine as the barium progresses. A better diagnostic tool would be SBE.

SBFT is poorly sensitive. It is limited by many factors as by the overlap of bowel loops, as previously written, but also by poor distension, flocculation of barium, intermittent barium filling,

G. Lo Re, PhD (✉) • F. Vernuccio • D. Picone
F. Midiri • M.C. Galfano • S. Salerno • R. Lagalla
M. Midiri
DIBIMED, Department of Biopathology and Medical
Biotechnology, University Hospital P. Giaccone –
University of Palermo, Palermo, Italy
e-mail: giuseppe.lore12@gmail.com;
massimo.midiri@unipa.it

© Springer International Publishing Switzerland 2016
G. Lo Re, M. Midiri (eds.), *Crohn's Disease: Radiological Features and Clinical-Surgical Correlations*,
DOI 10.1007/978-3-319-23066-5_9

and by the fact it is not possible to predict transit time [2]. For these reasons, small bowel enema, or enteroclysis, is the preferred method for detailed radiographic examination. The SBTF allows a better evaluation of small bowel transit time and the motility component of motor disorders compared to enteroclysis, but this latter is superior in showing the structural components of motor disorder and short lesions such as isolated adhesions [3].

9.2.2   Small Bowel Enteroclysis

For many years, conventional SBE has been considered the main imaging technique for the diagnosis of CD, given its high sensitivity and specificity. In Greek language, the word "entero" stands for intestine and "clysis" for washing out; hence, enteroclysis means washing out of the intestine.

SBE represents a low invasive radiographic technique: it requires firstly the positioning of a catheter into the small intestine and then a double-contrast examination is performed through the injection of both barium, which coats the intestine, and methylcellulose, which distends the bowel lumen [4].

Conventional enteroclysis is generally performed according to the technique proposed by Herlinger. An adequate preparation of the patient is mandatory and is obtained through a laxative the afternoon before the examination and fasting for at least 12 h. Moreover, about 20 min before the examination, a prokinetic drug is injected to accelerate the passage of the barium to the small intestine.

Visualization of the small bowel requires an adequate distension of the intestines in order to identify the configuration of bowel loops and to improve characterization of bowel wall with luminal contrast. This is achieved by positioning a nasojejunal tube into the proximal small bowel, beyond the duodenojejunal junction under fluoroscopic guidance [4].

Sedation is usually not recommended because the patient needs to cooperate and move during the examination.

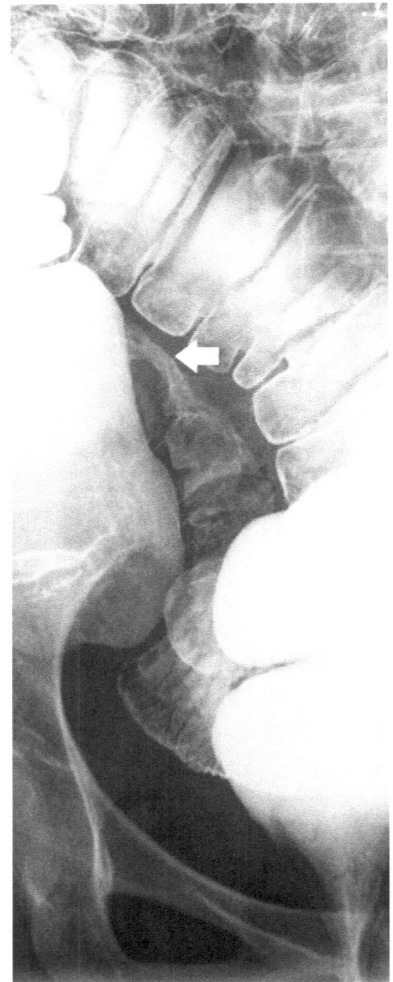

Fig. 9.1 Conventional small bowel enteroclysis clearly depicts the last ileal loop (*arrow*)

For the examination, a standard amount of barium (300 mL of barium 40/60 P/V) and 0.5 % methylcellulose solution (1.500 mL) or air is infused through the nasoenteric tube, achieving optimal double-contrast and small bowel distention [4].

Then, the patient is observed under fluoroscopic guidance both in a horizontal position, to better evaluate the proximal loops, then in right lateral decubitus, and finally after compression.

Thereafter, an additional bolus of barium is administered with the patient in the lateral decubitus position on the right side for about

10 minutes. This part of the examination is quite useful for the evaluation of all bowel loops, which are studied using targeted and gradual compressions and different degrees of rotation of the patient. The targeted and gradual compressions are used to evaluate also the mobility and flexibility of all small bowel loops, in order to differentiate Crohn's disease from tumoral and inflammatory stenosis [5]. The study ends when the last intestinal loop is documented (Fig. 9.1).

Its main limitations includes the high radiation dose, mainly due to the need of fluoroscopy guidance for placement of the nasojejunal tube, the invasiveness of the intubation procedure, and inability to provide direct information on possible extraparietal involvement and/or possible complications [1, 6, 7].

9.3 Normal Appearances of the Small Bowel

As widely known, a radiologist may diagnose on images just what he knows; moreover, to determine if there is an abnormality, he must be able to recognize normal findings.

The small bowel varies in length from 3 to 10 m, with an average length of 6 m, and occupies the central and lower abdomen, usually framed by the colon [8]. It begins where the intestine assumes a mesentery at the duodenojejunal flexure and ends at the ileocecal valve [8]. The ligament of Treitz lies to the left of the first part of the duodenum and marks the transition from the duodenum to small bowel [8].

Small bowel loops show a mesenteric border, which is the concave one, and is called mesenteric because it is where the mesentery attaches, and the antimesenteric border, which is the convex one and faces away from the mesentery [2].

On the conventional radiological methods used to evaluate the small bowel, SBTF and SBE, the barium forms a continuous column, thus defining the diameter of the small bowel [9]. Transverse folds of mucous membrane of small bowel appear as lucent filling defects of about 2–3 mm in width since barium lies between them [9].

Depending on bowel diameter, the appearance of these folds may change: when the small bowel is distended, they are called valvulae conniventes and are seen as lines traversing the barium column, while when it is contracted, they lie longitudinally, and when it is relaxed, the folds assume a feathery appearance [9].

The villi are fingerlike projections of mucosa that extend from the entire mucosal surface of the small bowel.

The morphological normality of the small bowel can be determined with good accuracy on the basis of the observation of many characteristics, as the abovementioned folds, the diameter of small bowel lumen, small bowel wall thickness, Peyer's patches, and arterial arcades as shown in Table 9.1 [8]. Though there are some differences between the jejunum and the ileum, the transition between these two tracts is gradual [2].

Table 9.1 Comparison between jejunum and ileum characteristics

Characteristics	Jejunum	Ileum
Mucosal folds	Thicker, (till 2 mm), and more numerous: 4–7 folds/2.5 cm	Thinner, less deep (about 1 mm), and less numerous: 2–4/2.5 cm
Lumen diameter	Wider (3–3.5 cm; in enteroclysis about 4.5 cm)	Narrower (2.5 cm; in enteroclysis about 3.5 cm)
Wall thickness[a]	Thicker	Thinner
Peyer's patches	Less numerous and bigger	More numerous
Arterial arcades	1–2 with fewer long branches	4–5 with many short branches

[a]Wall thickness is calculated in a radiogram taking as a reference two adjacent loops, which are parallel to each other for at least 5 cm, and measuring the distance between the two mucous-coated barium surfaces. This is the combined wall thickness; half of this value represents the thickness of a single small bowel loop wall (normal value: 1–2 mm)

9.4   Barium Findings in Crohn's Disease

The abnormalities encountered in barium studies in patients with Crohn's disease are numerous, depend upon the stage and location of the disease, and are expression of the pathological changes [10]. These abnormalities can be distinguished in functional and organic ones [10]:

- Functional signs: the inflammatory process may be responsible of either bowel hypermotility or hypomotility; in the acute phase, excessive luminal fluid and exudate may be responsible for barium flocculation or dilution, thus resulting at barium study as a blurred interface between the intraluminal barium and the mucosa.
- Organic signs: a coarser villous pattern together with thickening and distortion of mucosal fold (Fig. 9.2), which may appear straightened, fused, or nodular, due to mucosal and submucosal edema secondary to lymphatic obstruction; postinflammatory polyps, expression of a regenerated mucosa surrounded by healed epithelial surfaces, present as well-defined round or oval filling defects; and ulcerations, which may be responsible of an "ulceronodular pattern" in case of combination of intersecting longitudinal, transverse, and oblique linear ulcers that surround residual islands of mucosa, and that is expression of a more advanced stage of the disease.

To sum up, the major signs on barium examinations that may be seen in isolation or combination include [8]:

- Strictures (Fig. 9.3) and associated dilatation of the bowel proximal to narrowed areas. Strictures may vary in length and have to be differentiated from physiological narrowing due to peristaltic waves: the former do not contain normal mucosal folds and usually result in dilatation of the upstream bowel, while the latter are usually transient and smooth, with normal mucosal folds traversing them and the upstream bowel is normal. In presence of marked small bowel irritability

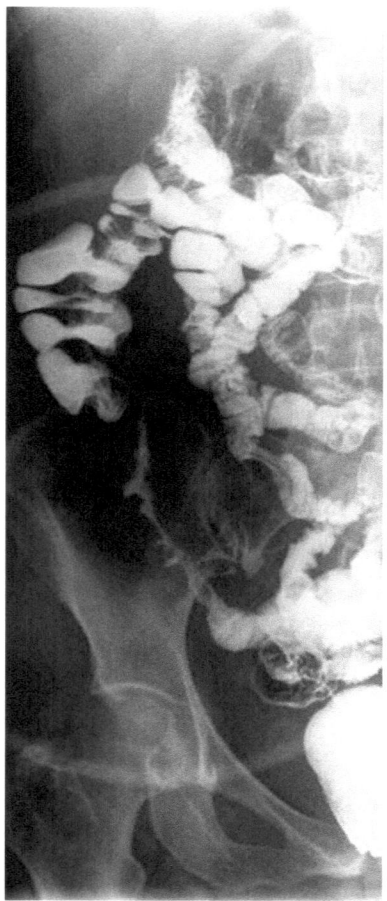

Fig. 9.2 Small bowel enteroclysis images show coarser villous pattern together with thickening and distortion of mucosal fold

and spasm "the string sign" may occur and the area of narrowing often widens as the peristaltic wave reaches the affected segment.

- Ulcers. "Aphthous ulcers" are erosions whose radiological appearance is that of shallow depressions, 1–2 mm in diameter, with a surrounding radiolucent halo. The presence of fine ulceration combined with mucosal edema is responsible of to the so-called cobblestone appearance.
- Thickening, distortion, or effacement of mucosal folds.
- Separation of bowel loops due to bowel wall thickening or an inflammatory mass.
- Signs of malabsorption.

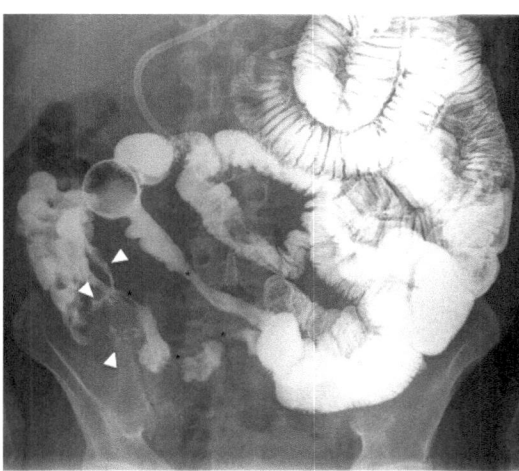

Fig. 9.3 SBE image shows fixed and angulated small bowel loops with multiple stenosis and skip lesions (*), determining a cobblestone pattern. Some ileocolic and enteroenteric fistulas can be noticed (*arrowheads*)

Concerning the evaluation of the most common complications of Crohn's disease, the main signs on barium studies are reported below [8]:

- Fistulae (Fig. 9.3) are due to transmural involvement of the disease in an advanced stage, and they link a small bowel loop to other small bowel loops, colon, bladder, or vagina. Prefistulas are seen as kissing lesions, while fistulas cause a premature filling of a fistulized organ, but when the fistula is between adjacent loops of the small intestine, it can be difficult to detect.
- Abscesses are the result of extension of inflammatory lesions beyond bowel wall, and their presence can be suggested on barium studies by mass effect.
- Stenoses are due to the worsening of the strictures. Enteroclysis helps in differentiating a true stenosis from a functional narrowing, since the resistance to lumen distention during the enema is a useful feature to confirm the presence of a true stenosis. Some patients may present with multiple stenoses, as an advanced and complicated stage of skip lesions.

Considering the above-described radiological signs and the pathological changes of Crohn's disease, it is possible to recognize a classification system from early lesions characterized by fold thickening, aphthous ulcerations, and coarse granularity of the villi, but with normal contraction of bowel wall, to intermediate and then advanced lesions, whose features are "ulceronodular" pattern ("cobblestone") in a narrowed segment, pronounced wall thickening and possible strictures; finally, the presence of complications due to Crohn's disease is indicative of the fourth and last stage [10].

Furthermore, conventional SBE may help in the diagnosis of Crohn's disease in patients with high clinical suspicioun of disease with a negative computed tomography enteroclysis examination [11, 12].

Moreover, during conventional enteroclysis, patient's ionizing radiation exposure is not negligible. Metter et al. [13] demonstrated that medium radiation dose exposure during the procedure is 8 mSv, including the fluoroscopic evaluation; this dose has to be compared with the exposure of 0.1 mSv for a posteroanterior and laterolateral chest x-ray.

Moreover, the chronicity of disease often leads to repeating the radiologic examination in these patients, and for this reason, the benefit/risk rate between utility of examinations and ionizing radiation exposure must be kept in mind, especially in young population.

References

1. Saibeni S, Rondonotti E, Iozzelli A, Spina L, Tontini GE, Cavallaro F, Ciscato C, de Franchis R, Sardanelli F, Vecchi M. Imaging of the small bowel in Crohn's disease: a review of old and new techniques. World J Gastroenterol. 2007;13:3279–87.
2. Brant WE, Helms CA, editors. Fundamentals of diagnostic radiology. 3rd ed. Philadelphia: Lippincott Williams & Wilkins; 2007.
3. Gore RM, Levine MS, Laufer I. Textbook of gastrointestinal radiology. Philadelphia: WB Saunders Co; 1995.
4. Gatta G, Di Grezia G, Di Mizio V, Landolfi C, Mansi L, De Sio I, Rotondo A, Grassi R. Crohn's disease imaging: a review. Gastroenterol Res Pract. 2012; 2012:816920.
5. Bret P, Cuche C, Schmutz G. Radiology of the small intestine. New York: Springer; 1989.

6. Ruiz-Cruces R, Ruiz F, Perez-Martinez M, Lopez J, Tort Ausina I, de los Rios AD. Patient dose from barium procedures. Br J Radiol. 2000;73:752–61.

7. Toms AP, Barltrop A, Freeman AH. A prospective randomized study comparing enteroclysis with small bowel follow-through examinations in 244 patients. Eur Radiol. 2001;11:1155–60.

8. Ryan S, McNicholas M, Eustace SJ. Anatomy for diagnostic imaging. 2nd ed. Edinburgh/New York: Saunders; 2004.

9. Rockall AG, Hatrick A, Armstrong P, Wastie M. Diagnostic imaging. 7th ed. Wiley-Blackwell; USA 2013.

10. Herlinger H. Anatomy of the small intestine. In: Herlinger H, Maglinte DDT, Birnbaum BA, editors. Clinical imaging of the small intestine. Berlin: Springer; 1999. p. 3–12.

11. Minordi LM, Vecchioli A, Guidi L, Mirk P, Fiorentini L, Bonomo L. Multidetector CT enteroclysis versus barium enteroclysis with methylcellulose in patients with suspected small bowel disease. Eur Radiol. 2006;16:1527–36.

12. Minordi LM, Vecchioli A, Guidi L, Poloni G, Fedeli G, Bonomo L. CT findings and clinical activity in Crohn's disease. Clin Imaging. 2009;33:123–9.

13. Mettler Jr FA, Huda W, Yoshizumi TT, Mahesh M. Effective doses in radiology and diagnostic nuclear medicine: a catalog. Radiology. 2008;248: 54–263.

US in Inflammatory Bowel Diseases

10

Di Grezia Graziella, Gatta Gianluca,
Berritto Daniela, Iacobellis Francesca,
Reginelli Alfonso, Gagliardi Giuliano,
Grassi Roberta, and Cappabianca Salvatore

Ultrasonography plays a multipurpose role in the different phases of idiopathic and non-idiopathic inflammatory bowel diseases. Even if abdominal ultrasound is most commonly used for the evaluation of parenchymatous abdominal organs, its utility in intestinal imaging tract has developed in the last years, thanks to improvements of technology and higher quality of images. The wide availability, joined with the absence of invasiveness and pain, makes it a clinically crucial imaging method in the diagnosis and follow-up of these complex and diffuse diseases.

Idiopathic inflammatory bowel diseases (Crohn's disease [CD], ulcerative colitis [UC], and indeterminate colitis [IC]) are probably related to an incongruous response of bowel mucosal immune system to gastrointestinal flora and/or ingested food antigens [1], typically present a peak of incidence during late adolescence and earlier adulthood and a second peak later in adulthood [2], and are characterized by similar clinical pictures and a lifelong relapses and remitting course that can deteriorate the quality of life [3, 4].

Crohn's patients can develop disease anywhere in the gastrointestinal tract, although the most frequent location is the terminal ileum; the earliest changes are hyperemia and edema involving the mucosa and submucosa; the progression of the disease can cause aphthoid or superficial ulcerations up to a fistulizing, fibrostenotic, or inflammatory pattern, often associated with extramural manifestations (fistulas, abscesses, adhesions, lymph node enlargement, fibrofatty proliferation).

UC exclusively affects the superficial layers of the colon with a continuous spreading from distal to proximal section; rectum can be involved or spared. The disease is characterized by small or large mucosal erosions with edema and/or thickening of submucosa, due to fat deposition.

In case of colonic features overlapping of CD and UC or diagnostic difficulties in differential diagnosis, the disease could be classified as IC; usually we can find the typical pattern of UC with transmural inflammation [4].

Clinical suspicion of IBD needs radiographic, endoscopic, and pathological confirmation, information about the extent of the disease, and long-term follow-up [6–9].

Di.G. Graziella (✉) • G. Gianluca • B. Daniela
I. Francesca • R. Alfonso • G. Giuliano • C. Salvatore
Radiology Department, Second University of Naples,
Naples, Italy
e-mail: graziella.digrezia@libero.it

G. Roberta
Radiology Department,
University of Sassari, Sassari, Italy
e-mail: roberto.grassi@unina2.it

© Springer International Publishing Switzerland 2016
G. Lo Re, M. Midiri (eds.), *Crohn's Disease: Radiological Features and Clinical-Surgical Correlations*,
DOI 10.1007/978-3-319-23066-5_10

10.1 Examination Performance Requirements

The main advantage of intestinal ultrasound is the low cost and the availability in all hospitals that provides real-time information in an expert radiologist [10].

The exam does require only 6 h of fasting to reduce postprandial peristalsis and luminal air; some authors suggest the injection of an oral contrast media, an isoosmolar polyethylene glycol solution (SICUS) that can mime the small bowel follow-through with high accuracy (100 % sensitivity, 97 % specificity) [11, 12].

The exam starts with a global evaluation of the abdomen using a convex multifrequency probe (3.5–5 MHz) applying an appropriate abdominal compression to move the intestinal content, such as stool and air, and to evaluate the stiffness of a tissue and the reaction after this maneuver. The exam continues with a focused high-resolution study (7–12 MHz) with high-quality images; in this case, due to the less penetration of the probe, the abdominal compression is required to decrease the distance between the transducer and the loops. The operator should do a gradual and not marked abdominal compression to improve the visualization of the layers and to avoid a change in the thickness of the intestinal wall and influence in the measurements [13].

10.2 Ultrasonographic Features of Small Bowel Anatomy

The small intestine can be differentiated from the colon, thanks to the arrangement of gas waves, conniventes valvulae (especially in the presence of fluid), and the peristaltic capacity; above and below the umbilical region, we can generally find, respectively, the jejunal and ileal loops.

The physiological appearance of the small bowel wall at ultrasonographic exam is of five concentric layers with different echogenicities; each layer does not correspond exactly to a histologic layer, but rather an interface between adjacent layers [14]. The first layer is the echogenic interface, followed by a hypoechoic mucosa, an echogenic submucosa, a hypoechoic muscular layer, and an echogenic interface between the serosa and the adjacent fatty mesentery [15]. However, there is evidence that the muscular and submucosal layers correspond to those identified on the ultrasonography [16, 17].

Many authors established the physiological range of the thickness of the intestinal wall from 1 to 5 mm, due to the equipment and frequencies used, the different scanning techniques, and the degree of abdominal compression during measurement (Fig. 10.1).

Currently, the majority of the authors consider normal a wall, using a midline abdominal compres-

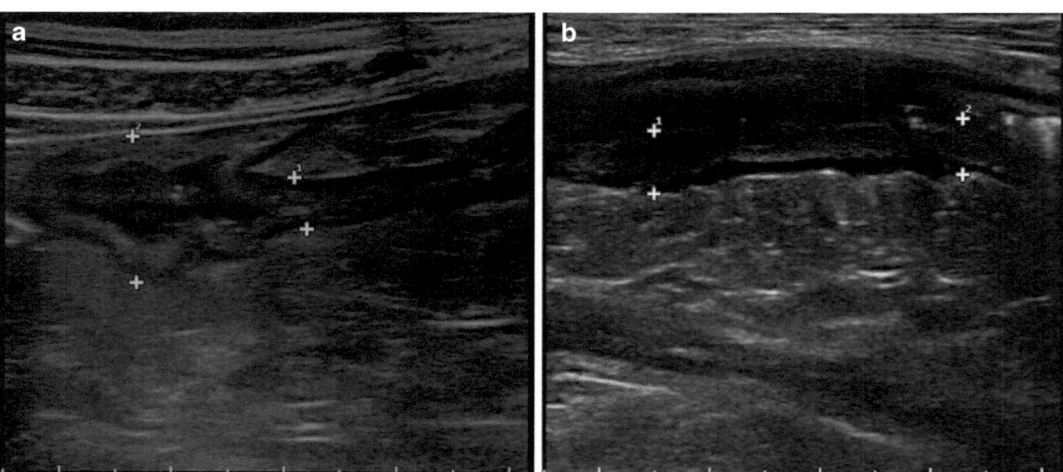

Fig. 10.1 (**a, b**) shows thickening and lack of compressibility of bowel loops (Courtesy of Giuseppe Cabibbo Gastroenterology Section Specialistic and Internal Medicine Biomedic Department - Palermo University)

sion, if the thickness is below 3 mm in the distended bowel and 5 mm in the nondistended bowel [18].

10.3   Ultrasonographic Features of Inflammatory Bowel Diseases

Intestinal ultrasonography allows to visualize the lack of compressibility, thickening, narrowing, and the loss of normal stratification and motility of the pathologic loops.

They can appear conglomerate and can coexist with mesenteric thickening, increased lymph nodes, abdominal fluid, and, in selected cases, abscess, fistulas, and stenoses related to dilations of the upper loops [19] (Fig. 10.2).

The location of the disease influences the diagnostic accuracy that is proportional to the accessibility of the anatomic area, such as the terminal ileum and left colon. The diagnostic accuracy is lower for upper small bowel and rectum [20] in overweight patients [21], in the detection of superficial lesions [22], and in case of proximal and anorectal involvement.

For these reasons, there is no cumulative value of diagnostic accuracy, but a range of sensitivity from 75 to 92 % and of specificity from 67 to 100 % [23].

In general, the magnitude of US changes has a high correlation with endoscopic and histological

magnitude of alterations and a weak correlation with indexes of clinical activity and biomarkers, especially in fistulas (sens. 71.4 %, spec. 95.8 %, acc. 85.2 %) and abscesses (acc. 88.5 %) evaluation [24].

10.4   IBD Differential Diagnosis

Differential diagnosis in inflammatory bowel disease is related to the localization of the disease and the involvement of terminal ileum rather than ultrasonographic features.

Terminal ileum is involved in Crohn's disease in over 70 % of cases, with transmural and discontinuous thickening of the wall with strictures and in some cases a linear path through all the bowel layers that can become a fistula [25] that, occasionally, can be complicated by an access.

Ulcerative colitis typically involves only the large intestine, from the rectum to the cecal region, and involves only the mucosal layer with the development of ulcers that only in selected cases can deepen, such as in toxic megacolon.

Other feature that can be distinguished between CD and UC from a specific or non-idiopathic inflammatory bowel disease is the involvement of mesenteric fat near the pathological loops.

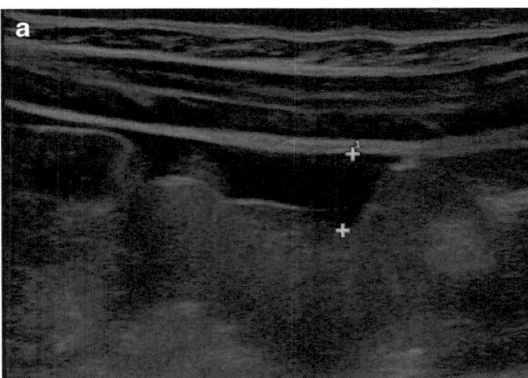 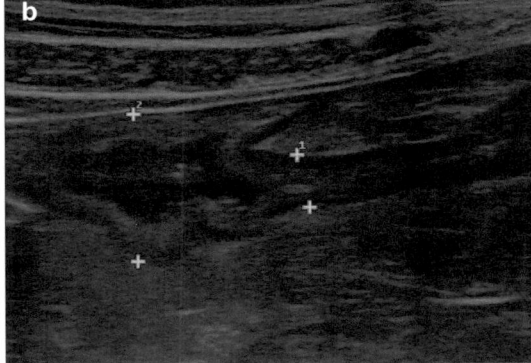

Fig. 10.2 (**a**) splenic flexure involvement of Crohn disease with (**b**) dilation of upper loops (Courtesy of Giuseppe Cabibbo Gastroenterology Section Specialistic and Internal Medicine Biomedic Department–Palermo University)

10.5 Advantages of Ultrasonography in IBD

In case of suspected inflammatory bowel disease, ultrasonography is the first-level examination that can provide general information on abdominal status, but its accuracy is very low, due to the inability to differentiate inflammatory, neoplastic, or infectious wall thickening [26].

Even if extraintestinal findings are present and can improve diagnostic accuracy, a histological examination is mandatory to confirm the presence of inflammatory bowel disease, to differentiate between idiopathic and non-idiopathic form, and to diagnose the kind of IBD [27].

The extension of disease can be evaluated with a good diagnostic accuracy if the disease involves the ileum, descending colon, and sigma; the diagnosis is very hard if there are localizations in the duodenum, proximal jejunum, and rectum [20].

Ultrasonography can help also in the evaluation of inflammatory bowel disease *complications*. Intra- or retroperitoneal *abscesses* usually are hypo-anechoic image with undefined borders and with or without echogenic content.

Fistulas are visualized as tracts or hypoechoic areas from a thickened intestinal loop. They can be classified as enteroenteric, enterovesical, and enteromesenteric [28, 29] with a sensitivity of 82 % if compared with entero-MRI [30].

For the detection of internal fistulas, the combination of small bowel enteroclysis and US significantly improved diagnostic accuracy (small bowel enteroclysis 84 %, US 85 %, combination 91 %) [19].

Ultrasonography has a high sensitivity in the detection and the characterization of thickened, narrowed, and aperistaltic loops and in the evaluation of prestenotic dilation, often associated to liquid distension or echogenic content [31].

10.6 Disease Activity

Inflammatory bowel disease activity can be determined by analyzing wall thickening, loss of echostructure wall, fibrofatty proliferation, and lymphadenopathy, but the main criterion is the degree of parietal vascularization [32, 33].

Color and power Doppler imaging usually is performed with parameters optimized to detect low-velocity and low-flow states (pulse repetition frequencies 800–1500 Hz, wall filter 40–50 Hz, maximal color signal gain immediately below the noise threshold, high levels of color versus echo priority, and color persistence) [34].

The intensity of the vascularity may be subjectively categorized as mild (small focal area of color signal), moderate (multiple areas of weak color signal), or marked (multiple areas of color signal) because some studies have found that increased vascularity of the diseased bowel wall correlates with the activity of the disease [35].

Doppler and sonographic parameters of the superior mesenteric artery are significantly correlated with disease activity in nonoperated and noncomplicated Crohn's disease [36].

The use of power Doppler US has been suggested to improve the diagnostic accuracy of US, particularly in discriminating inflammatory from fibrotic strictures, in better defining the presence of internal fistulas, and in differentiating these lesions from intra-abdominal abscesses [37].

The availability of dedicated contrast-specific techniques with microbubble contrast agents has enabled ultrasonography to obtain information regarding the perfusion behavior of the organs and their diffuse or focal diseases [38].

It might help in characterizing bowel wall thickening by differentiating inflammatory vascularization, edema, and fibrosis and may help to grade disease activity by assessing the presence and distribution of vascular perfusion within the layers of the bowel wall, although it is limited to the evaluation of a specific loop.

The high transmit power insonation produces extensive microbubble destruction with the production of a wideband irregular harmonic signal. Low transmit power insonation (about 30–70 KPa) produces microbubble resonance with production of regular harmonic frequencies and allows real-time scanning, and it is the technique of insonation which is usually in the clinical practice.

Four different perfusion patterns of bowel enhancement related to Crohn's activity have been recently proposed: (a) a complete enhancement of the entire wall section, from the mucosal to the serosal layer; (b) the absence of enhancement only in the outer border of the muscularis propria; (c) the absence of enhancement both in the outer and in the inner borders of the bowel wall and enhancement only in the intermediate layer; and (d) the complete absence of enhancement in the entire wall section [39].

CEUS can become the most useful imaging modality in the differential diagnosis between fibrotic and inflammatory thickening and in the detection of possible disease complications (abscess, phlegmons and fistulas). CEUS can assess the efficacy of medical therapy in reducing bowel wall vascularity in patients with chronic inflammatory disease and has a strong correlation with the CDAI (sens. 93.5 %, spec. 93.7 %, acc. 93.6 %, correlation coefficient 0.74; $P < 0.0001$) [40].

CEUS allows real-time assessment of the bowel wall perfusion with the highest temporal resolution of all imaging techniques and with a spatial and contrast resolution that rivals that of CT and MRI.

10.7 Recurrences and Follow-Up

Patients affected by inflammatory bowel disease should be monitored frequently to assess the response to medical treatment with a noninvasive and well-tolerated technique, without using ionizing radiation, and ultrasonography meets all these requirements.

Relapses in patients with a good clinical response have been related to the exacerbation of inflammatory activity; the residual hyperemia evaluated with color Doppler or with contrast agents can identify patients with incomplete histological remission reflecting subclinical inflammation, with increased susceptibility to relapse.

Quantitative techniques in ultrasonography with contrast agents can measure changes in the mural enhancement reflecting the response to therapy in monitoring the inflammatory disease. It has been proven that there is a significant reduction in the enhancement in patients with clinical response to biological treatments. However, to date there are no studies demonstrating that this assessment adds information to that provided by Doppler ultrasonography [41].

All studies showed a high accuracy of US for the diagnosis of postsurgical recurrence in CD, detecting almost all cases of severe or complicated recurrence, as well as high sensitivity and specificity in differentiating mild from severe recurrence, especially after giving oral contrast.

In conclusion, in known Crohn's disease following disease course and evaluating relapses and extramural manifestations, US is an excellent tool (sens. 88.4 %, 93.3 %, acc. 90.4 %) [42–44] (Table 10.1).

Table 10.1 Table shows the reliability of US, Doppler and CEUS in intra and extraintestinal findings of Inflammatory Bowel Diseases

			US	Doppler	CEUS
General features		Preparation	0	0	0
		Contrast media	0/1[a]	0	1
		Patient tolerance	2	2	1
		Costs	1	1	2
		Availability	2	2	1
		Pain	0	0	0
Gastrointestinal findings	*Mural*	Ulcers	0	0	0
		Erosions	0	0	0
		Aphthoid lesions	0	0	0
		Strictures	1	1	2
		Bowel wall thickening	1	1	2
		Bowel wall stratification	2	0	0
	Extramural	Fistulas	1[b]	2	0
		Abscesses	1	0	0
Extragastrointestinal findings		Lymph nodes	1	1	0
		Fibrofatty proliferation	0	0	0
		Attenuation of perivisceral fat	0	0	0
Other information		Localization	0/1	0	1
		Disease activity	1	1	2
		Degree activity	0	2	2
		Biopsies	0	0	0
		Therapy (bowel dilation)	0	0	0
		In case of risk of obstruction, perforation, or bleeding	1	1	0

0 not reliable, 1 somewhat or potentially reliable, 2 usually reliable
[a]Oral contrast media
[b]Endoscopic ultrasound

References

1. Baumgart DC, Carding SR. Inflammatory bowel disease: cause and immunobiology. Lancet. 2007; 369(9753):1627–40.
2. Loftus Jr EV. Clinical epidemiology of inflammatory bowel disease: incidence, prevalence and environmental influences. Gastroenterology. 2004;126(6): 1504–17.
3. Panes J et al. Imaging techniques for assessment of inflammatory bowel disease: joint ECCO and ESGAR evidence-based consensus guidelines. J Crohns Colitis. 2013;7(7):556–85.
4. Reginelli A, Pezzullo MG, Scaglione M, Scialpi M, Brunese L, Grassi R. Gastrointestinal disorders in elderly patients. Radiol Clin North Am. 2008;46(4):755–71.
5. Guindi M, Riddell RH. Inderterminate colitis. J Clin Pathol 2004;57(12):1233–44.
6. Di Mizio R, Rollandi GA, Bellomi M, Meloni GB, Cappabianca S, Grassi R. Multidetector-row helical CT enteroclysis. Radiol Med. 2006;111(1):1–10.
7. La Seta F, Buccellato A, Tesè L, Biscaldi E, Rollandi GA, Barbiera F, Cappabianca S, Di Mizio R, Grassi R. Multidetector-row CT enteroclysis: indications and clinical applications. Radiol Med. 2006;111(2): 141–58.
8. Grassi R, Rambaldi PF, Di Grezia G, Mansi L, Cuccurullo V, Cirillo A, Riegler G, Cappabianca S, Rotondo A. Inflammatory bowel disease: value in diagnosis and management of MDCT-enteroclysis and 99mTc labeled leukocyte scintigraphy. Abdom Imaging. 2011;36(4):372–81.
9. Iacobellis F, Berritto D, Fleischmann D, Gagliardi G, Brillantino A, Mazzei MA, Grassi R. CT findings in acute, subacute and chronic ischemic colitis: suggestions for diagnosis. Biomed Res Int. 2014;2014: 895248.
10. Joaquín P-C, Tomás R-G. Utility of abdominal ultrasonography in the diagnosis and monitoring of inflammatory bowel disease. Rev Esp Enferm Dig Madrid. 2014;106(6):395–408.
11. Pallotta N, Baccini F, Corazziari E. Small intestine contrast ultrasonography (SICUS) i the diagnosis of

small intestine lesions. Ultrasound Med Biol. 2001;27(3):335–41.

12. Parente F, Greco S, Molteni M, et al. Oral contrast enhanced bowel ultrasonography in the assessment of small intestine Crohn's disease. A prospective comparison with conventional ultrasound, x ray studies, and ileocolonoscopy. Gut. 2004;53(11):1652–7.

13. O'Malley ME, Wilson SR. US of gastrointestinal tract abnormalities with CT correlation. Radiographics. 2003;23(1):59–72.

14. Migaleddu V, Quaia E, Scano D, Virgilio G. Inflammatory activity in Crohn disease: ultrasound findings. Abdom Imaging. 2008;33(5):589–97.

15. Valette PJ, Rioux M, Pilleul F, Saurin JC, Fouque P, Henry L. Ultrasonography of chronic inflammatory bowel diseases. Eur Radiol. 2001;11(10):1859–66.

16. Kimmey MB, Martin RW, Haggitt RC, Wang KY, Franklin DW, Silverstein FE. Histologic correlates of gastrointestinal ultrasound images. Gastroenterology. 1989;96(2 Pt 1):433–41.

17. Wiersema MJ, Wiersema LM. High-resolution 25-megahertz ultrasonography of the gastrointestinal wall: histologic correlates. Gastrointest Endosc. 1993;39:499–504.

18. Fraquelli M, Colli A, Casazza G, Paggi S, Colucci A, Massironi S, et al. Role of US in detection of Crohn disease: meta-analysis. Radiology. 2005;236(1): 95–101.

19. Pan'es J, Bouzas R, Chaparro M, et al. Systematic review: the use of ultrasonography, computed tomography and magnetic resonance imaging for the diagnosis, assessment of activity and abdominal complications of Crohn's disease. Aliment Pharmacol Ther. 2011;34:125–45.

20. Parente F, Greco S, Molteni M, et al. Role of early ultrasound in detecting inflammatory intestinal disorders and identifying their anatomical location within the bowel. Aliment Pharmacol Ther. 2003;18: 1009–16.

21. Drews BH, Barth TFE, Hänle MM, et al. Comparison of sonographically measured bowel wall vascularity, histology, and disease activity in Crohn's disease. Eur Radiol. 2009;19(6):1379–86.

22. Di Mizio R, Maconi G, Romano S, D'Amario F, Porro GB, Grassi R. Small bowel Crohn disease: sonographic features. Abdom Imaging. 2004;29(1): 23–35.

23. Horsthuis K, Bipat S, Bennink RJ, Stoker J. Inflammatory bowel disease diagnosed with US, MR, scintigraphy, and CT: meta-analysis of prospective studies. Radiology. 2008;247(1):64–79.

24. Maconi G, Sanpietro GM, Parente F, et al. Contrast radiology, computed tomography and ultrasonography in detecting internal fistulas and intra-abdominal abscesses in Crohn's disease: a prospective comparative study. Am J Gastroenterol. 2003;98(7):1545–55.

25. Kunihiro K, Hata J, Haruma K, Manabe N, Tanaka S, Chayama K. Sonographic detection of longitudinal ulcers in Crohn disease. Scand J Gastroenterol. 2004;39:322–6.

26. Truong M, Atri M, Bret PM, Reinhold C, Kintzen G, Thibodeau M, et al. Sonographic appearance of benign and malignant conditions of the colon. AJR Am J Roentgenol. 1998;170:1451–5.

27. Maconi G, Radice E, Greco S, Bianchi Porro G. Bowel ultrasound in Crohn's disease. Best Pract Res Clin Gastroenterol. 2006;20:93–112.

28. Maconi G, Bollani S, Bianchi Porro G. Ultrasonographic detection of intestinal complications in Crohn's disease. Dig Dis Sci. 1996;41:1643–8.

29. Gasche C, Moser G, Turetschek K, Schober E, Moeschl P, Oberhuber G. Transabdominal bowel sonography for the detection of intestinal complications in Crohn's disease. Gut. 1999;44:112–7.

30. Martínez MJ, Ripollés T, Paredes JM, Blanc E, Martí-Bonmatí L. Assessment of the extension and the inflammatory activity in Crohn's disease: comparison of ultrasound and MRI. Abdom Imaging. 2009;34:141–8.

31. Parente F, Maconi G, Bollani S, Anderloni A, Sampietro G, Cristaldi M, et al. Bowel ultrasound in assessment of Crohn's disease and detection of related small bowel strictures: a prospective comparative study versus x ray and intraoperative findings. Gut. 2002;50:490–5.

32. Hata J, Haruma K, Yamanaka H, Fujimura J, Yoshihara M, Shimamoto T, et al. Ultrasonographic evaluation of the bowel wall in inflammatory bowel disease: comparison of in vivo and in vitro studies. Abdom Imaging. 1994;19:395–9.

33. Maconi G, Di Sabatino A, Ardizzone S, Greco S, Colombo E, Russo A, et al. Prevalence and clinical significance of sonographic detection of enlarged regional lymph nodes in Crohn's disease. Scand J Gastroenterol. 2005;40:1328–33.

34. Ciáurriz-Munuce A, Fraile-González M, León-Brito H, Vicuña-Arregui M, Miquélez S, Uriz-Otano J, et al. Ionizing radiation in patients with Crohn's disease. Estimation and associated factors. Rev Esp Enferm Dig. 2012;104:452–7.

35. Maconi G, Parente F, Bollani S, et al. Factors affecting splanchnic haemodynamics in Crohn's disease: a prospective controlled study using Doppler ultrasound. Gut. 1998;43(5):645–50.

36. Karoui S, Nouira K, Serghini M, et al. Assessment of activity of Crohn's disease by Doppler sonography of superior mesenteric artery flow. J Crohn's Colitis. 2010;4(3):334–40.

37. Robotti D, Cammarota T, Debani P, Sarno A, Astegiano M. Activity of Crohn disease: value of color-power- Doppler and contrast-enhanced ultrasonography. Abdom Imaging. 2004;29(6):648–52.

38. Migaleddu V, Quaia E, Scanu D, et al. Inflammatory activity in Crohn's disease: CE-US. Abdom Imaging. 2010;36:142–8.

39. Serra C, Menozzi G, Labate AMM, et al. Ultrasound assessment of vascularization of the thickened terminal ileum wall in Crohn's disease patients using a low-mechanical index real-time scanning technique with a second generation ultrasound contrast agent. Eur J Radiol. 2007;62(1):114–21.

40. Migaleddu V, Scanu AM, Quaia E, et al. Contrast-enhanced ultrasonographic evaluation of inflammatory activity in Crohn's disease. Gastroenterology. 2009;137(1):43–52.

41. Quaia E, Migaleddu V, Baratella E, Pizzolato R, Rossi A, Grotto M, et al. The diagnostic value of small bowel wall vascularity after sulfur hexafluoride-filled microbubble injection in patients with Crohn's disease. Correlation with the therapeutic effectiveness of specific antiinflammatory treatment. Eur J Radiol. 2009;69:438–44.

42. Panes J, Gasche C, Moser G, et al. Transabdominal bowel sonography for the detection of intestinal complications in Crohn's disease. Gut. 1999;44(1):112–7.

43. Tarjian Z, Toth G, Gyorke T, et al. Ultrasound in Crohn's disease of the small bowel. Eur J Radiol. 2000;35(3):176–82.

44. Gatta G, Di Grezia G, Di Mizio V, Landolfi C, Mansi L, De Sio I, Rotondo A, Grassi R. Crohn's disease imaging: a review. Gastroenterol Res Pract. 2012; 2012:816920.

MDCT Enteroclysis and Enterography

11

Giuseppe Lo Re, Federica Vernuccio,
Dario Picone, Fabrizio Rabita, Antonio Lo Casto,
Massimo Galia, Roberto Lagalla,
and Massimo Midiri

11.1 Introduction

Since the first studies suggesting its possible role in the management of Crohn's disease (CD) patients [1], multidetector computed tomography (MDCT) has usually been considered a useful diagnostic technique in CD for the detection of extraenteric complications, as intra-abdominal abscesses, the study of strictures, prestenotic dilatations, fistulas, and postsurgical complications [2]. Moreover, it is a widely available technique and is considered the gold standard in emergency.

Conventional enteroclysis has been the most widely used technique for identifying the sites of disease (often multifocal) and assessing possible complications for years [3]. However, many limits pertained to this technique as its inability to provide direct information on the degree of extramural involvement and the presence of complications [3].

To overcome these limitations, investigators proposed the use of MDCT enteroclysis (EC-MDCT) that can be obtained by means of a

fairly large amount (1500–2000 mL or more) of contrast agent administered orally or by the positioning of a nasojejunal tube; this technique usually allows the evaluation of the colon as well [2]. However, the need for nasojejunal intubation made MDCT enteroclysis poorly tolerated by patients, so its use was precluded in some cases [3]. Hence, MDCT enterography (EG-MDCT) was introduced [4] in 1997: for this technique, patients are required to drink approximately 1.5–2 l of oral contrast over 45–60 min. Computed Tomography (CT) is largely used in CD population, so that Brenner et al. demonstrated that CT studies are accountable for 51 % of the effective dose in CD patients [5].

Moreover, EC-MDCT has shown to be able to modify clinical management of CD in 62 % of patients with symptomatic disease [6].

11.2 MDCT Enteroclysis

The introduction of MDCT technology has allowed the evaluation of organs, such as the small intestine, that have a tortuous course, obtaining isotropic or near-isotropic resolution voxels of the abdomen and pelvis with 16-section or higher MDCT scanners in a reasonable breath hold, thus allowing the creation of coronal and sagittal reformations of similar resolution as transverse images [7].

G. Lo Re, PhD (✉) • F. Vernuccio • D. Picone
F. Rabita • A. Lo Casto • M. Galia • R. Lagalla
M. Midiri
DIBIMED, Department of Biopathology and Medical Biotechnology, University Hospital P. Giaccone – University of Palermo, Palermo, Italy
e-mail: giuseppe.lore12@gmail.com; massimo.midiri@unipa.it

© Springer International Publishing Switzerland 2016
G. Lo Re, M. Midiri (eds.), *Crohn's Disease: Radiological Features and Clinical-Surgical Correlations*,
DOI 10.1007/978-3-319-23066-5_11

In the 1980s and 1990s, considering the high diagnostic accuracy of CT studies of the small bowel for identifying the typical signs of disease on the bowel wall and possible complications [8–11], it was suggested to combine the conventional enteroclysis technique, involving nasojejunal intubation and methylcellulose administration, with CT [12–14]. To distend the bowel loops, several types of intraluminal contrast media have been used: positive, such as iodinated contrast agents [9]; negative, such as 0.5 % methylcellulose [4]; or water or lipid contrast media [15].

Patients have to do cathartic bowel preparation the day before the examination.

The *neutral contrast media* include water and methylcellulose and have attenuation similar to that of water; when neutral agents are used, intravenous contrast medium is also administered [3, 7, 16]. These neutral contrast media allow better assessment of mucosal enhancement, mural thickness, and mesenteric vasculature.

Concerning the nasojejunal intubation, the balloon tip should be positioned at the level of the Treitz, and the balloon inflated with 30 mL of air [7]. Thereafter, the rapid pressurized infusion of enteral contrast material and the use of an antiperistaltic agent allow an adequate bowel distension; on the other hand, the amount and rate of administration of intravenous contrast medium depends on the radiologist's individual preference [7, 16].

If our aim is to distend large bowel, we failed since enteroclysis is aimed at distending just the small bowel while the distension of both small and large bowel requires also the retrograde bowel distension [17]. The distension of both small and large bowel raises the diagnostic accuracy of the examination because the reflux of water from the cecum through the ileocecal valve into the terminal ileum combined with the orally ingested contrast material results in excellent luminal distension of both sides of the ileocecal area [18].

The *positive enteral contrast material*, as 4–15 % water-soluble solution or a dilute (1 %) barium solution, does not require intravenous contrast medium injection and is mainly used to detect lower grades of small bowel obstruction and internal fistula [3, 7, 16].

11.3 MDCT Enterography

Intravenous contrast material-enhanced abdominopelvic MDCT following ingestion of a large volume of neutral oral contrast agent, typically 1.5–2 L, is termed EG-MDCT [7]. Actually, EG-MDCT has a consolidated role in the management of CD, and, in referral centers, the number of EG-MDCT has continued to grow while the number of barium examinations decreased [19].

EG-MDCT provides practical advantages: EG-MDCT requires less time and no direct radiologists' exposure to ionizing radiation and is not invasive because it does not require intubation. Though increasing concern has been recently expressed about radiation exposure, especially in young women, children, and adolescents, submitted to repeat exams, EG-MDCT is easily accessible even in non-specialized centers and district hospitals while MR, which has the advantages of avoiding radiation exposure and providing excellent depiction of soft tissues and of perianal fistulas, is more expensive and time-consuming since it has longer acquisition times and is not available in all radiological departments [19].

Concerning the technique, all patients have to do a cathartic preparation the day before the examination. The day of the examination, it is important to obtain an adequate small bowel distension, and this is achieved through oral administration of approximately 1.5–2 l of oral contrast over 45–60 min prior to scanning.

The optimal volume of oral contrast that should be ingested has been extensively evaluated by many authors; Maglinte [20] stated that a volume of <1.5 l is unlikely to be sufficient to adequately distend the small bowel without active inflammation. In pediatric patients and patients with history of previous small bowel resection, smaller volumes of oral contrast may be sufficient, mainly considering patient tolerance [21].

Boudiaf et al. [22] classified small bowel distension using a grading system based on diameters of jejunum and ileum grades 0–3 (where 0 was for no distension and 3 was optimal distension). The evaluation of the small bowel is obtained just through oral contrast material, while the good evaluation of the colon can be achieved through rectal water enema. Optimal distension of both small and large bowel raises the diagnostic capability, thanks to a better distension that can be obtained in case of ileocecal valve incontinence and to the less progression of oral contrast material caused by the presence of colon enema. The water enema can also improve the ileal distension in patients with ileocolostomy.

Before MDCT scan, all patients are usually injected with an i.v. anticholinergic drug (except in case of contraindication to the drugs) to minimize potential artifacts due to peristaltic bowel movement, to obtain homogeneous small bowel distension, and to reduce abdominal discomfort [19]. Thereafter, EG-MDCT is performed before and after i.v. administration of iodinated nonionic

contrast medium, with the patient in the supine position from the diaphragm to the perineum during a single breath hold.

CD predominantly involves the mesenteric border of the small bowel, frequently leading to asymmetric inflammation and fibrosis, with pseudosacculation of the antimesenteric border [21]. The most common EC/EG-MDCT signs of CD in the affected bowel loops are (Fig. 11.1) [3, 19] the following:

- Mural ulceration and mucosal pseudopolyps that lead to the cobblestone aspect of endoscopy examination
- Bowel wall thickening, defined as pathological if ≥4 mm on an adequately distended loop
- Mural hyperenhancement (Fig. 11.2) , defined

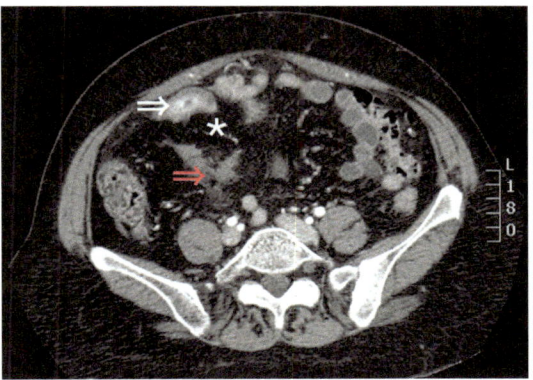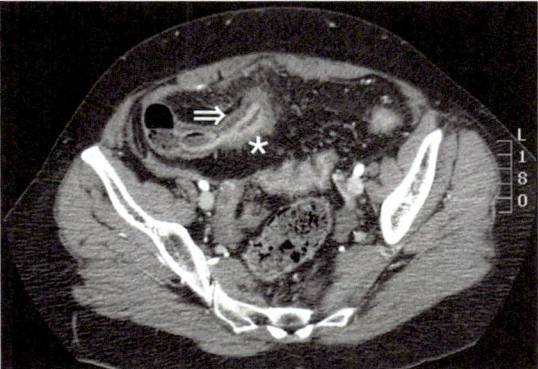

Fig. 11.1 Axial CT images in a patient with Crohn's disease show the bowel wall thickening with mural stratification (*white arrows*) and comb sign, creeping fat (*), and fistula between the ileal loops (*red arrow*)

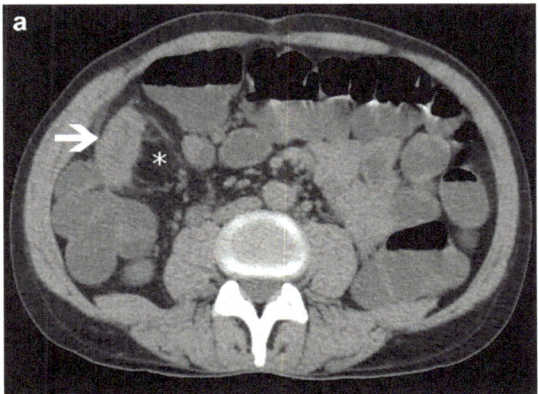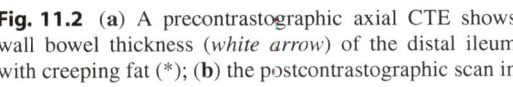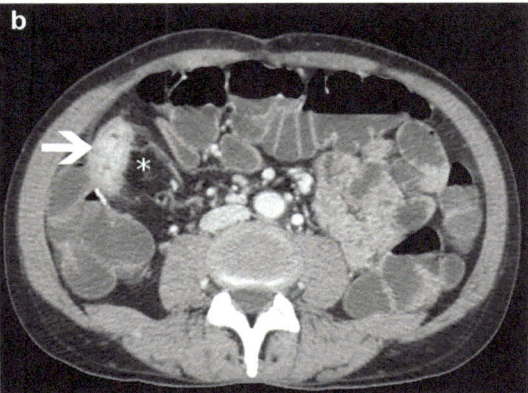

Fig. 11.2 (**a**) A precontrastographic axial CTE shows wall bowel thickness (*white arrow*) of the distal ileum with creeping fat (*); (**b**) the postcontrastographic scan in

the same patient better shows the bowel wall stratified thickness with marked mural hyperenhancement (*white arrow*), creeping fat (*), and engorgement of vasa recta

as segmental greater enhancement in all or part (in the case of mural stratification) of the small bowel wall
- Stenotic bowel segments (diameter <3 cm) with prestenotic dilatation

The cobblestone pattern is due to transmural ulcerations that are detected by discontinuity of the mucosa, associated with "clefts" in the thickened wall; these features are also recognized at the histologic evaluation [21]. Moreover, these ulcerations may penetrate through the wall forming a small periluminal abscess.

Mural stratification is due to the visible layers of the inflamed wall of the small bowel loops that is demonstrated after intravenous contrast medium injection in the enteric phase [21]. The mucosa and serosa show an intense enhancement, but the intervening bowel wall enhances to a varying degree, either due to intramural edema, indicating active disease, or intramural fat, indicating chronic inflammation [21].

Another important sign is the enhancement and thickening of the perivisceral fat [3]. Fibrofatty proliferation (known as "creeping fat" of the mesentery) (Figs. 11.1 and 11.2) refers to fatty deposition along the mesenteric border of bowel segments affected by CD. Increased fat density refers to fluid density in the fat surrounding thickened or abnormally enhancing bowel resulting from inflammatory infiltration of the perienteric adipose tissue. The "comb sign" (Figs. 11.1 and 11.2) refers to the hypervascularity of the involved mesentery because of the presence of dilated and tortuous vasa recta that penetrate the bowel wall perpendicular to the bowel lumen, mimicking the appearance of a comb. Mesenteric lymphoadenopathies located near the affected intestinal segments are usually considered pathological if their transverse diameter is >15 mm.

Moreover, enlarged lymph nodes can be detected along the course of the ileocolic vein and mesenteric root, but just in few cases, their maximum transverse diameter exceeds 15 mm [3]. In most of the patients, the mucosa of the thickened loops shows intense contrast enhancement after contrast medium injection, with engorgement of the mesenteric vasa recta (comb sign) [3].

However, considering that focal small bowel spasm is frequently encountered mimicking short strictures, despite the use of antiperistaltic agent, it is important to identify lack of mucosal hyperenhancement and absence of mesenteric abnormality to distinguish spasm from true pathology.

Concerning the radiological evaluation of response to therapy in patients with CD, an assessment of the disease activity is useful considering that efficacious therapies for CD that may modify the natural history of the disease are available [19]; hence, there is increasing clinical

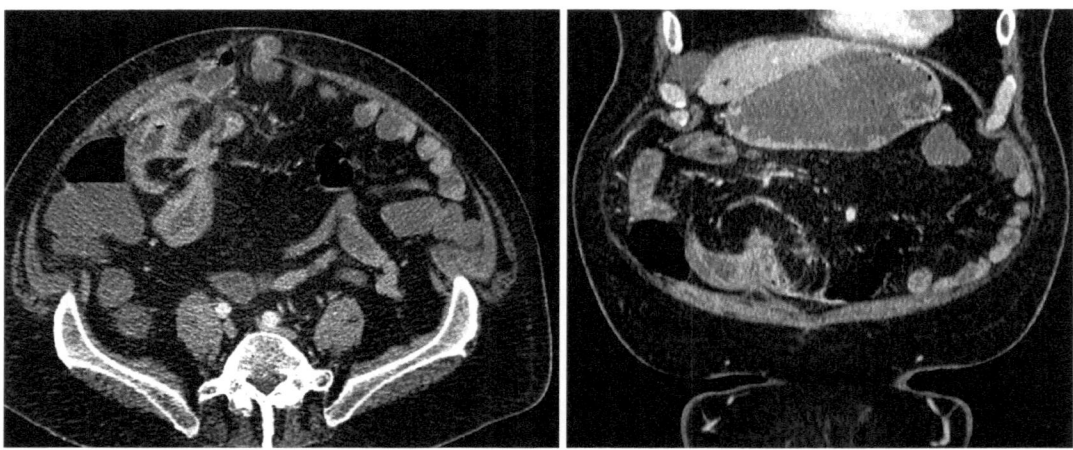

Fig. 11.3 A-axial and B-coronal CTE images of an enteroenteric fistula with perivisceral fat involvement

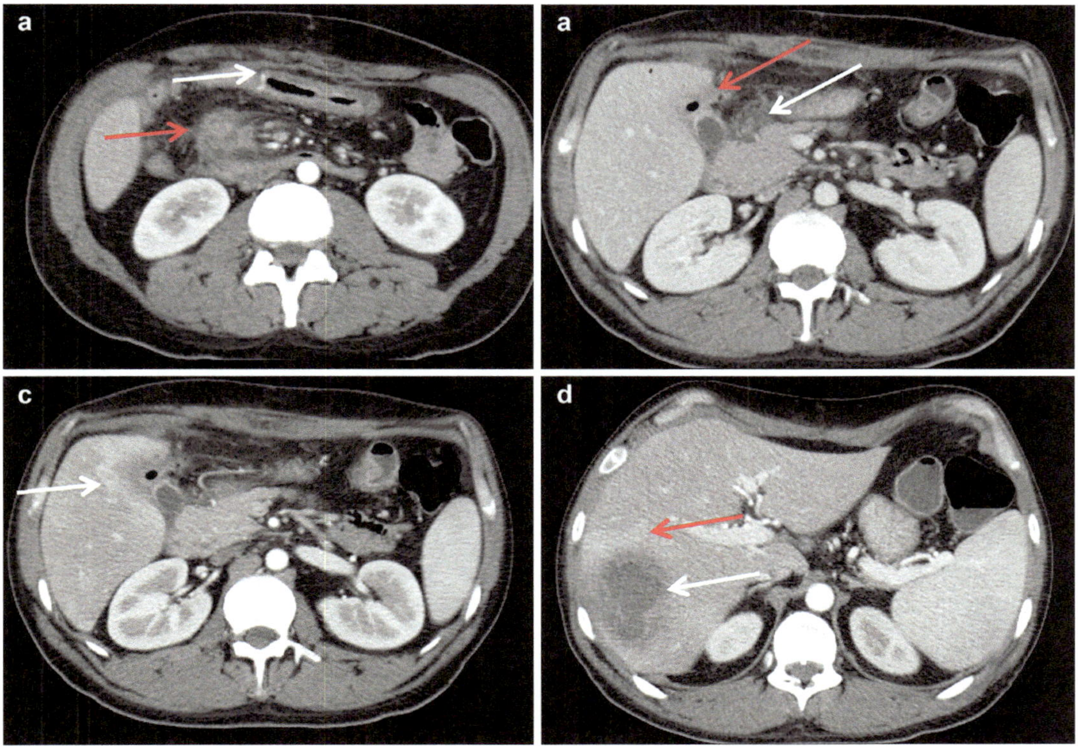

Fig. 11.4 Patient with advanced stage fibrostenotic Crohn's disease who had undergone viscerolysis, right hemicolectomy, ileotransverse anastomosis 3 years before CT. (**a**) The colonic side of anastomosis shows thickened walls (*white arrow*) for a length of about 13 cm with marked postcontrastographic mucosal enhancement; pseudopolyps and interspersed minute undermined ulcerations are visible in the mucosa, as a typical localization of Crohn's disease. In the same figure part, it can be noticed on the right paramedian region of the mesenterial root a newly formed inflammatory fluid collection (*red arrow*), with thick walls that are hyperdense after contrast medium injection; this abscess is in contiguity with mesenteric vessels of the right abdomen, with the duodenum and the uncinate process of the pancreas. (**b**) From the abovementioned fluid collection, many fistulous tracks origin; these latter connect the abscess in the mesenterial root with other two inflammatory fluid collections: the first (*white arrow*) is at the level of the duodenum and of the head of the pancreas and has air bubbles within and the second (*red arrow*) is a pericholecystic abscess (maximum diameter 4 cm) which is in contiguity with the surrounding liver parenchyma. The involvement of liver presents with a postcontrastographic heterogeneous density of the parenchyma near the pericholecystic abscess (**c**) and with an hepatic abscess (*white arrow*) that is also responsible of postcontrastographic heterogeneous density of the near parenchyma (**d**)

and research need for a reproducible and validated activity scoring system to quantify inflammatory activity over time [23]. Lymph node enlargement and free abdominal fluid have been recognized in active phase of CD [20] and even if Minordi et al. [24] tried to create a semiquantitative score system (CTE0–CTE3) using the endoscopic Rutgeerts score, actually , there is not a widely accepted scoring system for CD severity assessment [23].

Finally, the presence of abdominal free fluid and other complications related to the disease are assessed in patients with CD. The MDCT study after distension of bowel loops is also useful in depicting fistulas (Fig. 11.3) and other extraintestinal complications of CD [25], such as abscesses (Fig. 11.4), and in patients suspected of having small bowel obstruction, proved to be superior to conventional MDCT for the diagnosis of lower grades of bowel obstruction [26].

Another important complication of CD is bowel obstruction caused by fibrostenotic or inflammatory pattern; moreover, if there is a history of abdominal surgery, adhesions are also a possible cause [7].

When CD is located in the large bowel, it must be distinguished from the chronic inflammatory disease due to ulcerative colitis (UC). This differential diagnosis is more easily performed through the distension of both small and large bowel (oral anterograde and bowel retrograde distension) which allows also a better evaluation of the disease.

UC mainly affects the rectum, and then it can extend proximally to the descending, transverse, ascending colon, and cecum. Lesions in UC are characterized by inflammation of the mucosal layer, which is hyperemic and slightly thickened without or with low submucosal and muscle layers involvement and with lower mesentery fat stranding compared to CD.

It is also important to underline that, as firstly described in 1949 by McCready et al., about 10 % of patients with UC inflammatory findings can be found in the terminal ileum, termed as backwash ileitis, with inflammation adjacent to the ileocecal valve [27].

Differential diagnosis that should be kept in mind in CD patients is Meckel's diverticulum, which is about 40–60 cm from the ileocecal valve and may contain heterotopic gastric mucosa, small bowel GISTs, which may show an inhomogeneous intestinal bowel thickening, ileal endometriosis, which appear in female patients as nodular wall thickening and whose presence has to be related to patient's symptoms, and adenocarcinoma or metastases in oncologic patients.

Moreover, some typical MDCT signs of IBD may be encountered in other diseases:

- Comb sign without skip lesions in small bowel carcinoid
- Distal ileal loop hyperemia without thickened and layered bowel wall in infectious ileitis
- Thickened distal ileal loop hyperemia but without layered bowel wall or inhomogeneously and poor enhancing asymmetric bowel wall thickening in lymphoma

- Inhomogeneously enhancing and asymmetric bowel wall thickening in metastases from melanoma
- Bowel wall thickening extended for longer bowel segment without skip lesions in Cytomegalovirus enteritis
- Stenotic thickening of bowel wall in graft-versus-host disease

The evaluation of the severity of the abdominal disease is improved by the use of latest generation of workstations that are particularly useful to exceed an intrinsic limit of the technique which is the absence of multiplanarity. In particular, the use of MPR, slabMPR, slabMIP, slabVR, and VR allows a better assessment of potential fistulas and abscesses as well as their relationships with the surrounding anatomical structures. The use of curvilinear MPR (CPR) could theoretically put in one plane the entire affected intestinal tract, thus allowing a better assessment of its extension.

11.4   EC-MDCT Versus EG-MDCT

Regarding EC-MDCT, nasojejunal intubation is poorly tolerated by patients, precluding execution of the examination in some cases. The discomfort associated with nasoenteric tube placement may be alleviated with the use of conscious sedation and smaller tubes [28]. However, the limits of MDCT enteroclysis are not just related to patients' discomfort but also to the increased costs related to the addition of MDCT to enteroclysis, the additional radiologist time required for catheter placement and the highest exposure of patients and staff to radiation during the nasojejunal intubation, even if MDCT technology has improved dose efficiency [29]. Furthermore, the invasiveness of the procedure raises concern for complications such as bowel perforation, enteral contrast material aspiration, or respiratory depression from sedation [7]. In some patients, enteroclysis cannot be performed because of inability to place the tube in an adequate position [7].

The main advantages of EG-MDCT over imaging alternatives are its widespread access, together with rapid scan times and high-quality diagnostic images, even in claustrophobic patients who are unable to lie flat for long periods and/or reliably hold their breath [23].

However, some limitations pertain to EG-MDCT since it is currently unable to match the exquisite soft tissue contrast afforded by magnetic resonance enterography and does not provide functional motility information as it is possible using ever-improving cinematic MRI techniques/sequences [23].

Furthermore, there are some clinical scenarios in which EG-MDCT cannot be considered the appropriate examination as in CD patients with recurrent small bowel obstructions and in whom a previous EG-MDCT has been performed or in patients who cannot receive intravenous iodinated contrast medium due to chronic kidney disease [30].

The ionizing radiation exposure of CD patients in an important question in world literature; in fact Brenner et al. [5], demonstrated that the median total effective dose in a population of 103 patients was of 26.6 mSv, greater than in a UC population.

References

1. Berliner L, Redmond P, Purow E, Megna D, Sottile V. Computed tomography in Crohn's disease. Am J Gastroenterol. 1982;77:548–53.
2. Saibeni S, Rondonotti E, Iozzelli A, Spina L, Tontini GE, Cavallaro F, Ciscato C, de Franchis R, Sardanelli F, Vecchi M. Imaging of the small bowel in Crohn's disease: a review of old and new techniques. World J Gastroenterol. 2007;13:3279–87.
3. Lo Re G, Galia M, Bartolotta TV, Runza G, Taibbi A, Lagalla R, De Maria M, Midiri M. Forty-slice MDCT enteroclysis: evaluation after oral administration of isotonic solution in Crohn's disease. Radiol Med. 2007;112:787–97.
4. Raptopoulos V, Schwartz RK, McNicholas MM, Movson J, Pearlman J, Joffe N. Multiplanar helical CT enterography in patients with Crohn's disease. AJR Am J Roentgenol. 1997;169:1545–50.
5. Brenner DJ, Hall EJ. Computed tomography–an increasing source of radiation exposure. N Engl J Med. 2007;357:2277–84.
6. Turetschek K, Schober E, Wunderbaldinger P, et al. Findings at helical CT-enteroclysis in symptomatic patients with Crohn disease: correlation with endoscopic and surgical findings. J Comput Assist Tomogr. 2002;26:488–92.
7. Maglinte DD, Sandrasegaran K, Lappas JC, Chiorean M. CT enteroclysis. Radiology. 2007;245:661–71.
8. Furukawa A, Saotome T, Yamasaki M, et al. Cross-sectional imaging in Crohn disease. Radiographics. 2004;24:689–702.
9. Goldberg HI, Gore RM, Margulis AR, et al. Computed tomography in the evaluation of Crohn disease. AJR Am J Roentgenol. 1983;140:277–82.
10. Gore RM, Cohen MI, Vogelzang RL, et al. Value of computed tomography in the detection of complications of Crohn's disease. Dig Dis Sci. 1985;30:701–9.
11. Frick MP, Feinberg SB, Stenlund RR, et al. Evaluation of abdominal fistulas with computed body tomography (CT). Comput Radiol. 1982;6:17–25.
12. Sailer J, Peloschek P, Schober E, et al. Diagnostic value of CT enteroclysis compared with conventional enteroclysis in patients with Crohn's disease. AJR Am J Roentgenol. 2005;185:1575–81.
13. Rollandi GA, Curone PF, Crespi G, et al. Spiral CT and transparent small bowel enema; correlation between imaging and CDAI (Crohn Disease Activity Index). Radiology. 1996;201(P):381.
14. Rollandi GA, Curone PF, Biscaldi E, et al. Spiral CT of the abdomen after distention of small bowel loops with transparent enema in patients with Crohn's disease. Abdom Imaging. 1999;24:544–9.
15. Mako EK, Mester AR, Tarjan A, et al. Enteroclysis and spiral CT examination in diagnosis and evaluation of small bowel Crohn disease. Eur J Radiol. 2000;35:168–75.
16. Maglinte DD, Bender GN, Heitkamp DE, et al. Multidetector-row helical CT enteroclysis. Radiol Clin North Am. 2003;41:249–62.
17. Paparo F, Bacigalupo L, Garello I, Biscaldi E, Cimmino MA, Marinaro E, Rollandi GA. Crohn's disease: prevalence of intestinal and extraintestinal manifestations detected by computed tomography enterography with water enema. Abdom Imaging. 2012;37:326–37.
18. Paparo F, Revelli M, Puppo C, Bacigalupo L, Garello I, Garlaschi A, Biscaldi E, Rollandi L, Binda GA, Rollandi GA. Crohn's disease recurrence in patients with ileocolic anastomosis: value of computed tomography enterography with water enema. Eur J Radiol. 2013;82:e434–40.
19. Lo Re G, Cappello M, Tudisca C, Galia M, Randazzo C, Craxì A, Cammà C, Giovagnoni A, Midiri M. CT enterography as a powerful tool for the CDAI and acute-phase reactants. Radiol Med. 2014;119:658–66.
20. Maglinte D. Invited commentary. Radiographics. 2006;26:657–62.
21. Ilangovan R, Burling D, George A, Gupta A, Marshall M, Taylor SA. CT enterography: review of technique and practical tips. Br J Radiol. 2012;85:876–86.
22. Boudiaf M, Jaff A, Soyer P, Bouhnik Y, Hamzi L, Rymer R. Small-bowel diseases: prospective evaluation of multidetector helical CT enteroclysis in 107 consecutive patients. Radiology. 2004;233:338–44.

23. Bruining DH, Bhatnagar G, Rimola J, Taylor S, Zimmermann EM, Fletcher JG. CT and MR enterography in Crohn's disease: current and future applications. Abdom Imaging. 2015;40:965–74.

24. Minordi LM, Vecchioli A, Poloni G, et al. Enteroclysis CT and PEG-CT in patients with previous small-bowel surgical resection for Crohn's disease: CT findings and correlation with endoscopy. Eur Radiol. 2009;19:2432–40.

25. Kloppel R, Thiele J, Bosse J. The Sellink CT method. Rofo. 1992;156:291–2.

26. Bender GN, Timmons JH, Williard WC, Carter J. Computed tomographic enteroclysis: one methodology. Invest Radiol. 1996;31:43–9.

27. McCready FJ, Bargen JA, Dockerty MB, Waugh JM. Involvement of the ileum in chronic ulcerative colitis. N Engl J Med. 1949;240:119–27.

28. Maglinte DD, Lappas JC, Heitkamp DE, Bender GN, Kelvin FM. Technical refinements in enteroclysis. Radiol Clin North Am. 2003;41:213–29.

29. Kalra MK, Maher MM, Toth TL, et al. Techniques and applications of automatic tube current modulation for CT. Radiology. 2004;233:649–57.

30. Baker ME, Hara AK, Platt JF, Maglinte DD, Fletcher JG. CT enterography for Crohn's disease: optimal technique and imaging issues. Abdom Imaging. 2015;40:938–52.

Giuseppe Lo Re, Federica Vernuccio,
Fabrizio Rabita, Dario Picone, Giuseppe La Tona,
Sergio Salerno, Massimo Galia,
and Massimo Midiri

Magnetic resonance imaging (MRI) is actually the most complete and less invasive imaging technique in the evaluation of Crohn's disease (CD). Compared to CT and US, MRI allows both a morphological and qualitative evaluation of the disease at the same time, thus allowing an evaluation of its extension in the gastrointestinal tract and of its grade of activity, obtaining an accurate relation with the clinical status of the patient.

This is possible thanks to its intrinsic characteristics, as multiplanarity, high contrast resolution, and the possibility to make a functional assessment; moreover, there is no use of ionizing radiation. For all these reasons, this technique has a high diagnostic potential.

Even if the costs are still moderately elevated (both in economic terms and in terms of acquisition time) and the accessibility is partially limited, to date MRI should be considered the first choice examination in the study of patients with CD and the gold standard in the follow-up of young patients [1].

G. Lo Re, PhD (✉) • F. Vernuccio • F. Rabita
D. Picone • G. La Tona • S. Salerno • M. Galia
M. Midiri
DIBIMED, Department of Biopathology and Medical
Biotechnology, University Hospital P. Giaccone –
University of Palermo, Palermo, Italy
e-mail: giuseppe.lore12@gmail.com;
massimo.midiri@unipa.it

MRI is actually used to study both small and large bowel, and the perianal region, whose pathological aspects and imaging will be discussed in the next chapter.

12.1 Technical Aspects

Technical aspects can be easily divided in two key moments: patient preparation and MR images acquisition.

12.1.1 Patient Preparation

Scientific literature agrees on the need for an adequate cathartic preparation of the whole intestine before performing a MRI study of the small and/or large bowel.

In our institution, the cathartic preparation is performed asking the patient to drink a water solution with laxative effect the day before the exam together with a low-residue diet for the preceding 3 days to reduce fecal matter in the colon and to allow an easier distension of the bowel necessary for the MRI study.

Table 12.1 shows the most used scheme for patients' cathartic preparation. Although in some centers an adequate preparation is not considered mandatory, we strongly believe that no intestinal tract, mainly the large bowel, can be evaluated in absence of an adequate cathartic preparation.

Table 12.1 Cathartic preparation recommended for patients who have to be submitted to CT- or MR- enteroclysis/enterography

Starting from 3 days before examination	Low fiber diet	Patients should avoid fried foods, sausage, bacon and hot dogs, nuts and seeds, luncheon meats, peas, lentils, legumes, dried beans, sushi, whole grain breads, pancakes, waffles, high fiber cereal, popcon, brown and wild rice, all raw and undercooked vegetables, cooked greens and spinach and gas forming vegetables, dried fruit, coconut, jams, marmalades
Starting from 12 h before	Cleansing solution	A semiliquid diet and 2 L of water and polyethylene glycol solution
Starting from 6 h before examination	Don't eat or drink anything	

Regarding patient's preparation, another important point is the distension with an endoluminal contrast medium. MRI evaluation is done with two kinds of contrast media, an endoluminal and an intravenous one (gadolinium). As already known in the literature, CD may affect all the digestive tract, from mouth to anus; excluding the proximal tracts (as oropharynx, esophagus, and stomach), which are usually less affected by the disease, MRI evaluation can evaluate both small bowel (MR enterography) and large bowel (colonography-MR), with the possibility to simultaneously distend with different techniques both the small and large bowel. Obviously, small bowel distension is the most performed one since ileal location of the disease (last ileal loop) is the most common one.

The type of endoluminal contrast medium used for the study depends on several factors as costs, availability, tolerability, and intensitometric characteristics. According to the signal intensity they produce on T1- and T2-weighted images, the endoluminal contrast medium is classified in negative, positive, or biphasic.

The positive ones are represented by paramagnetic agents (e.g., Gd, Mn); they are called positive agents because they produce high signal intensity on T1- and T2-weighted images ("bright lumen"). These agents facilitate the identification of pathological wall thickening, but they can easily interfere with the assessment of the degree of wall enhancement; however, though being widely available, their use is limited by high costs.

Negative contrast media are superparamagnetic agents (e.g., iron oxides, Ba). These agents are characterized by low signal intensity on T1- and T2-weighted sequences ("dark lumen") thus improving the identification of wall edema; unfortunately, they are too expensive and have an unpleasant taste.

Biphasic contrast agents (e.g., water, methylcellulose and polyethylene glycol (PEG)) give high signal intensity on one sequence and low signal intensity on the opposite sequence. Thanks to this intrinsic feature, their low costs, good patient compliance, and wide availability, biphasic agents are now the most used intraluminal contrast agent for MR enterography [2–4].

As previously said, the optimal distension of small bowel plays a pivotal role in the evaluation of CD; this distension can be achieved through two techniques, enteroclysis and enterography.

In enteroclysis, the patient is firstly submitted to nasojejunal intubation under fluoroscopic guidance, and the balloon tip is ideally positioned at the level of the Treitz. Afterward, the patient is transferred to the MRI room; here, endoluminal contrast medium is injected under MR dynamic fluoroscopic sequence guide (single-shot T2W sequence, high slice thickness)

Endoluminal injection can be performed with a monophasic or a biphasic technique.

The first technique is performed with a continuous infusion of 1.5–2 L of endoluminal contrast medium trough a manual pump (compatible with MR imaging), until the ileocecal valve is reached; then the distension is stopped and a spasmolytic agent is injected.

In the biphasic technique, the distension is obtained with a flow rate of 80–150 mL/min dur-

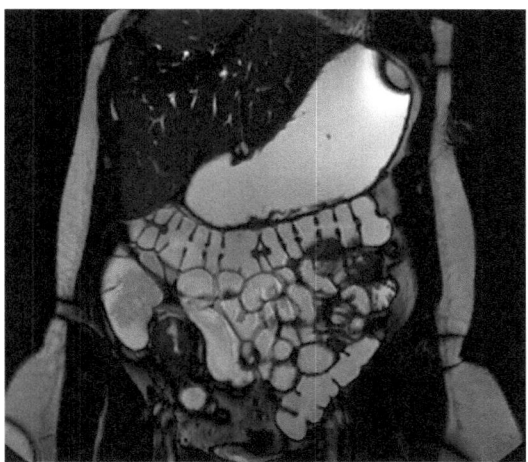

Fig. 12.1 Coronal SSFP MR image shows a good ileal loops distension during an MR enterography; last ileal loop is easily detectable

ing the first phase, until the contrast medium reaches the terminal ileum. During the second phase, reflex atony is created with an increase in the flow rate to 200 mL/min; hence, it is not necessary to inject any spasmolytic agent [5].

MR enterography is performed after oral administration of the endoluminal contrast medium. The patient is invited to drink approximately 1.5–2 L of a solution with usually water and PEG [6] continuously and in a short span of time (in about 20 min).

Thereafter, no later than 30–40 min since the beginning of the ingestion of the contrast agent, MR images acquisition begins (Fig. 12.1).

Both MR enteroclysis and enterography can be completed with large bowel distension to accurately evaluate all the bowel [7]. Large bowel distension is achieved in our department through an enema containing about 2000 ml of warm water.

Comparing MR enteroclysis and enterography, many studies agree that enteroclysis allows a better bowel distension, while enterography may not turn into a complete and homogeneous distension of the bowel loops, mainly of the jejunal ones.

For this reason, it is recommended to the patient to drink the oral contrast medium continuously and as fast as he can, since an adequate distension

determines a better accuracy in the detection of intestinal mucosal abnormalities.

However, considering diagnostic sensitivity and sensibility, both the techniques do not significantly differ, mainly in the diagnosis and the characterization of the "stenoses" and "fistulous tracks," which are common in CD [8].

Another key point is the use of ionizing radiation for the correct positioning of the tip of nasojejunal tube, thus exposing patients to a minimal biological invasivity and to a discomfort caused by the intubation.

For the abovementioned reasons, many patients who were submitted to both MR enteroclysis and enterography prefer the latter one.

Lastly, MR enterography is less time consuming: nasojejunal intubation, x-ray evaluation of the correct position of the tip, and the contrast medium injection through MR fluoroscopic guidance significantly lengthen the duration of the entire MRI.

On the other hand, using the enterography technique, the patient drinks the contrast medium and enters the magnet room ready for MR images acquisition.

12.1.2 MR Imaging Acquisition

After the bowel distension, MR images are acquired. Nowadays, it is recommended to use high-field MR scanners (at least 1.5 T).

The patient is usually placed in a prone position; such a position facilitates separation of small bowel loops, and their ascent from the pelvic cavity decreases the volume of the peritoneal cavity and thus the number of imaging sections needed and reduces the abdominal wall movement during breathing [9]. If patients do not tolerate this position, it is possible to place them in the supine one.

MR exam is performed using surface multichannel body coils (12 channels) that can increase the signal/noise ratio.

The following sequences are considered mandatory in our protocol: steady-state free-precession (SSFP), single-shot fast spin echo (SS-FSE), 3D spoiled gradient echo (GE), and DWI.

Except for DWI, all the other sequences are acquired on axial and coronal plane, including the whole abdomen and pelvic cavity.

The SSFP sequences (e.g., FIESTA, BFFE, TrueFISP) are acquired before contrast medium injection and without fat saturation and are not affected by bowel movements. They show a high contrast between the hyperintense mesenteric fat and the hypointensity of vessels, bowel wall, and lymph nodes. These sequences are usually acquired during a single respiratory apnea and usually show the typical chemical shift artifact which is sometimes responsible of disturbance in the evaluation of wall thickness. The SSFP sequences are useful in the extra-enteric evaluation of CD.

SSFP sequences may be used for the "cine loop" technique [10], acquiring 15/25 phases of a single coronal section thus allowing the differential diagnosis between functional or mechanical stenosis. In this case it is important the spasmolytic agent has not been previously injected [10].

The single-shot-FSE sequences are acquired before contrast medium injection and with fat suppression (FAT-SAT); they are ultrafast sequences not affected by respiratory movement artifacts. They enhance tissues thanks to long T2 relaxation time, increasing their spatial resolution. However, there are flow void artifacts due to the vessel blood movement. Fat suppression is used to enhance the "enteric" findings as wall edema and ulcerations but also "extra-enteric" findings as the presence of free fluid or the thickness and edematous stranding of mesenteric fat.

3D spoiled GE sequences are used before and after contrast medium injection. These sequences are T1 weighted, volumetric, and FAT-SAT, and they are affected by bowel peristaltic movements. For this reason, it is suggested the i.v. injection of a spasmolytic agent. Excluding contraindications, we suggest the intravenous injection of single or double dose of hypotonizing drug as hyoscine N-butylbromide or glucagon when the patient is already positioned on the scanning table, before the acquisition of the precontrastographic 3D spoiled GE sequence. It is usually then acquired a single coronal precontrastographic scan. After contrast medium injection

(gadolinium), three coronal scans after 25, 40, and 70 s (arterial, enterographic, and portal phase) and a delayed axial scan centered on the pathological findings are made; thanks to these scans, it will be possible a multiplanar evaluation. These sequences provide important information on wall thickness, grade of activity of the disease, and presence of fistulous tracks and abscesses.

More recently, DWI sequences have been more and more used in the routine evaluation of CD. Many clinical studies underlined that on DWI, the presence of hyperintense bowel walls (due to restriction of the diffusivity of water molecules) is related to a high inflammatory activity [11, 12].

For this reason, we recommend to acquire at least images at two b values, between 400 and 1000 s/mm^2. If possible, it is useful to acquire images with the multi-b technique. Clinical studies demonstrate that this latter allow to create a unique ADC map with a possible increase of sensibility, also reducing acquisition time.

12.2   MR Findings

Crohn's disease can be active or inactive and may present chronic fibrotic changes.

The objective of MRI is to diagnose CD, to assess the location, mural and extramural extent, and severity of disease, and to assess for complications such as strictures, bowel tethering, obstruction, or abscess.

During the active phase of CD, the most common finding we can delineate is the typical cobblestone pattern, which is due to the simultaneous presence of both wall thickening greater than 3 mm (Fig. 12.2), which is best assessed on single-shot TSE/FSE to avoid chemical shift artifact on True FISP sequences, and transmural ulcerations, which are best accessed on single-shot TSE/FSE sequences and whose evaluation is highly dependent on the quality of luminal distention; however, early and superficial ulceration cannot be adequately demonstrated even with full luminal distention [3].

The cobblestone pattern is best assessed on True FISP as fast spin-echo T2-weighted images are particularly prone to intraluminal flow artifact

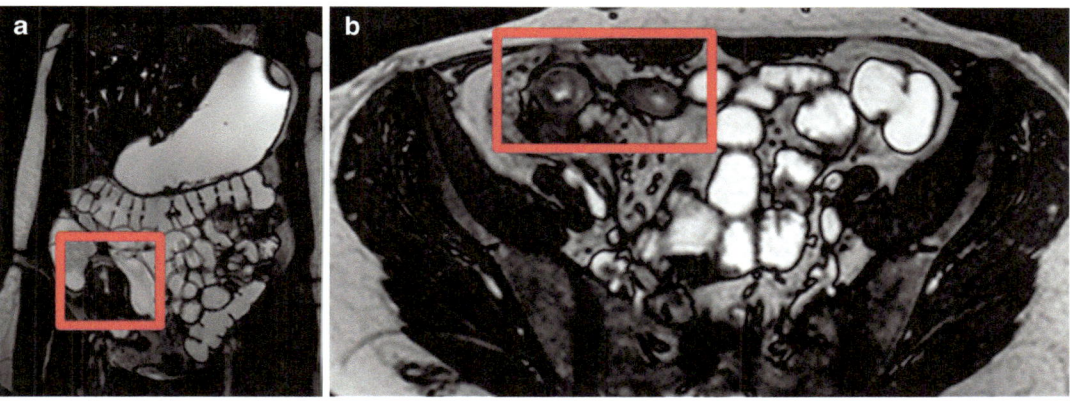

Fig. 12.2 Coronal (**a**) and axial (**b**) SSFP MR images show concentric bowel wall thickening with bowel wall edema and substenotic lumen

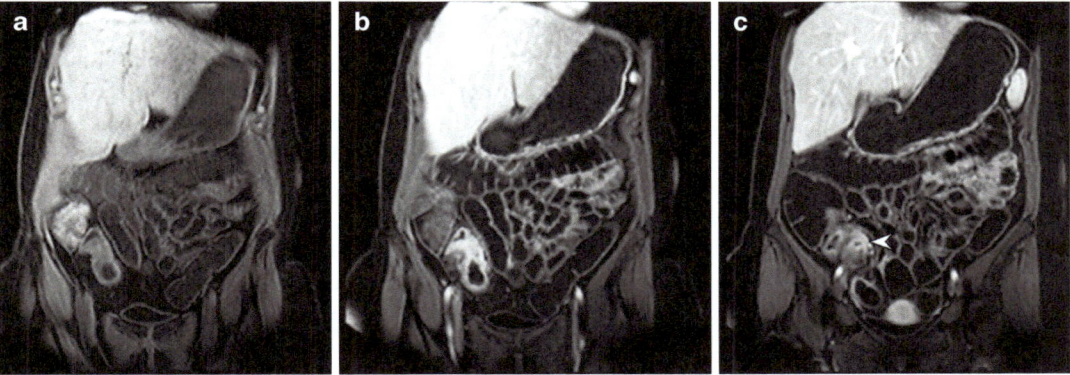

Fig. 12.3 3D-GE coronal MR images. (**a**, **b**) Show an extensive location of Crohn's disease in the last ileal loops with bowel wall involvement; (**c**) shows a small abscess (*arrowhead*) in the contiguous mesentery

and may be mistaken for cobblestoning (antispasmodic agents are used to reduce fluid flow in the lumen) [3].

The acute inflammatory changes associated are responsible of a hyperintense bowel wall on T2 FAT-SAT-weighted images due to mucosal and submucosal edema and increased enhancement in bowel wall relative to adjacent loops on post contrastographic T1-weighted fat suppressed sequences, due to mucosal hyperemia.

Regarding this latter characteristic, three main patterns of mucosal enhancement have been described, and these may help determine the likely level of disease activity [3]:

1. Stratified contrast enhancement pattern, which results from an inner enhancing ring (hyper-

emic mucosa), poor submucosal enhancement (submucosal edema), and an outer enhancing ring (hyperemic serosa)
2. Transmural contrast enhancement, which results from an intense homogeneous enhancement affecting the entire wall (Fig. 12.3)
3. Low level inhomogeneous contrast enhancement, due to fibrosis

The mesentery adjacent to the affected bowel wall shows many abnormalities (Fig. 12.4) [3]:

- Mesenteric edema (intermediate to high signal intensity of the mesenteric fat tissue on fat sat T2WI)
- Creeping fat or fat wrapping due to an increased mesenteric fat producing a mass

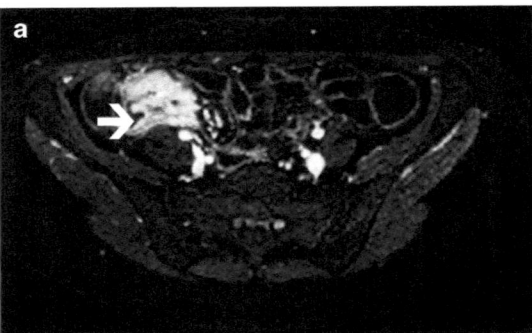 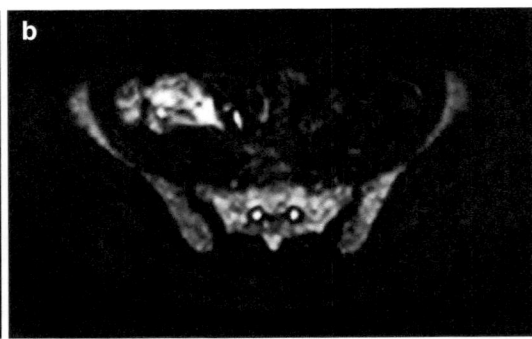

Fig. 12.4 (a) 3D GE axial MR image shows a severe bowel wall thickening (*arrow*) with mesenteric involvement (comb sign and inflammatory mesenteric lymph nodes) and a small abscess that has a marked a reduction in the water molecules diffusion, as it can be seen in the DWI sequence (**b**)

effect (slightly decreased signal intensity of the fat adjacent to the affected bowel segment on single-shot TSE/FSE sequences)

- Inflammatory mesenteric lymph nodes, demonstrated by fat saturated sequences
- Increased mesenteric vascularity and engorgement of the vasa recta (comb sign) seen as short parallel lines with low signal intensity on true FISP sequences and high signal intensity on post contrast T1 (Volume Interpolated GRE sequences).

Another important goal of MR in CD is the assessment of its complications. MRI proved to be equal or superior to CT at characterizing extraenteric complications [13]. According to the occurring complication, we can distinguish three subtypes of CD, fistulizing, fibrostenotic, and reparative one [14].

The fistula forming subtype of disease is characterized by severe inflammation with progression to transmural ulcers or fissures that then penetrate the bowel muscle layer involving the adjacent mesenteric tissue and thus leading to formation of blind-ending sinus tracts [15]. These sinus tracts appear as high-signal-intensity tracts on T2-weighted images and may result in fluid collections, phlegmon, and abscesses; moreover, they may extend and communicate through the wall of an adjacent hollow organ and form a fistula [15]. Fistulas are seen on MRI as high-signal-intensity tubular tracts between bowel loops on T2-weighted sequences with strong peripheral enhancement on post contrastographic T1-weighted images [3]. Fistulas can be enteroenteric, entero-colonic, enterovesical, enterovaginal, or enterocutaneous among others, but the anal ones are the most common [3]. Complicated fistulas with abscesses or severe underlying bowel disease have to be adequately treated and followed up because they can lead to spontaneous intestinal perforation.

Regarding the fibrostenotic subtype of CD, we have to keep in mind that during the chronic phase of CD, the signs of acute inflammatory disease moderately change since inflammation leads to fatty infiltration of the bowel wall, fibrofatty proliferation in adjacent mesenteric fat, and wall fibrosis. This latter may be responsible of strictures and consequent bowel obstruction with marked prestenotic dilatation. However, this subtype should be differentiated from small bowel obstruction secondary to spasm associated with active inflammatory disease [14]. Actually this differential diagnosis can be solved through the "cine loop" technique: an inflammatory stenosis should open on cine imaging, while a fibrotic stricture does not [16].

The evaluation of the involvement of mesentery in CD plays a key role since the presence of creeping fat, comb sign, and extraparietal findings as fistulas tracks and/or abscesses may result in an advanced stage of the disease. Due to its high contrast resolution and to multiplanarity, MRI is actually the most useful technique in the evaluation of mesenteric involvement of CD.

Lastly, the inactive phase of CD is characterized by mucosal atrophy with focal areas of sparing and regenerative polyps that do not show significant hyperemia or mural edema, leading to the reparative or regenerative disease subtype [14, 15]. Luminal narrowing may be seen, but usually there are no signs of inflammation or obstruction [15].

However, the most common clinical scenario is the coexistence of the different patterns in the same patient, differentiating the active, fistulizing, fibrostenotic and reparative subtypes depending on the predominant pattern of involvement [14].

References

1. Leyendecker JR, Bloomfeld RS, DiSantis DJ, et al. MR enterography in the management of patients with Crohn disease. Radiographics. 2009;29:1827–46.
2. Laghi A, Carbone I, Catalano C, et al. Polyethylene glycol solution as an oral contrast agent for MR imaging of the small bowel. AJR Am J Roentgenol. 2001;177(6):1333–4.
3. Tolan DJ, Greenhalgh R, Zealley IA, Halligan S, Taylor SA. MR enterographic manifestations of small bowel Crohn disease. Radiographics. 2010;30:367–84.
4. Ramalho M, Heredia V, Cardoso C, et al. Magnetic resonance imaging of small bowel Crohn's disease. Acta Med Port. 2012;25:231–40.
5. Prassopoulos P, Papanikolaou N, Grammatikakis J, Rousomoustakak M, Maris T, Gourtsoyiannis N. MR enteroclysis imaging of Crohn disease. Radiographics. 2001;21:S161–72.
6. Lo Re G, Galia M, Bartolotta TV, Runza G, Taibbi A, Lagalla R, De Maria M, Midiri M. Forty-slice MDCT enteroclysis: evaluation after oral administration of isotonic solution in Crohn's disease. Radiol Med. 2007;112:787–97.
7. Ajaj W, Lauenstein TC, Langhorst J, et al. Small bowel hydro-MR imaging for optimized ileocecal distension in Crohn's disease: should an additional rectal enema filling be performed? J Magn Reson Imaging. 2005;22:92–100.
8. Masselli G, Casciani E, Polettini E, Gualdi G. Comparison of MR enteroclysis with MR enterography and conventional enteroclysis in patients with Crohn's disease. Eur Radiol. 2008;18:438–47.
9. Cronin CG, Lohan DG, Mhuircheartaigh JN, et al. MRI small-bowel follow-through: prone versus supine patient positioning for best small-bowel distention and lesion detection. AJR Am J Roentgenol. 2008;191(2):502–6.
10. Froehlich JM, Waldherr C, Stoupis C, Erturk SM, Patak MA. MR motility imaging in Crohn's disease improves lesion detection compared with standard MR imaging. Eur Radiol. 2010;20(8):1945–51.
11. Hordonneau C, Buisson A, Scanzi J, Goutorbe F, Pereira B, Borderon C, Da Ines D, Montoriol PF, Garcier JM, Boyer L, Bommelaer G, Petitcolin V. Diffusion-weighted magnetic resonance imaging in ileocolonic Crohn's disease: validation of quantitative index of activity. Am J Gastroenterol. 2014;109(1): 89–98.
12. Kiryu S, Dodanuki K, Takao H, Watanabe M, Inoue Y, Takazoe M, Sahara R, Unuma K, Ohtomo K. Ree-breathing diffusion-weighted imaging for the assessment of inflammatory activity in Crohn's disease. J Magn Reson Imaging. 2009;29(4):880–6.
13. Horsthuis K, Bipat S, Bennink R. Inflammatory bowel disease diagnosied with US, MR, scintigraphy and CT: meta-analysis of prospective studies. Radiology. 2008;247:64–79.
14. Maglinte DD, Gourtsoyiannis N, Rex D, Howard TJ, Kelvin FM. Classification of small bowel Crohn's subtypes based on multimodality imaging. Radiol Clin North Am. 2003;41:285–303.
15. Sinha R, Verma R, Verma S, Rajesh A. MR enterography of Crohn disease: part 2, imaging and pathologic findings. AJR. 2011;197:80–5.
16. Griffin N, Grant LA, Anderson S, Irving P, Sanderson J. Small bowel MR enterography: problem solving in Crohn's disease. Insights Imaging. 2012;3:251–63.

Anal Fistula in Crohn's Disease

13

Giuseppe Lo Re, Daniela Berritto,
Federica Vernuccio, Alfonso Reginelli,
Dario Picone, Francesca Iacobellis,
Maria Cristina Galfano, Roberto Luca,
Roberto Grassi, and Massimo Midiri

13.1 Introduction

Transmural bowel inflammation in Crohn's disease (CD) is associated with the development of fistulas, which are tracts or communications that connect two epithelial-lined organs. Common sites for fistulas connect the intestine to bladder (enterovesical), to skin (enterocutaneous), to bowel (enteroenteric), and to the vagina (enterovaginal).

Anorectal fistulas (often called fistula in ano or cryptogenic fistulas) represent one of the major perianal complications of CD.

The lifetime risk for developing a fistula in CD patients is approximately 25–50 %, while rectovaginal fistulas accounted for 9 % [1–6].

The development of perianal fistulas can result in considerable morbidity and inaccurate diagnosis before treatment may lead to irreversible functional consequences. Fistula is defined by an abnormal communication between the epithelialized surface of the anal canal and (usually) the perianal skin. They develop in approximately

20–30 % percent of patients [7–9] and in up to 45 % of these patients they develop before the diagnosis of CD [10]. However, when perianal fistulas are the initial presentation of CD, it may be difficult to distinguish from the ones seen in patients who do not have CD.

The pathogenesis of the fistula in ano is controversial and there have been several theories for its explanation. The most cogent theory has a long history of advocacy starting in 1878 with Chiari [11], who suggested the origin from an infection of the anal glands, which are located between the two layers of the anal sphincters and which drain into the anal canal. These glands were found to occur in the anal canal and to discharge their contents into the anus at the dentate line. It was postulated that infection of these glands was the cause of anal abscesses and fistulas.

With anal fistulas as with all other conditions, it is important to evaluate history and physical examination. Usually, patients refer a history of previous pain, swelling, and spontaneous or planned surgical drainage of an anorectal abscess, while clinical symptoms are usually perianal discharge, pain, external opening, swelling, and drainage [12]. If not adequately drained, fistulas may lead to overwhelming soft tissue and fascial infection.

The classification of the area involved with the fistula is helpful in planning surgical intervention.

However, a knowledge of perianal anatomy is mandatory in order to better understand how perianal fistulas develop and to more accurately classify fistulas.

G. Lo Re (✉) • F. Vernuccio • D. Picone
M.C. Galfano • M. Midiri
DIBIMED, Department of Biopathology and Medical Biotechnology, University Hospital P. Giaccone – University of Palermo, Palermo, Italy
e-mail: giuseppe.lore12@gmail.com

D. Berritto • A. Reginelli • F. Iacobellis • R. Luca
R. Grassi
Department of Radiology, Second University of Naples, Caserta, Italy

© Springer International Publishing Switzerland 2016
G. Lo Re, M. Midiri (eds.), *Crohn's Disease: Radiological Features and Clinical-Surgical Correlations*,
DOI 10.1007/978-3-319-23066-5_13

There are two major muscular groups found in the anorectum (see Fig. 13.1) [12]:

- The inner muscle group, which is a circular smooth muscle that hypertrophies distally and develops into the internal sphincter muscle.
- The external sphincter muscles, which are composed, starting distally, of the subcutaneous, superficial, and deep sections, followed by the puborectalis. The puborectalis muscle is the level of what is anatomically described as the anorectal ring and has been described as the "key to continence (Fig. 13.2)."

The intersphincteric space is the surgical plane of dissection between the internal and external sphincters and is most frequently found between the longitudinal muscle and external sphincter, where it exists as a sheet of fat containing loose areolar tissue [13].

The dentate line lies approximately 2 cm proximal to the anal verge and is a crucial landmark in fistula in ano because the anal glands empty into the crypts that lie proximal to the valves [13].

Considering the above anatomic prerequisites, it is important to distinguish between the anatomical anal canal, which extends from the perineal skin to the linea dentata, and the surgical anal canal, which extends from the perineal skin to the anorectal ring.

As reported in a recent consensus on perianal fistulizing Crohn's disease [14], several classification and scoring systems have been developed in an attempt to quantify disease extent and severity of pCD. In this consensus, the World Gastroenterology Organization, International Organization for Inflammatory Bowel Diseases IOIBD, European Society of Coloproctology and Robarts Clinical Trials propose that a distinction is made between a detailed anatomic description

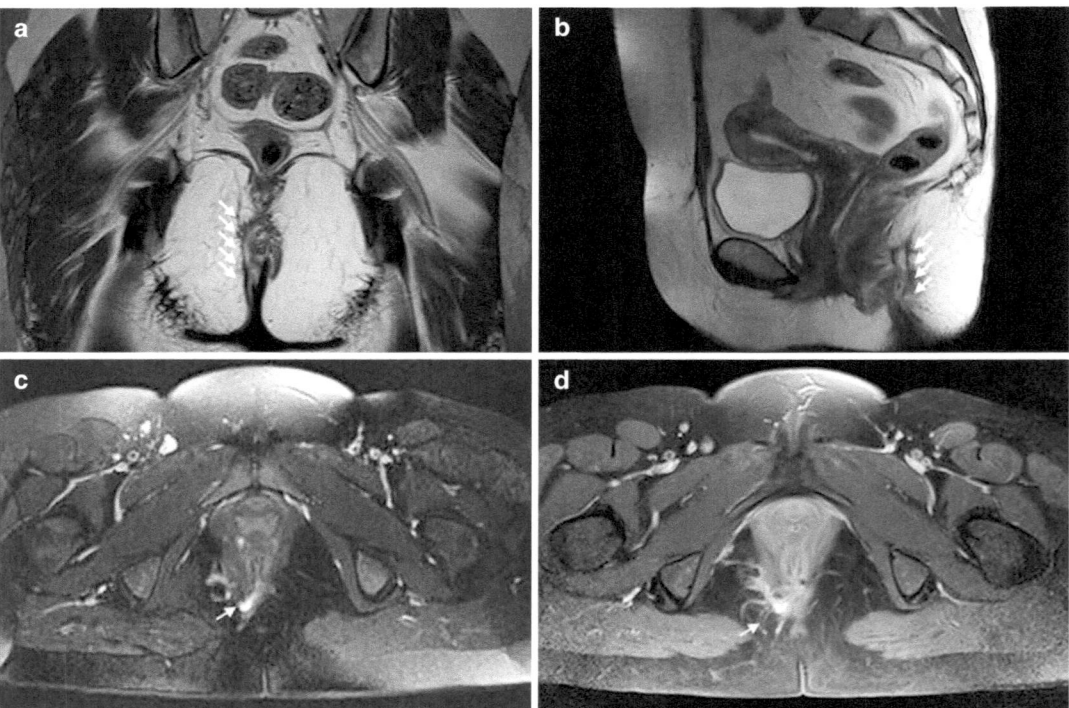

Fig. 13.1 Transsphincteric perianal fistula. The first MRI examination reveals a transsphincteric perianal fistula at 9 o'clock with abscess in right ischioanal space. T2-W images on paracoronal (**a**) and parasagittal (**b**) planes show deposition of fistulous tract (*white arrows*). Hyperintense signal on T2-W images (**c**) corresponds to the local inflammatory activity of fistula (*white arrow*), while on gadolinium-enhanced T1-weighted images (*white arrow* in **c**), an increase in signal intensity of inflammatory tissue can be seen because of increased tissue perfusion

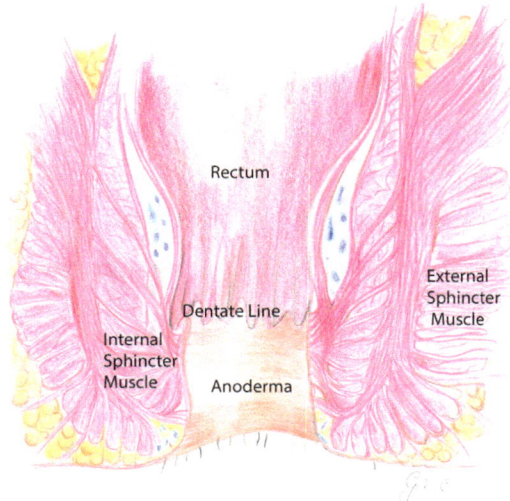

Rectum

External
Sphincter
Muscle

Dentate Line

Internal
Sphincter
Muscle

Anoderma

Fig. 13.2 Coronal section of the anal canal demonstrating the external and internal sphincters and the longitudinal muscle bundles

of perianal fistulas and the assessment of fistula activity (scoring), a dynamic measure that is sensitive to change under treatment.

Regarding the anatomic description, it is important to evaluate both the ends of any fistula, the epithelialized surface of the anal canal, and the perianal skin.

The relationship of the cutaneous opening to the expected site of the enteric opening has been described by Goodsall [15]: usually, cutaneous openings anterior to the transverse anal line are associated with direct radial fistulous tracks into the anal canal, while the posterior ones have tracks that enter the canal in the midline posteriorly. Exceptions are external openings more than 3 cm from the anal verge. However, the cutaneous opening is evident to the surgeon and the role of the radiologist is not its demonstration.

In 1934, Milligan and Morgan [16] classified anorectal fistulas according to their relationship to the anorectal ring, formed by the puborectalis muscle, as follows:

- Subcutaneous
- Low anal (below the dentate line)
- High anal (above the dentate line but below the anal ring)

- Anorectal below the levator ani muscle (ischiorectal or infralevator)
- Anorectal above the levator ani muscle (pelvirectal or supralevator)
- Submucous (high intermuscular between the internal and external anal sphincters)

In 1976, Parks et al. proposed a more anatomically precise classification system describing the course and relationship of perianal fistulas to the sphincter mechanism with reference to the coronal plane [6]; Parks identified four main types of fistulas (see Fig. 13.3) but numerous variations of each occur:

- *Intersphincteric* (most common; ~70 %): are confined to the intersphincteric space and internal sphincter. They result from perianal abscesses.
- *Transsphincteric* (25 %): are the result of ischiorectal abscesses, with extension of the tract through the external sphincter; it crosses both internal and external sphincters.
- *Suprasphincteric* (5 %): are the result of supralevator abscesses. They pass through the levator ani muscle, over the top of the puborectalis muscle, and into the intersphincteric space, without relationship with anal sphincter.
- *Extrasphincteric* (1 %): bypass the anal canal and sphincter mechanism, passing through the ischiorectal fossa and levator ani muscle, and open high in the rectum (Fig. 13.4).

An easier classification used in clinical practice is the one proposed by the American Gastroenterological Association (AGA) [17]: it distinguishes between simple fistulas, which are low, including superficial, intersphincteric, or intrasphincteric fistulas below the dentate line, with a single external opening, and are characterized by the absence of perianal complications, and complex fistulas that are high, arriving above the dentate line, with many external openings, and may be associated with perianal abscesses, rectal stricture, proctitis, or connection with the bladder or vagina.

The MR imaging-based St. James's University Hospital classification is an easy-to-use classification that uses axial anatomic landmarks, which

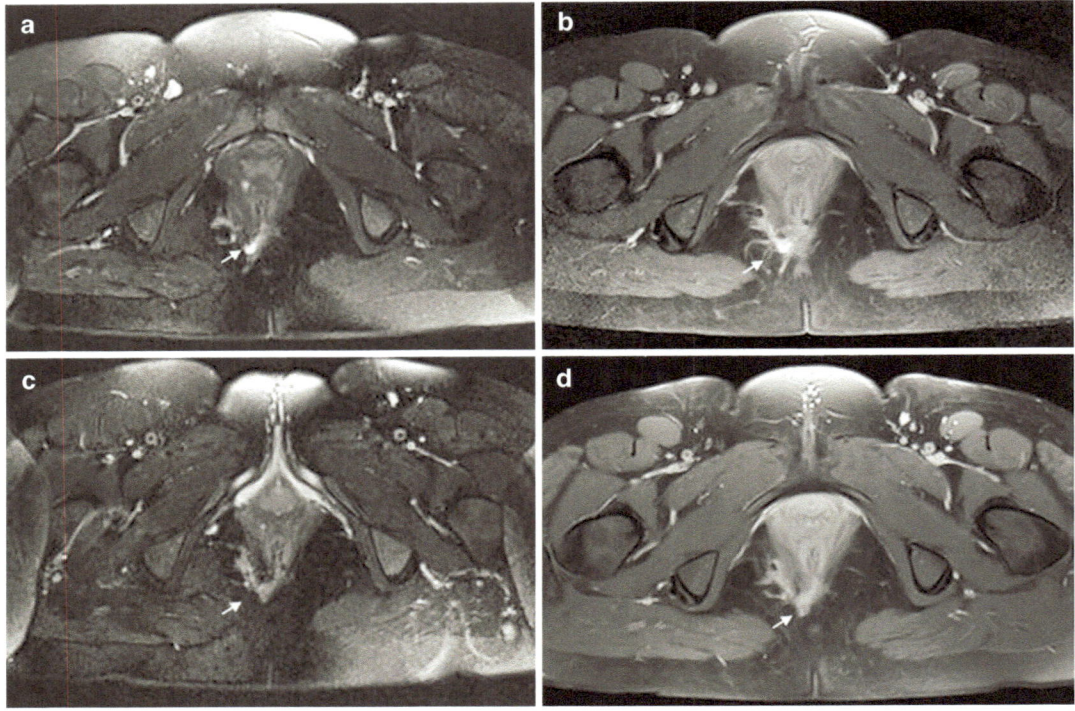

Fig. 13.3 On (**a, b**) same exam of Fig. 13.1; on (**c, d**) follow-up after 3 months demonstrated reduction of the local inflammatory activity of fistula (*arrow*) as well as of the signal intensity of inflammatory tissue

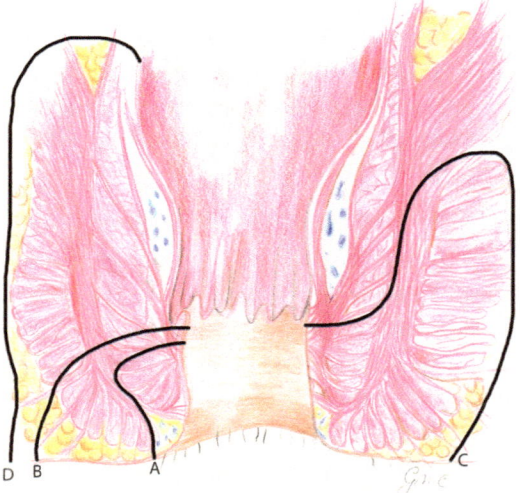

Fig. 13.4 Anatomic classification of anal fistulas according to Parks classification: *A* intersphincteric fistula; *B* transsphincteric fistula; *C* suprasphincteric fistula; *D* extrasphincteric fistula

are familiar to radiologists, and consists of five grades and relates the Parks surgical classification to anatomy seen at MR imaging in both axial and coronal planes:

- *Grade 1* – simple linear intersphincteric
- *Grade 2* – intersphincteric with abscess or secondary track
- *Grade 3* – transsphincteric
- *Grade 4* – transsphincteric with abscess or secondary track within the ischiorectal fossa
- *Grade 5* – supralevator and translevator extension

Considering the assessment of fistula activity, it is recommended to consider both clinical and radiological features. The Perianal Disease Activity Index (PDAI) is based on the assessment of quality of life (pain/restriction of activities and restriction of sexual activities) and perianal disease severity (fistula discharge, type of perianal disease, and degree of induration) [18, 19].

Concerning the diagnosis of anal fistulas in CD, physical examination remains the mainstay. The examiner should observe the entire perineum, looking for an external opening and eventual spontaneous discharge of pus or blood through it. Digital rectal examination may reveal a fibrous tract or cord beneath the skin.

Radiologic studies are not performed for routine evaluation since the anatomy of most anal fistulas can be determined in the operating room, and, until very recently, surgeons have operated without preoperative imaging [20].

13.2   Anal Endosonography

Anal endosonography (AES), with or without hydrogen peroxide, is safe, rapid, and well tolerated by patients [21], and its accuracy compared to clinical assessment of fistulas has been proved [22].

AES uses high-frequency sound wave probes (with a frequency between 5–16 MHz) to produce detailed high spatial resolution images of the sphincter muscles and other structures of the pelvic floor [14]. At AES, although a breach in the subepithelial layer of the anal canal is occasionally present, it is more common for the position of the internal opening to be revealed as a hypoechoic focus in the intersphincteric space that abuts the internal sphincter, often with a small corresponding defect in the internal sphincter [13].

Using a high-resolution 3D endoanal ultrasound, some perianal fistulas in patients with CD, unlike conventional fistula tracks, show a hypoechogenic fistula tract surrounded by a well-defined hyperechogenic area with a thin hypoechogenic edge in patients with Crohn's disease, and this has been called "Crohn's ultrasound fistula sign." The histological explanation of this sign is unknown, but it might be due to a deep inflammatory process associated with Crohn's fistula, with the hyperechoic component

of the sign being a reflection of inflammatory debris [23].

The accuracy of AES ranges between 86 and 95 % for correct classification of fistulas and 62–94 % for identification of internal openings [14]. Moreover, the Crohn's ultrasound fistula sign can differentiate between Crohn's related and cryptogenic fistulae in ano with a positive and negative predictive value of 87 and 93 %, respectively [23].

Even if sphincter mechanism and intersphincteric plane are usually well visualized with endosonography, some limits are inherent to this techniques as the difficulty to assess the external sphincter in some individuals, the difficulty in entering the probes in case of luminal stenosis, the inability in distinguishing infection from fibrosis, and failure to identify secondary ramifications and more distant sepsis because of an insufficient depth penetration [20].

13.3   Fistulography

Fistulography consists in the catheterization with a fine cannula of the external opening of the fistula and in the injection of a water-soluble contrast agent in order to establish the direction and openings of a fistula. However, many limits pertain to this radiologic technique as the difficulty or failure in the identification of the primary track if it is plugged in with debris, the absence of visualization of sphincter muscles, and of the levator plate [13].

13.4   Computed Tomography

Computed tomography (CT), performed with rectally and intravenously administered contrast media, may depict fistula in ano and initial reports were encouraging [24, 25].

However, CT cannot be used for fistula classification since the attenuation values for the sphincters, levator ani, fibrotic fistulous tracks, and active fistulas are quite similar resulting in a difficult characterization of these structures on

CT, unless the track contains gas or leaked contrast material [13, 20].

However, CT may be helpful in the setting of perirectal inflammatory because it is better for delineating fluid pockets that require drainage than for delineating small fistulas.

Potentially, the disadvantages of CT might be overcome by using multidetector row CT fistulography, but the widespread of this technique is limited by radiation exposure and the ready availability of MR imaging, which is a radiation-free technique [13].

However, in the acute setting, MR is not always immediately available; hence, it has been recently proposed to perform a CT scan after rectal administration of a contrast (gastrografin or barium) through a catheter in the anal canal and intravenous administration of an iodinated contrast [26, 27]. Using this technique, a fistulous tract appears as a well-defined tubular, soft tissue, or fluid-/air-filled structure that arises from the anal sphincter, while an infected fistula will typically have a thick, enhancing wall along with surrounding inflammatory changes [26]. Furthermore, advances in CT hardware and software enable scans to be performed with a much lower radiation dose than conventional CT scans [27].

13.5   Magnetic Resonance

Pelvic MRI has become the gold standard imaging technique for perianal CD. Considering all imaging techniques available, magnetic resonance (MR) proved to have a more important diagnostic role in patients with rectal/pelvic CD, showing a significant superiority [28]; this is due to its multiplanarity, spatial and contrast resolution, which allows a satisfactory depiction of fistulas and other possible pathological findings (abscesses) of inflammatory bowel disease [29].

MR imaging examinations performed using a body coil do not require patient preparation and are well tolerated, while endoanal coils are poorly tolerated in symptomatic patients, and

though providing an excellent anatomic detail of the anal sphincters, they fail to provide the overview required for surgical management and are susceptible to motion artifact [13, 30, 31]. Moreover, endoanal coils have not an adequate depth penetration; hence, it does not allow a good visualization of distant organs or inflammatory manifestation of perianal CD.

Spasmolytics administered intramuscularly may help to reduce motion-induced artifact. However, the choice of coil depends mainly on personal preference, availability, patient group studied, and the clinical question in each patient; when circumstances allow, an optimal examination will be achieved by using both external and endoluminal coils [13].

MR imaging accurately visualizes the anal sphincter and the pelvic floor muscles, as well as the fistula tracts and abscesses, with an accuracy ranging from 76 to 100 % [14].

The combined analysis of axial, coronal, and sagittal images allows an accurate study of the fistula tracks evaluating their course, extension, their relationships, and, in particular, the relations between fistulae, the anal sphincter complex, and the surrounding pelvic structures.

Axial and coronal MR images help in identifying the relations of the fistula with the sphincteric apparatus, the levator ani, and the ischial rectal fossa; on the other hand, sagittal images are useful in the evaluation of rectovesical and rectovaginal fistulae and of presacral disease.

13.5.1 MR Sequences and Image Plans

Considering the MR sequences to image fistula in ano, various investigators have adopted different strategies [32–35]. Anatomic precision is needed to adequately assess the course of the fistula with respect to adjacent structures.

Most of the radiologists prefer use of the rapid and convenient fast spin-echo T2-weighted sequence, due to its good contrast between hyperintense fluid in the tract and the hypointense fibrous wall of the fistula and the good discrimination between the several layers of the anal sphincter [32, 34].

Others use T1-weighted sequences, before and after intravenous contrast material injection [33]. Fat suppression is applied to both T2-weighted and T1-weighted, before and after gadolinium-enhanced sequences.

Unenhanced T1-weighted (T1W) images provide an excellent anatomic overview of the sphincter complex, levator plate, and the ischiorectal fossae, while on T2-weighted (T2W) and STIR images; pathologic processes including fistulas, secondary fistulous tracks, and fluid collections are clearly depicted as areas of high signal intensity in contrast with the lower signal intensity of the sphincters, muscles, and fat [20].

Recently, Horsthuis et al. [36] investigated the role of dynamic contrast-enhanced MR imaging in the diagnosis of disease activity in perianal CD and concluded that rapid enhancement and maximum enhancement during dynamic series correlate to disease activity.

Furthermore, gradient-echo T1-weighted dynamic intravenous contrast material-enhanced MR imaging combined with T2-weighted imaging proved to be useful to assess perianal fistulas and their complications, clearly demonstrating active fistulous tracks, secondary ramifications, and abscesses [20, 33].

STIR images can also be used in replacement of T1W images after contrast medium due to their high capacity of detecting the walls of the fistulae and their degree of inflammation.

Diffusion-weighted images display information based on diffusion of water molecules. As inflammatory tissues have a high signal intensity on diffusion-weighted images, DWI may be of value for evaluating perianal fistula activity [37].

With regard to imaging planes, a localizer in three directions is needed in order to align the T2W sequences axial and coronal to the anal canal. It is central to success that imaging planes are correctly aligned with respect to the anal canal; hence, oblique transverse and coronal planes oriented orthogonal and parallel, respectively, to the anal sphincter, are needed and they are most easily planned by using a midline sagittal image [13].

13.5.2 MR Interpretation

The visualization of the fistulae is related to the degree of inflammation and consequently to their content and to the sequences used in the study. In the active phases of the disease, the fistula shows both walls containing granulation tissue and fluid or mucin in its lumen; furthermore, it presents itself as a stria or as a band of tissue with high signal intensity, well contrasted compared to the muscles and to the surrounding fat. On T1W images, acquired with fat suppression and after the use of paramagnetic contrast agents (gadolinium and its chelates), the walls of fistulae – containing granulation tissue – as well as the areas of active inflammation, exhibit intense postcontrastographic enhancement.

Active fistulas are filled with pus and granulation tissue, thus appearing as longitudinal structures hyperintense on T2W images and on STIR sequences. In the STIR images, the signal suppression of adipose tissue provides a good contrast between fistula and adjacent tissues and makes easier its identification.

On T1W FSE sequences, active granulation tissue is hyperintense after contrast medium injection, while the fluid in the lumen remains hypointense.

At axial DWI, fistula exhibits spotty slightly high signal intensity [37].

The fistulae in the active phase are often surrounded by hypointense fibrous walls, which can be relatively thin, particularly in patients with recurrent disease, or with a recent surgical operation; however, in case of edema, the walls may appear hyperintense, and this hyperintensity can spread into the surrounding parenchyma.

The external anal sphincter is moderately hypointense and its wall contrasts with the fat of the ischioanal fossa, both in STIR and FAT-SAT sequences. It is therefore relatively easy to distinguish the presence of a fistula in the ischioanal fossa.

The main advantage of the MR is its ability in recognizing the extension associated to the primary fistulous tract, which is hyperintense both on T2W and STIR sequences, and shows contrast enhancement. It is also important to recognize the relationships with the elevator ani muscle and the extensions above it.

13.5.3 MR Report

When reporting an anal canal fistula in MR reports, it is important to assess:

• Internal opening: this is the starting point of the fistula from the anal canal. Most of anal fistulas open into the anal canal at the level of the dentate line, but unfortunately, the dentate line cannot be identified as a discrete anatomic entity on MR, even when endoanal receiver coils are used. However, the general position of the dentate line can be estimated with sufficient precision for the imaging assessment: it is probably best appreciated on coronal views at approximately the mid-anal canal level, between the superior border of the puborectalis muscle and the most caudal extent of the subcutaneous external sphincter [13].
• External opening and track of the fistula: this corresponds to the position of the mucosal opening on axial images (using the anal clock). Surgeons describe the site and direction of fistulous tracks by referring to the "anal clock," which is, the view of the anal region with the patient in the lithotomy position. At 12 o'clock is the anterior perineum and at 6 o'clock, the natal cleft; 3 o'clock refers to the left lateral aspect, and 9 o'clock, to the right of the anal canal [20]. These descriptions correspond exactly with the view of the anal canal on axial MR images.

Moreover, thanks to MR imaging, it is possible to demonstrate extensions associated with a primary tract, as secondary fistulas and abscesses.

In particular, it is useful to delineate the course of the fistula tracks with respect to the ischiorectal fossa and to assess any confluence of different fistulas and/or of fistulae and abscesses and/or of fistulae and nearby organs.

13.5.4 Pitfalls

Few concepts should be kept in mind to avoid pitfalls: veins can be mistaken for fistulas, but veins usually are thin-walled, tortuous, symmetric structures; a pilonidal sinus may resemble a fistula, but several findings, as extension to the intersphincteric space in fistulas, help one to discriminate between the two [38].

13.6 Follow-Up of Perianal Fistulas in Crohn's Disease

Approximately one-third of the patients who have Crohn's disease have perianal involvement [39].

Perianal involvement is seen in a significant proportion of children with Crohn's disease [17, 40] and is a significant source of symptoms and extraluminal disease complications. A number of medical and surgical treatment strategies have been developed to treat Crohn's perianal disease, but a unique challenge in perianal fistulizing Crohn's disease is to monitor the response to the treatment. The most common clinical parameter used is cessation of drainage of the fistulas [41]. The healing of fistulas occurs from the skin (external orifice) to inside (internal orifice); therefore, cessation of drainage from the external orifice may not be the best indicator of complete healing of the fistula.

3D endoanal ultrasound (3D-EAUS) and pelvic magnetic resonance imaging (MRI) are the imaging modalities commonly used in adults to evaluate this disease [20, 42, 43].

3D-EAUS is a valuable tool to represent the normal anatomy of the anal canal resulting in simple, cheap, readily available, and less demanding for the patient and reaching high diagnostic accuracy. It allows rapid evaluation for specialized equipment, is easy to perform and easily reproducible, is painless, and does not require patient preparation.

This method can be very useful also in the follow-up of anal diseases, both to study surgical drainages and in the postoperative study of anal fistulae, providing excellent imaging of the rectal wall, of the internal and external sphincters, and of the intersphincteric plane, and of the position of the internal opening and of fistulous tract.

3D-EAUS is more accurate in comparison to MRI in the individuation of intersphincteric/submucosal fistulas, better depicting the intersphincteric plane and both the internal and external sphincters. In fact, the introduction of 3D technique has optimized US evaluation.

However, above all in patients with Crohn's disease, where in most cases perianal involvement results complicated, 3D technique has limited ability to resolve ischioanal and supralevator infections and it does not allow a reliable distinction between infection and fibrosis [13, 44–48].

MRI is more accurate in comparison to 3D-EUAS in the individuation of suprasphincteric and extrasphincteric fistulas and has the advantage of an excellent intrinsic soft tissue resolution, thus showing the fistula tract in the context of the surrounding structures. It has a wider FOV than 3D-EAUS and results more suited for the assessment of complex branching tracts, the lateral extension into the perianal spaces, and the cranial extension above the levator ani [49].

It is useful for successful treatment by correct assessment of the extent of disease, in the treatment response monitoring of perianal fistulas, especially in Crohn's disease, in the differential diagnosis between infection from fibrosis, ischioanal from supralevator infections, and, in coronal plane, between supra- and infralevator extension. It could be a valid second-level examination, especially in the case of abscesses or when complex tracts where internal opening cannot be confidently shown and tracts seen going up across the pelvic diaphragm [28, 31, 49–52].

MRI of the pelvis has been shown to be useful, not only in defining the anatomy of the pelvic region in perianal fistula but also in measuring inflammatory activity of the fistula [53, 54].

The follow-up MRI is generally obtained from 3 months to up to 2 years after the baseline MR examination (Fig. 13.3).

Despite various studies have been conducted, the precise role of pelvic MRI in monitoring therapy is still being investigated [53, 55].

Various parameters such as number of fistulas, complexity of fistulas, presence of abscesses, rectal wall involvement, and T2 hyperintensity have been used to monitor disease activity [56].

The most common MRI-based score used in literature is the Van Assche which gives a particular score to each anatomical and inflammatory parameter.

The anatomical parameters include the number of fistulas, the extension of fistulas, and the location of fistulas, whereas the inflammatory parameters include hyperintensity on T2 images, presence of collections, and rectal wall involvement. The most important parameter of local inflammatory activity is T2 hyperintensity.

Few prior studies in adults have shown a significant decrease in Van Assche score with treatment [54, 57], whereas there are other studies that did not show a decrease in Van Assche score with treatment [55, 56]. In the study of Kulkarni et al., the only inflammatory parameter that decreased with decreasing severity of disease was the presence of collections.

According to Shenoy-Bhangle et al. [58], the length of a perianal fistula on the first MR study is a significant predictor of treatment response on the follow-up MR study.

Maximum single fistula length of <2.5 cm predicts treatment response, while aggregate length ≥2.5 cm predicts disease progression. Small abscesses (<1 cm^3) respond to medical therapy at a rate comparable to surgical treatment of larger abscesses and often do not require surgical intervention.

Villa et al. [69] were the first to adopt the gadolinium-enhanced T1W images as indicators of fistula activity. On gadolinium-enhanced T1W images, a marked increase in signal intensity of inflammatory tissue can be seen because of increased tissue perfusion [60]. Villa et al. used percentage increase of fistula activity after contrast administration [P.I.], which is the signal intensity of the fistula compared with the signal

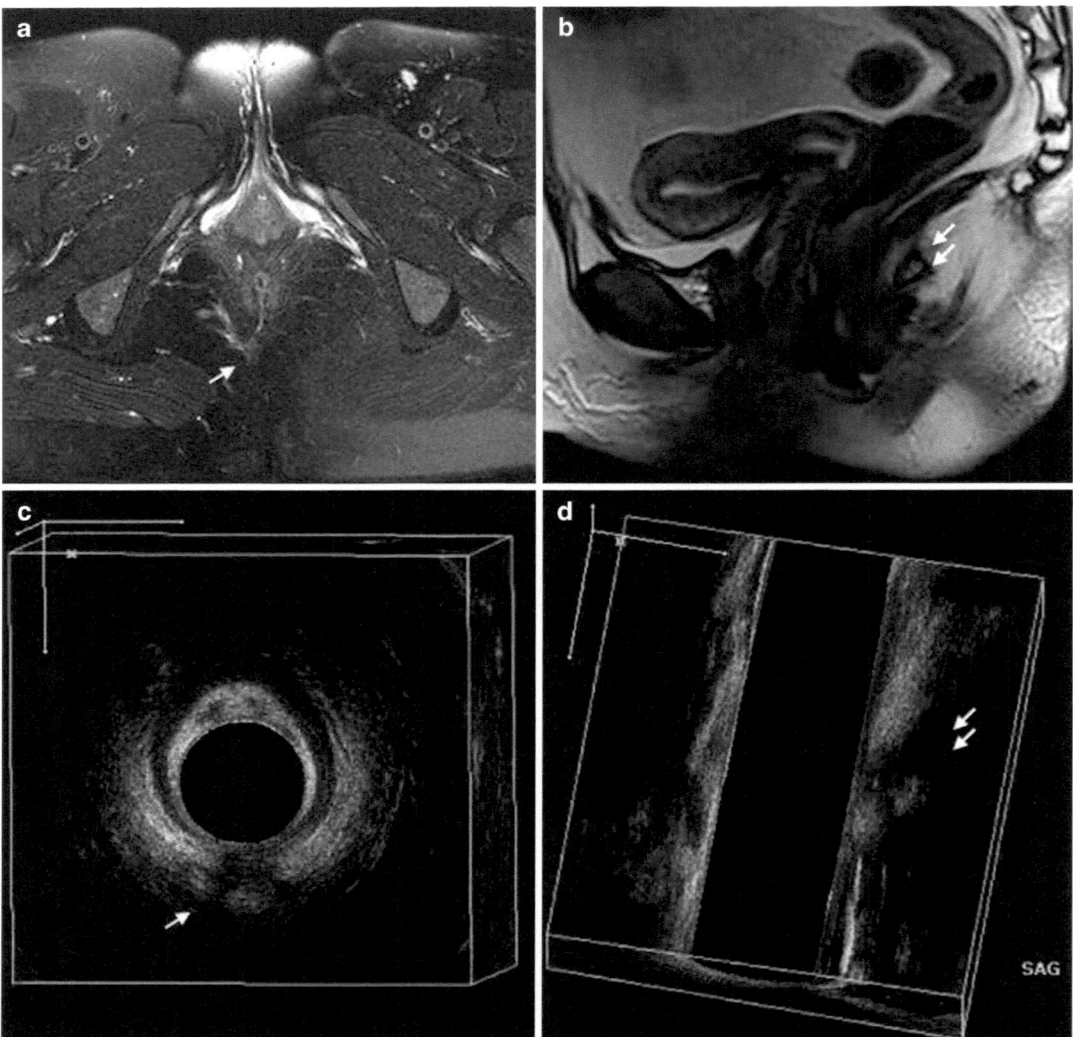

Fig. 13.5 Same patient of Figs. 13.1 and 13.2; follow-up after 3 months from Fig. 13.2 showing a reduction of inflammatory activity of fistula and of adjacent adipose tissue. 3D-EAUS on axial plane (**c**, **d**) better depicts the involvement of the contact of fistula with internal anal sphincter than axial MRI image (**a**, **b**); on the contrary, MRI is more accurate in comparison to 3D-EUAS in the definition of extension into the perianal spaces

intensity of adjacent healthy fat, to determine the disease activity of the fistula.

The measurement of PI is not time consuming and could be done in every MRI station. PI = ([signal intensity of fistula – signal intensity of healthy fat] × 100/signal intensity of healthy fat).

Although the PI did not decrease significantly with treatment, further prospective studies may be required to study the role of this parameter in follow-up during treatment of perianal Crohn's disease.

References

1. Hellers G, Bergstrand O, Ewerth S, Holmström B. Occurrence and outcome after primary treatment of anal fistulae in Crohn's disease. Gut. 1980;21:525.
2. Farmer RG, Hawk WA, Turnbull Jr RB. Clinical patterns in Crohn's disease: a statistical study of 615 cases. Gastroenterology. 1975;68:627.
3. Rankin GB, Watts HD, Melnyk CS, Kelley Jr ML. National Cooperative Crohn's Disease Study: extraintestinal manifestations and perianal complications. Gastroenterology. 1979;77:914.

4. Schwartz D, Loftus E, Tremaine W, et al. The natural history of fistulizing Crohn's disease: a population based study. Gastroenterology. 2000;118:A337.

5. Mc CI. The comparative anatomy and pathology of anal glands. Arris and Gale lecture delivered at the Royal College of Surgeons of England on 25th February 1965. Ann R Coll Surg Engl. 1967;40:36–67.

6. Parks AG, Gordon PH, Hardcastle JD. A classification of fistula-in-ano. Br J Surg. 1976;63:1–12.

7. McKee RF, Keenan RA. Perianal Crohn's disease – is it all bad news? Dis Colon Rectum. 1996;39:136.

8. van Dongen LM, Lubbers EJ. Perianal fistulas in patients with Crohn's disease. Arch Surg. 1986;121:1187.

9. Schwartz DA, Loftus Jr EV, Tremaine WJ, et al. The natural history of fistulizing Crohn's disease in Olmsted County, Minnesota. Gastroenterology. 2002;122:875.

10. Lichtenstein GR, Hanauer SB, Sandborn WJ. Practice Parameters Committee of American College of Gastroenterology. Management of Crohn's disease in adults. Am J Gastroenterol. 2009;104:465.

11. Chiari H. Uber die analen divertikel der rectumschleimahut und ihre beziehung zu den anal fisteln. Wien Med Press. 1878;19:1482–3.

12. Robinson AM, DeNobile JW. Anorectal abscess and fistula-in-ano. J Natl Med Assoc. 1988;80:1209–13.

13. Halligan S, Stoker J. Imaging of fistula in ano. Radiology. 2006;239:18–33.

14. Gecse KB, Bemelman W, Kamm MA, Stoker J, Khanna R, Ng SC, Panés J, van Assche G, Liu Z, Hart A, Levesque BG, D'Haens G, World Gastroenterology Organization, International Organisation for Inflammatory Bowel Diseases IOIBD, European Society of Coloproctology and Robarts Clinical Trials; World Gastroenterology Organization International Organisation for Inflammatory Bowel Diseases IOIBD European Society of Coloproctology and Robarts Clinical Trials. A global consensus on the classification, diagnosis and multidisciplinary treatment of perianal fistulising Crohn's disease. Gut. 2014;63:1381–92.

15. Goodsall DH, Miles WE. Diseases of the anus and rectum. London: Longmans, Green; 1900.

16. Milligan ET, Morgan CN. Surgical anatomy of the anal canal with special reference to anorectal fistulae. Lancet. 1934;2:1213.

17. Sandborn WJ, Fazio VW, Feagan BG, Hanauer SB. AGA technical review on perianal Crohn's disease. Gastroenterology. 2003;125:1508–30.

18. Allan A, Linares L, Spooner HA, Alexander-Williams J. Clinical index to quantitate symptoms of perianal Crohn's disease. Dis Colon Rectum. 1992;35:656–61.

19. Irvine EJ. Usual therapy improves perianal Crohn's disease as measured by a new disease activity index. McMaster IBD Study Group. J Clin Gastroenterol. 1995;20:27–32.

20. Morris J, Spencer JA, Ambrose NS. MR imaging classification of perianal fistulas and its implications for patient management. Radiographics. 2000;20:623–35; discussion 635–7.

21. Pomerri F, Dodi G, Pintacuda G, Amadio L, Muzzio PC. Anal endosonography and fistulography for fistula-in-ano. Radiol Med. 2010;115:771–83.

22. Buchanan GN, Halligan S, Bartram CI, et al. Clinical examination, endosonography, and MR imaging in preoperative assessment of fistula in ano: comparison with outcome-based reference standard. Radiology. 2004;233:674–81.

23. Zawadzki A, Starck M, Bohe M, Thorlacius H. A unique 3D endoanal ultrasound feature of perianal Crohn's fistula: the 'Crohn ultrasound fistula sign'. Colorectal Dis. 2012;14(9):e608–11.

24. Guillaumin E, Jeffrey RB, Shea WJ, et al. Perirectal inflammatory disease: CT findings. Radiology. 1986;161:153–7.

25. Yousem DM, Fishman EK, Jones B. Crohn disease: perirectal and perianal findings at CT. Radiology. 1988;167:331–4.

26. Khati NJ, Sondel Lewis N, Frazier AA, Obias V, Zeman RK, Hill MC. CT of acute perianal abscesses and infected fistulae: a pictorial essay. Emerg Radiol. 2015;22:329–35.

27. Liang C, Lu Y, Zhao B, Du Y, Wang C, Jiang W. Imaging of anal fistulas: comparison of computed tomographic fistulography and magnetic resonance imaging. Korean J Radiol. 2014;15(6):712–23.

28. Lunniss PJ, Barker PG, Sultan AH, Armstrong P, Reznek RH, Bartram CI, Cottam KS, Phillips RK. Magnetic resonance imaging of fistula-in-ano. Dis Colon Rectum. 1994;37(7):708–18.

29. Llauger J, Pllmer J, Pèrez C, et al. The normal and pathologic ischiorectal fossa at CT and MR imaging. Radiographics. 1998;18:61–82.

30. Hussain SM, Stoker J, Schouten WR, Hop WCJ, Lameris JS. Fistula-in-ano: endoanal sonography versus endoanal MR imaging in classification. Radiology. 1996;200:475–81.

31. Halligan S, Bartram CI. MR imaging of fistula-in-ano: are endoanal coils the gold standard? AJR Am J Roentgenol. 1998;171:407–12.

32. Stoker J, Rociu E, Zwamborn AW, Schouten WR, Laméris JS. Endoluminal MR imaging of the rectum and anus: technique, applications, and pitfalls. RadioGraphics. 1999;19:383–98.

33. Spencer JA, Ward J, Beckingham IJ, Adams C, Ambrose NS. Dynamic contrast-enhanced MR imaging of perianal fistulas. AJR Am J Roentgenol. 1996;167:735–41.

34. Maier AG, Funovics MA, Kreuzer SH, et al. Evaluation of perianal sepsis: comparison of anal endosonography and magnetic resonance imaging. J Magn Reson Imaging. 2001;14:254–60.

35. Halligan S, Healy JC, Bartram CI. Magnetic resonance imaging of fistula-in-ano: STIR or SPIR? Br J Radiol. 1998;71:141–5.

36. Horsthuis K, Lavini C, Bipat S, Stokkers PC, Stoker J. Perianal Crohn disease: evaluation of dynamic contrast-enhanced MR imaging as an indicator of disease activity. Radiology. 2009;251(2):380–7.

37. Yoshizako T, Wada A, Takahara T, Kwee TC, Nakamura M, Uchida K, Hara S, Luijten PR, Kitagaki H. Diffusion-weighted MRI for evaluating perianal fistula activity: feasibility study. Eur J Radiol. 2012;81:2049–53.

38. Horsthuis K, Stoker J. MRI of perianal Crohn's disease. AJR Am J Roentgenol. 2004;183:1309–15.

39. American Gastroenterological Association Clinical Practice Committee. American Gastroenterological Association medical position statement: perianal Crohn's disease. Gastroenterology. 2003;125:1503–7.

40. Essary B, Kim J, Anupindi S, et al. Pelvic MRI in children with Crohn disease and suspected perianal involvement. Pediatr Radiol. 2007;37:201–8.

41. Present DH, Rutgeerts P, Targan S, et al. Infliximab for the treatment of fistulas in patients with Crohn's disease. N Engl J Med. 1999;340:1398–405.

42. Schwartz DA, White CM, Wise PE, et al. Use of endoscopic ultrasound to guide combination medical and surgical therapy for patients with Crohn's perianal fistulas. Inflamm Bowel Dis. 2005;11:727–32.

43. Koelbel G, Schmiedl U, Majer MC, et al. Diagnosis of fistulae and sinus tracts in patients with Crohn disease: value of MR imaging. AJR Am J Roentgenol. 1989;152:999–1003.

44. Sun MR, Smith MP, Kane RA. Current techniques in imaging of fistula in ano: three-dimensional endoanal ultrasound and magnetic resonance imaging. Semin Ultrasound CT MR. 2008;29(6):454–71.

45. Siddiqui MR, Ashrafian H, Tozer P, Daulatzai N, Burling D, Hart A, Athanasiou T, Phillips RK. A diagnostic accuracy meta-analysis of endoanal ultrasound and MRI for perianal fistula assessment. Dis Colon Rectum. 2012;55(5):576–85.

46. Sahni VA, Ahmad R, Burling D. Which method is best for imaging of perianal fistula? Abdom Imaging. 2008;33(1):26–30.

47. Reginelli A, Mandato Y, Cavaliere C, Pizza NL, Russo A, Cappabianca S, Brunese L, Rotondo A, Grassi R. Three-dimensional anal endosonography in depicting anal-canal anatomy. Radiol Med. 2012;117:759–71.

48. Brunese L, Amitrano M, Gargano V, Pinto A, Vallone G, Grassi R, Rotondo A, Smaltino F. Role of anal endosonography in inflammation and trauma of the anal canal. Radiol Med. 1996;92(6):742–7.

49. Panes J, Bouhnik Y, Reinisch W, Stoker J, Taylor SA, Baumgart DC, Danese S, Halligan S, Marincek B, Matos C, Peyrin-Biroulet L, Rimola J, Rogler G, van Assche G, Ardizzone S, Ba-Ssalamah A, Bali MA, Bellini D, Biancone L, Castiglione F, Ehehalt R, Grassi R, Kucharzik T, Maccioni F, Maconi G, Magro F, Martín-Comín J, Morana G, Pendsé D, Sebastian S, Signore A, Tolan D, Tielbeek JA, Weishaupt D, Wiarda B, Laghi A. Imaging techniques for assessment of inflammatory bowel disease: joint ECCO and ESGAR evidence-based consensus guidelines. J Crohns Colitis. 2013;7(7):556–85. doi:10.1016/j.crohns.2013.02.020.

50. Grassi R, Rotondo A, Catalano O, Amitrano M, Vallone G, Gargano V, Fanucci A. Endoanal ultrasonography, defecography, and enema of the colon in the radiologic study of incontinence. Radiol Med. 1995;89(6):792–7. Review. Italian.

51. Taylor SA, Halligan S, Bartram CI. Pilonidal sinus disease: MR imaging distinction from fistula in ano. Radiology. 2003;226(3):662–7. Epub 2003 Jan 15.

52. Nelson R. Anorectal abscess fistula: what do we know? Surg Clin North Am. 2002;82(6):1139–51.

53. Ng SC, Plamondon S, Gupta A, et al. Prospective evaluation of anti- tumor necrosis factor therapy guided by magnetic resonance imaging for Crohn's perineal fistulas. Am J Gastroenterol. 2009;104:2973–86.

54. Karmiris K, Bielen D, Vanbeckevoort D, et al. Long-term monitoring of infliximab therapy for perianal fistulizing Crohn's disease by using magnetic resonance imaging. Clin Gastroenterol Hepatol. 2011;9:130–6.

55. Tougeron D, Savoye G, Savoye-Collet C, et al. Predicting factors of fistula healing and clinical remission after infliximab-based combined therapy for perianal fistulizing Crohn's disease. Dig Dis Sci. 2009;54:1746–52.

56. Horsthuis K, Ziech ML, Bipat S, et al. Evaluation of an MRI-based score of disease activity in perianal fistulizing Crohn's disease. Clin Imaging. 2011;35:360–5.

57. Van Assche G, Vanbeckevoort D, Bielen D, et al. Magnetic resonance imaging of the effects of infliximab on perianal fistulizing Crohn's disease. Am J Gastroenterol. 2003;98:332–9.

58. Shenoy-Bhangle A, Nimkin K, Goldner D, Bradley WF, Israel EJ, Gee MS. MRI predictors of treatment response for perianal fistulizing Crohn disease in children and young adults. Pediatr Radiol. 2014;44(1):23–9.

59. Villa C, Pompili G, Franceschelli G, et al. Role of magnetic resonance imaging in evaluation of the activity of perianal Crohn's disease. Eur J Radiol. 2012;81:616–22.

60. Weinmann H-J, Brasch RC, Press W-R, et al. Characteristics of gadolinium-DTPA complex: a potential NMR contrast agent. AJR Am J Roentgenol. 1984;142:619–24.

Extraintestinal Findings in Crohn's Disease Patients

14

Gian Andrea Rollandi, Riccardo Piccazzo, and Francesco Paparo

Crohn's disease is a chronic inflammatory bowel disease with a relapsing and remitting course that may affect any part of the gastrointestinal tract, often with multiple discontinuous involvements [1–3].

This pathology involves all the layers of the bowel, with the first localization in the submucosal layer, which becomes filled of hyperplastic lymphoid tissue and, being associate with lymphatic stasis, develop with dystrophy and fissuration of the superior mucosal layer [4, 5]. These alterations lead to the development of aphtoid ulcers, alternated with normal mucosal tracts, in a pattern described as "cobblestone."

The inflammatory process can extend also toward the muscular layer, reaching the serosal surface, stimulates fibrin production, causing adhesions between adjacent bowel loops, and to parietal and visceral peritoneum. Disease progression into the mesentery produces typical alteration such as fibro-fatty proliferation, extraenteric fistulae, and abscesses.

Over intestinal alterations, Crohn's disease can be associated with pathological processes affecting organs and systems outside the gastrointestinal tract, generally known as extraintestinal manifestations (Table 14 1).

Starting from the pathogenetic mechanism and the relationship with the underlying disease, these alterations can be classified in four categories [6–8] (Table 14.1).

Extraintestinal manifestations are often the onset symptomatology, producing greater morbidity than the intestinal disease. The presence of extraintestinal manifestations leads to a higher risk to develop other complications [9].

Table 14.1 Extraintestinal manifestation related to Crohn's disease, classified on the basis of the pathogenetic mechanism and the relationship with the underlying disease

Related to active inflammation, with a self-immune-like pathogenetic mechanism
Arthropathies
Skin pathologies
Ocular and oral alterations
Primary sclerosing cholangitis
Related to small bowel alterations, based on metabolic dysfunction
Cholelithiasis
Nephrolithiasis and obstructive uropathy
Related to therapeutic drugs
Osteopenia
Osteoporosis
Nonspecific manifestations
Amyloidosis
Pulmonary alterations
Risk of neoplastic degeneration (adenocarcinoma, lymphoma)

G.A. Rollandi (✉) • R. Piccazzo • F. Paparo
Radiodiagnostic Unit, E.O. Ospedali Galliera,
Mura della Cappuccine 14, Genoa 16128, Italy
e-mail: gianandrea.rollandi@galliera.it

© Springer International Publishing Switzerland 2016
G. Lo Re, M. Midiri (eds.), *Crohn's Disease: Radiological Features and Clinical-Surgical Correlations*,
DOI 10.1007/978-3-319-23066-5_14

Many extraintestinal manifestations of Crohn's disease have a symptomatic behavior synchronous with intestinal pathology, sensibility to therapy included. Some others, such as primary sclerosing cholangitis and ankylosing spondylitis, have a course independent from the bowel disease activity [10].

While the correlation of the different extraintestinal manifestations with inflammatory bowel diseases (IBD) is known, the specific pathogenic mechanisms are not clear. Some systemic disorders may be based on immunologic processes, being likely related to the pathophysiology of the underlying intestinal disease. Others seem to be caused by intestinal bacterial overgrowth, or being direct iatrogenic complications of the therapy [9, 11, 12].

In this context, it is useful to maintain a focus on extraintestinal manifestations, which are an important source of decreased quality of life for affected patients. Imaging plays an important role in early recognition of extraintestinal manifestations, guiding therapy and reducing overall morbidity. Therefore, the ideal technique should provide not only information about gastrointestinal tract but also about the other organs at the same time.

Bowel *ultrasonography* is often used for an initial screening in cases of suspected Crohn's disease [13], but it lacks panoramic view of the whole abdominal cavity, resulting in a difficult detection of extraintestinal manifestations [14, 15]. So it could be a valid option only in the follow-up of specific pathological bowel loops, but not for general restaging.

Conversely, cross-sectional imaging techniques optimized for small bowel evaluation (*computed tomography (CT)* and *magnetic resonance imaging (MRI)*) should allow a combined and simultaneous demonstration of both intestinal lesions and extramural complications [16, 17].

Currently, the advantages of CT over MR imaging include higher spatial resolution, greater availability, and, in particular, the possibility depict together bowel wall inflammation and extraenteric complications in shorter examination times. The most important limiting factor of this technique is the x-rays exposition, but the new technologies of dose reduction are significantly reducing its importance in the risk-benefits assessment.

MRI provides important information such as quantitative contrast-enhancement parameters and time–signal intensity curves, derived from dynamic MRI, enabling to differentiate between active and inactive disease [18]. MRI is more expensive, time consuming, and less available than CT, but it should be considered the imaging method of choice in young patients.

CT enterography technique (CTe) used in association with *colon water enema* (CTe-WE) results in excellent luminal distension of both sides of the ileocecal area, allowing a simultaneous and constant distension of both small and large bowel. Moreover, it is possible to study adjacent organs and their enhancement, ensuring a complete evaluation of the abdomen, that could be extended to the rest of the body, if any doubts arise during the examination [17, 19–22].

14.1 Arthropathies

IBD-related arthropathies are classified as nonspinal (or peripheral) and spinal.

Non-spinal arthropathies are differentiated according to the pattern of articular involvement [9]:

- Type I: large joint pauciarticular arthropathy, occurring during phases of IBD activity
- Type II: small joint polyarticular arthropathy, independent from IBD activity

Type I arthropathy is defined pauciarticular because it affects fewer than five joints. It involves weight-bearing joints such as ankles, knees, and hips. Symptoms are usually acute, self-limiting, and linked with disease activity. It decreases in few weeks, leaving no permanent joint damage. Clinical examination reveals painful, tender, swollen joints. The differential diagnosis includes rheumatoid arthritis, osteoarthritis, gout, septic arthritis, and pyrophosphate arthropathy.

Type II arthritis is defined polyarticular because more than five joints are affected. It involves the small joints of both hands as a symmetrical arthropathy. Pain is usually not proportionate to the signs of arthritis. It is not related to IBD activity, persisting for months or years, even after colectomy. To perform a correct differential diagnosis some different conditions must be considered, such as osteoarthritis, mesalazine- or azathioprine-induced arthropathy, and even side effects of treatment such as steroid-induced pseudorheumatism [23].

Spinal arthritis is represented by sacroiliitis and ankylosing spondylitis, which diagnosis is based on clinical setting and supported by characteristic radiological findings. HLA B-27 is not considered of diagnostic value even if it is overrepresented in IBD-related spinal arthritis. Its association is found in a majority of patients, but is less common than in patients with ankylosing spondylitis not associated with IBD [24–26].

Sacroiliitis is one of the most frequent Crohn's disease extraintestinal complications [3]. Symptomatic sacroiliitis is characterized by pelvic pain, which improves with movement. This condition must be suspected if the patient refers discomfort in the sacroiliac joints during pressure on the pelvic brim.

However, symptomatic sacroiliitis is common, and up to 50 % of Crohn's patients have abnormal radiography (Fig. 14.1) [27, 28].

The principal symptom of ankylosing spondylitis is persistent low back pain, affecting people before the age of 30. At the clinical examination, it is possible to observe limited spinal flexion and loss of the lumbar lordosis. In the early stages, conventional radiographs are usually normal, while CT scans and radionuclide bone scans are more sensitive [29, 30]. In advanced cases, the classical condition of

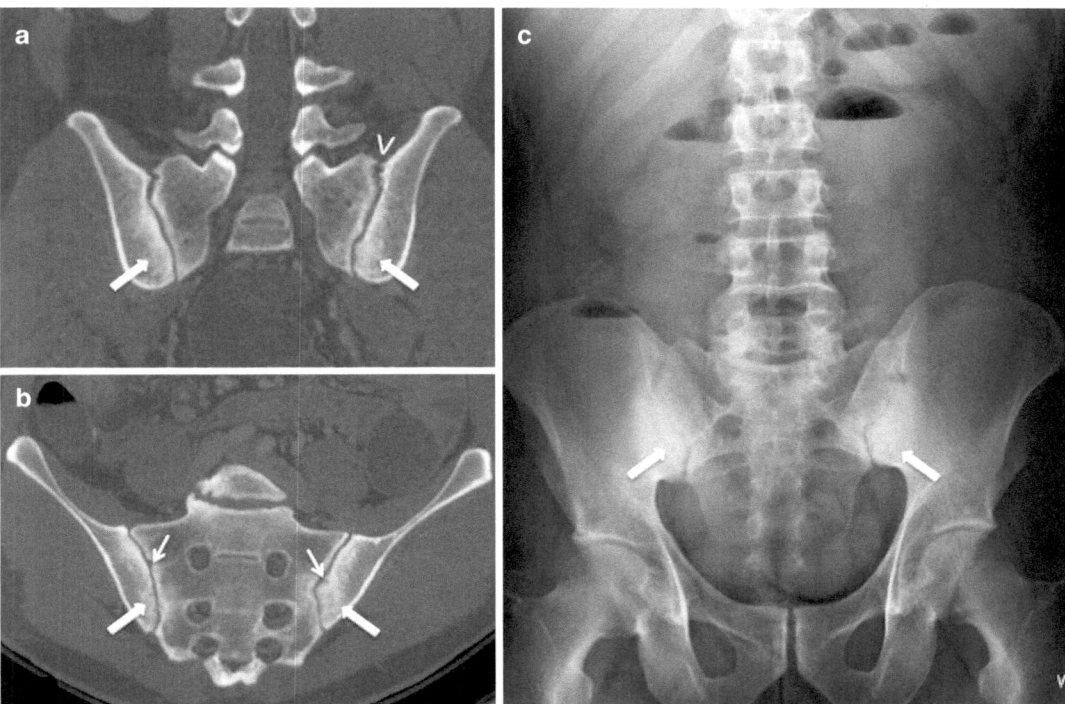

Fig. 14.1 Bilateral sacroiliitis in a patient affected by Crohn's disease. CT oblique reconstruction (**a**) and oblique coronal reconstruction oriented parallel to the sacral promontory (**b**). Specific findings of sacroiliitis are visible in CT scans using bone window: spongiosclerosis, which is more evident along the iliac side of sacroiliac joints (*arrows*); erosions (*small arrows*); irregular bony bridges crossing the joint space (*arrowhead*). Anteroposterior radiograph (**c**) shows diffuse subchondral sclerosis involving the iliac portion (anteroinferior) of both sacroiliac joints (*arrows*)

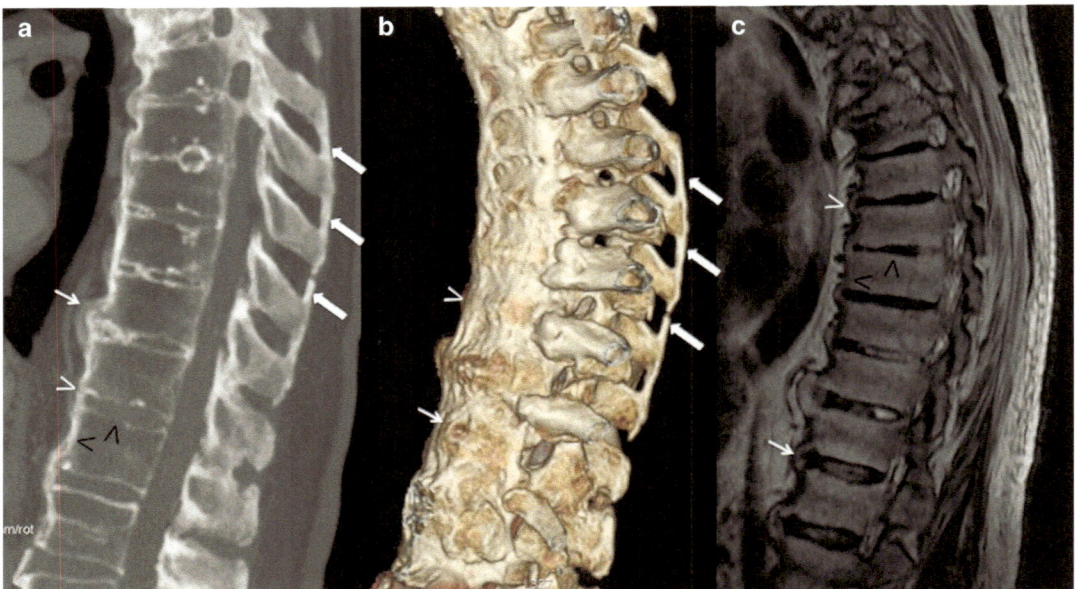

Fig. 14.2 Crohn's disease related to ankylosing spondy- litis. Sagittal multiplanar reformation (**a**) and correspond- ing surface-rendered (**b**) CT scan, and T1-weighted sagittal MRI image (**c**) of the dorsal spine, clearly define some specific findings: the ossification of the supraspi- nous ligaments (*arrows* in **a**, **b**); syndesmophytes (*thin arrows* in **a–c**); ossification of the anterior longitudinal ligament (*white arrowheads* in **a–c**); "squaring" of the vertebral body endplates, with loss of the normal concav- ity (*black arrowheads* in **a**, **c**). These alterations are observable in all figures, and in **b** it is possible to see how the chronic inflammation of the discovertebral junction leads to the onset of an osteoproliferative process, con- necting together the anterior portion of vertebral bodies. In advanced stages, the ossification of vertebral (longitu- dinal, supraspinous, and interspinous) ligaments may occur, leading to ankylosis

"bamboo spine" may be observed, characterized by vertebral bodies squaring, marginal syndes- mophytes, and bony proliferation with ankylosis (Fig. 14.2) [24–26, 31].

Even if MRI is considered as the gold stan- dard, CT is an appropriate diagnostic tool for the evaluation of structural changes of the sacroiliac joints in seronegative spondyloarthropathies. The spinal involvement in Crohn's disease is not eas- ily differentiable from that of ankylosing spondy- litis, and it is not correlated with the activity of intestinal inflammation [3].

Treatment is based almost entirely on extrapo- lation from other forms of arthritis, including the use of different classes of drugs: analgesics, non- steroidal anti-inflammatory agents, sulfasalazine, local steroid injections, and even infliximab in ankylosing spondylitis. Physiotherapy is an important element common to these treatments.

14.2 Cutaneous Manifestations

The diagnosis of IBD-related cutaneous manifestations is based on clinical signs and their characteristic features, once excluded the presence of specific skin disorders. The fre- quency of these pathologies in patients affected by Crohn's disease is greater than in the normal population.

14.2.1 Pyoderma Gangrenosum

Pyoderma gangrenosum is a pathological condi- tion characterized by cutaneous lesions often preceded by trauma, which may occurred several years before. The lesions are localized in the same position of the trauma, due to the pathoge- netic phenomenon known as pathergy.

Lesions appear more frequently in the shins, but they can affect the whole body. Starting from single or multiple erythematous papules, these lesions develop with necrosis of the dermis, leading to ulcerations that contain purulent material (sterile on culture) with the possibility of subsequent secondary infection.

Steroids, with topical and systemic administration, were considered the best treatment for pyoderma gangrenosum, with cyclosporin or tacrolimus reserved for selected cases [32]. The biologic drug infliximab has changed the management of this pathology, starting to be used only in specific cases and becoming, nowadays, a first-line treatment [33].

14.2.2 Erythema Nodosum

Erythema nodosum is characterized by raised, tender, red, or violet subcutaneous nodules up to 5 cm in diameter. It usually affects the extensor surfaces of the extremities, particularly the anterior tibial aspect, being related to the intestinal disease activity. Due to these specific characteristics, the diagnosis is normally done by the clinical presentation.

Because of its relationship to disease activity, treatment is based on that of the underlying colitis, requiring systemic steroid administration. Even in these cases, infliximab is showing promising results [34].

14.2.3 Sweet's Syndrome

Sweet's syndrome is a neutrophilic dermatosis, like pyoderma gangrenosum, that has been recognized as an extraintestinal manifestation of IBD only recently.

It is characterized by tender, red nodules or papules, commonly affecting the upper limbs, neck, or face.

The rash is usually associated with active disease, but may precede the onset of intestinal symptoms, or it could appear several months after proctocolectomy for ulcerative colitis [35].

14.3 Ocular Manifestations

Different ocular complications have been reported in patients with IBD, and they are commonly associated with articular symptoms. Uveitis and iritis are more common in ulcerative colitis (UC), while episcleritis affects more frequently patients with Crohn's disease [36].

Uveitis and episcleritis are probably the most common extraintestinal manifestations of IBD [37, 38].

14.3.1 Episcleritis

Episcleritis has a wide range of clinical presentation. In fact, it may be painless, showing only hyperemic sclera and conjunctiva, or it could present with acute burning sensations. The differential diagnosis must be made with different features of uveitis and usually does not require specific treatment other than for underlying disease activity, providing the use of topical steroids in most painful cases [39].

14.3.2 Uveitis

Uveitis is less common than episcleritis, but has potentially more severe consequences, with the possibility of vision loss.

Most frequent symptoms are blurred vision, pain, photophobia, and headaches, and, after clinical examination, slit lamp will confirm the diagnosis.

The normal treatment is based on steroid administration, sometimes with both topical and systemic routes. Even in these cases, infliximab has showed to be rapidly effective [39, 40].

14.4 Hepatobiliary Disease

Hepatobiliary diseases are relatively common in patients affected by IBD, including a wide spectrum of different pathological conditions.

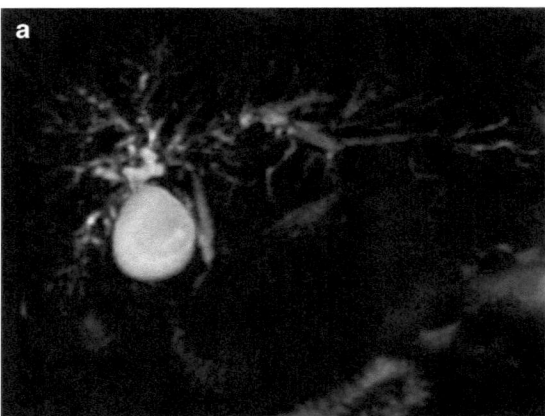

Fig. 14.3 Crohn's disease related to primary sclerosing cholangitis. 3D MIP reconstruction of magnetic resonance cholangiography, anterior (**a**) and lateral view (**b**). In these figures, it is possible to observe typical alteration of the biliary tree, represented by multiple and diffuse segmental strictures alternate with biliary dilatations and diverticula

The most common presentation is the finding of abnormal liver function tests. So diagnostic flowchart usually proceeds with ultrasound (US) examination and serology tests to exclude infective or autoimmune causes, up to liver biopsy.

In a clinical setting of biliary-type pain, US could show the presence of gallstones, steatosis, cholangitis, cirrhosis, chronic hepatitis, or abnormal anatomy of biliary ducts suggestive of primary sclerosing cholangitis (PSC). This last pathological condition is the most important and relatively specific manifestation to the underlying IBD.

However, clinicians should always consider the possibility of hepatotoxicity due to drugs used for colitis, although it usually presents within 3 weeks from starting therapy [41].

14.4.1 Primary Sclerosing Cholangitis

Primary sclerosing cholangitis is a chronic cholestatic liver disease characterized by fibrosis and inflammation of the bile ducts, resulting in cirrhosis and causing a reduced life expectancy. Moreover, it is associated with an increased risk of both cholangio- and colorectal carcinoma.

PSC is the most specific hepatobiliary complication of IBD with a reported frequency up to 10 %, affecting primarily young and middle-aged men, and a wider number of cases described in patients affected by UC [9, 42].

This pathological condition has not a correlation with the activity of colitis, and it could precede the clinical manifestation of the underlying IBD. Moreover, liver alterations may appear even several years after therapeutic procedure such as colectomy [36]. The etiology of primary sclerosing cholangitis includes self-immune mechanisms and elements of undefined nature [43].

Often it is possible to reach only an exclusion diagnosis, thinking to PSC in all that cases of patients affected by IBD, with specific symptoms, but without diagnostic or serological alterations for primary liver diseases.

Magnetic resonance cholangiography (MRC) is now considered as the first-line imaging modality in cases of suspected PSC, avoiding potential adverse effects of radiation exposure and contrast media reactions associated with examination like endoscopic retrograde cholangiopancreatography (ERCP) [42]. MRC examination demonstrates typical features of markedly distorted biliary tract, characterized by multiple segmental strictures alternating with dilation or diverticula (Fig. 14.3). In advanced stages, it is possible to observe atrophy of the entire liver with the exception of the caudate lobe that results hypertrophied in almost all cases (68–98 %) [44].

If PSC is still suspected, after instrumental and laboratory negative examinations, the last diagnostic step to reach a definitive diagnosis is represented by liver biopsy.

Several drugs have been evaluated in the treatment of PSC, but none of them has convincing benefits, and some are associated with significant side effects.

So several combination therapies, such as ursodeoxycholic acid and methotrexate, have been studied to normalize liver biochemistries of these patients, showing promising results. However, nowadays, there are no effective medical therapies to halt the progression of disease. The only definitive therapy for PSC is liver transplantation [45].

14.4.2 Cholelithiasis

Cholesterol-based gallbladder cholelithiasis is more common in individuals with Crohn's disease than in the general population, and it is thought to be related to a decreased reabsorption of bile salts due to terminal ileitis [3].

Starting from this physiopathological background, it has been shown that intestinal resections are significantly associated with cholelithiasis. In fact, patients undergoing ileal resection run a higher risk to develop gallstones in comparison with those not receiving ileal resection [46].

Ultrasonography is the first-line imaging modality for the evaluation of cholelithiasis, and gallstones appear as echoic findings with posterior acoustic shadowing, mobile when patient changes decubitus.

In CT examination, gallstones are either hypoattenuating or hyperattenuating filling defects within the gallbladder lumen, depending on composition.

14.5 Metabolic Bone Disease

The relationship between bone loss and IBD is well known and studied from several years.

Osteopenia and osteoporosis are common in these patients (20–50 %), with a similar prevalence in ulcerative colitis and Crohn's disease, in men and women.

These pathological alterations lead to an increased risk of bone fracture, but the risk is only moderately above normal population [47].

Pathogenetic mechanism of bone loss in patients affected by IBD seems to develop on two different levels:

- Intestinal: were inflammation mediators produced during disease activity alter osteoblast function and bone formation.
- Therapeutic: caused by corticosteroids, drugs with multiple adverse effects on bone metabolism. In fact, they impair osteoblast function, reducing intestinal calcium absorption, while increasing renal calcium excretion, inducing secondary hyperparathyroidism.

The final effect of these two mechanisms is a pattern of low turnover, with reduced bone formation. These alterations correlate with current corticosteroid dose and duration of the therapy [48].

Dual-energy x-ray absorptiometry (DEXA) scanning must be performed in selected IBD patients to evaluate their bone mineral density (BMD), in addition to measurement of albumin and calcium levels at diagnosis.

The diagnosis of osteoporosis is an indication for therapy. However, the correct therapeutic approach in these cases remains unclear, but the early use of vitamin D and calcium supplementation is widely recommended [21, 43].

14.6 Other Extraintestinal Manifestations

Other pathological conditions associated with IBD can be observed: nephrolithiasis, obstructive uropathy, pulmonary manifestations, avascular necrosis (AVN), deep vein thrombosis, and amyloidosis.

All these conditions can reduce patients' quality of life, influencing their care and therapy [3, 17].

The prevalence of nephrolithiasis in patients affected by Crohn's disease compared to the

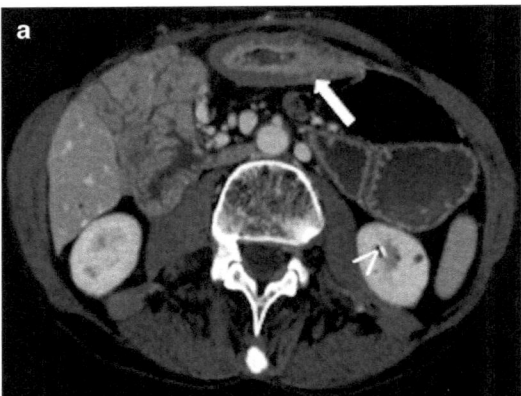

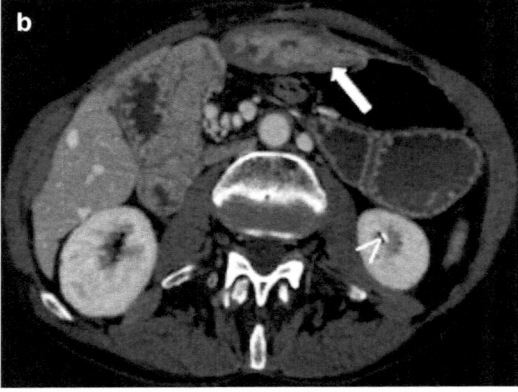

Fig. 14.4 Nephrolithiasis in a patient affected by Crohn's disease. Axial CT scan with abdominal window (**a**, **b**) two consecutive slices. In each image, it is possible to observe a renal calculus in the inferior part of the left kidney (*arrowheads*) and a pathological bowel loop (transverse colon), characterized by wall thickening and submucosal involvement (*arrows*)

general population is increased and is estimated to be more prevalent than in patients affected by ulcerative colitis (Fig. 14.4) [3, 10]. Dehydration associated with chronic diarrhea, decreased urine volume, aciduria, bowel resection, and abnormal metabolism of oxalic acid is pathological condition typical of IBD and can lead to the development of kidney stones. Calcium oxalate renal calculi commonly arise in the setting of terminal ileitis because of a relative increase in oxalate to calcium absorption from the GI tract [3].

To prevent this complication, patients undergo regular urological examination and ultrasonography.

Excepting drug-related disease, pulmonary manifestations of IBD remain nonspecific. In fact, tuberculosis reactivation due to infliximab and eosinophilic pneumonia, induced by mesalamine and sulfasalazine, is important complication observable in these patients. Other conditions such as sarcoidosis, bronchiolitis obliterans, and bronchiectasis have been reported in association with IBD, but there are no evidences for a definitive association.

Colobronchial and esophagobronchial fistulae may occur rarely in Crohn's disease [8].

Moreover, patients with inflammatory bowel disease have an increased risk to develop colorectal cancer. Although colorectal cancer complicating IBD represents only 1–2 % of all cases in the general population, it is a serious complication and accounts for approximately 15 % of all deaths in inflammatory bowel disease patients.

The risk of colon cancer increases by 0.5–1.0 % yearly and 8–10 years after diagnosis. The magnitude of the risk increases with early age of the inflammatory bowel disease diagnosis, extent of the pathological alterations, and longer duration of symptoms [49]. Foci of high-grade epithelial dysplasia, adjacent to adenocarcinoma, suggest a dysplasia–carcinoma sequence promoted by chronic mural inflammation, while sporadic small bowel adenocarcinoma is thought to develop following the adenoma–carcinoma sequence [50, 51].

Ulcerative colitis and Crohn's disease can degenerate mainly in two different kinds of neoplasms: adenocarcinoma and lymphoma. Starting directly from the mucosal layer, ulcerative colitis involves principally the adenomatous structures subjected to neoplastic degeneration. Differently, Crohn's disease has its development in the submucosal layer, involving lymphatic structure. So the frequency and the kind of neoplastic degeneration reflect the underlying pathological process of the intestinal disease. Patients with long-standing ulcerative colitis have an increased risk of developing colorectal adenocarcinoma, while in Crohn's disease, there is an increased risk of developing lymphoma and a rare share of adenocarcinoma [52].

Conclusions

IBD may be considered systemic disorders predominantly affecting the gastrointestinal tract, but with different kinds of extraintestinal associations, which reduce patient's quality of life [9].

Disease management and therapy planning are mainly based on information regarding pathology extent, so early recognition of these extraintestinal manifestations should help to guide therapy reducing overall morbidity [3].

References

1. Freeman HJ. Natural history and clinical behavior of Crohn's disease extending beyond two decades. J Clin Gastroenterol. 2003;37(3):216–9.
2. Soyer P, Boudiaf M, Sirol M, et al. Suspected anastomotic recurrence of Crohn disease after ileocolic resection: evaluation with CT enteroclysis. Radiology. 2010;254(3):755–64.
3. Paparo F, Bacigalupo L, Garello I, Biscaldi E, Cimmino MA, Marinaro E, Rollandi GA. Crohn's disease: prevalence of intestinal and extraintestinal manifestations detected by computed tomography enterography with water enema. Abdom Imaging. 2012;37(3):326–37.
4. Soyer P, Hristova L, Boudghene F, Hoeffel C, Dray X, Laurent V, Fishman EK, Boudiaf M. Small bowel adenocarcinoma in Crohn disease: CT-enterography features with pathological correlation. Abdom Imaging. 2012;37(3):338–49.
5. Morson BC. Histopathology of Crohn's disease. Proc R Soc Med. 1968;61(1):79–81.
6. Juillerat P, Mottet C, Pittet V, Froehlich F, Felley C, Gonvers JJ, Vader JP, Michetti P. Extraintestinal manifestations of Crohn's disease. Digestion. 2007;76(2): 141–8.
7. Christodoulou DK, Katsanos KH, Kitsanou M, Stergiopoulou C, Hatzis J, Tsianos EV. Frequency of extraintestinal manifestations in patients with inflammatory bowel disease in Northwest Greece and review of the literature. Dig Liver Dis. 2002;34(11): 781–6.
8. Storch I, Sachar D, Katz S. Pulmonary manifestations of inflammatory bowel disease. Inflamm Bowel Dis. 2003;9(2):104–15.
9. Ardizzone S, Puttini PS, Cassinotti A, Porro GB. Extraintestinal manifestations of inflammatory bowel disease. Dig Liver Dis. 2008;40 Suppl 2:S253–9.
10. Trikudanathan G, Venkatesh PG, Navaneethan U. Diagnosis and therapeutic management of extraintestinal manifestations of inflammatory bowel disease. Drugs. 2012;72(18):2333–49.
11. Das KM. Relationship of extraintestinal involvement in inflammatory bowel disease. Dig Dis Sci. 1999;44: 1–13.
12. Urlep D, Mamula P, Baldassano R. Extraintestinal manifestations of inflammatory bowel disease. Minerva Gastroenterol Dietol. 2005;51(2):147–63.
13. Fraquelli M, Colli A, Casazza G, Paggi S, Colucci A, Massironi S, Duca P, Conte D. Role of US in detection of Crohn disease: meta-analysis. Radiology. 2005;236(1):95–101.
14. Calabrese E, La Seta F, Buccellato A, Virdone R, Pallotta N, Corazziari E, Cottone M. Crohn's disease: a comparative prospective study of transabdominal ultrasonography, small intestine contrast ultrasonography, and small bowel enema. Inflamm Bowel Dis. 2005;11(2):139–45.
15. Parente F, Greco S, Molteni M, Anderloni A, Sampietro GM, Danelli PG, Bianco R, Gallus S, Bianchi Porro G. Oral contrast enhanced bowel ultrasonography in the assessment of small intestine Crohn's disease. A prospective comparison with conventional ultrasound, x ray studies, and ileocolonoscopy. Gut. 2004;53(11):1652–7.
16. Siddiki HA, Fidler JL, Fletcher JG, Burton SS, Huprich JE, Hough DM, Johnson CD, Bruining DH, Loftus Jr EV, Sandborn WJ, Pardi DS, Mandrekar JN. Prospective comparison of state-of-the-art MR enterography and CT enterography in small-bowel Crohn's disease. AJR Am J Roentgenol. 2009;193(1): 113–21.
17. Bruining DH, Siddiki HA, Fletcher JG, Tremaine WJ, Sandborn WJ, Loftus Jr EV. Prevalence of penetrating disease and extraintestinal manifestations of Crohn's disease detected with CT enterography. Inflamm Bowel Dis. 2008;14(12):1701–6.
18. Giusti S, Faggioni L, Neri E, Fruzzetti E, Nardini L, Marchi S, Bartolozzi C. Dynamic MRI of the small bowel: usefulness of quantitative contrast-enhancement parameters and time-signal intensity curves for differentiating between active and inactive Crohn's disease. Abdom Imaging. 2010;35(6): 646–53.
19. Paparo F, Garlaschi A, Biscaldi E, Bacigalupo L, Cevasco L, Rollandi GA. Computed tomography of the bowel: a prospective comparison study between four techniques. Eur J Radiol. 2013;82(1):e1–10.
20. Ridereau-Zins C, Aubé C, Luet D, Vielle B, Pilleul F, Dumortier J, Gandon Y, Heresbach D, Beziat C, Bailly F, Debilly M, Carbonnel F, Pierredon-Foulongne MA, Bismuth M, Chretien JM, Lebigot J, Pessaux P, Valette PJ. Assessment of water enema computed tomography: an effective imaging technique for the diagnosis of colon cancer: colon cancer: computed tomography using a water enema. Abdom Imaging. 2010;35(4):407–13.
21. Soyer P, Sirol M, Dray X, Placé V, Pautrat K, Hamzi L, Boudiaf M. Detection of colorectal tumors with water enema-multidetector row computed tomography. Abdom Imaging. 2012;37(6):1092–100.

22. Laghi A, Rengo M, Graser A, Iafrate F. Current status on performance of CT colonography and clinical indications. Eur J Radiol. 2013;82(8):1192–200.

23. Orchard TR, Wordsworth BP, Jewell DP. Peripheral arthropathies in inflammatory bowel disease: their articular distribution and natural history. Gut. 1998;42:387–91.

24. Bjarnason I, Helgason KO, Geirsson AJ, Sigthorsson G, Reynisdottir I, Gubjartsson D, et al. Subclinical intestinal inflammation and sacroiliac changes in relatives of patients with ankylosing spondylitis. Gastroenterology. 2003;125:1598–605.

25. Braun J, Sieper J. The sacroiliac joint in the spondyloarthropathies. Curr Opin Rheumatol. 1996;8(4): 275–87.

26. Steer S, Jones H, Hibbert J, Kondeatis E, Vaughan R, Sanderson J, et al. Low back pain, sacroiliitis, and the relationship with HLA-B27 in Crohn's disease. J Rheumatol. 2003;30:518–22.

27. Fornaciari G, Salvarani C, Beltrami M, Macchioni P, Stockbrugger RW, Russel MG, et al. Musculoskeletal manifestations in inflammatory bowel disease. Can J Gastroenterol. 2001;15:399–403.

28. Heuft-Dorenbosch L, Landewe R, Weijers R, Wanders A, Houben H, van der Linden S, et al. Combining information obtained from magnetic resonance imaging and conventional radiographs to detect sacroiliitis in patients with recent onset inflammatory back pain. Ann Rheum Dis. 2006;65:804–8.

29. Braun J, Baraliakos X, Golder W, Hermann KG, Listing J, Brandt J, et al. Analysing chronic spinal changes in ankylosing spondylitis: a systematic comparison of conventional x rays with magnetic resonance imaging using established and new scoring systems. Ann Rheum Dis. 2004;63:1046–55.

30. Geijer M, Sihlbom H, Göthlin JH, Nordborg E. The role of CT in the diagnosis of sacroiliitis. Acta Radiol. 1998;39(3):265–8.

31. Paparo F, Revelli M, Semprini A, Camellino D, Garlaschi A, Cimmino MA, Rollandi GA, Leone A. Seronegative spondyloarthropathies: what radiologists should know. Radiol Med. 2014;119(3):156–63.

32. Brooklyn T, Dunnill G, Probert C. Diagnosis and treatment of pyoderma gangrenosum. BMJ. 2006;333: 181–4.

33. Agarwal A, Andrews JM. Systematic review: IBD-associated pyoderma gangrenosum in the biologic era, the response to therapy. Aliment Pharmacol Ther. 2013;38(6):563–72.

34. Trost LB, McDonnel JK. Important cutaneous manifestations of inflammatory bowel disease. Postgrad Med J. 2005;81:580–5.

35. Cohen PR, Kurzrock R. Sweet's syndrome revisited: a review of disease concepts. Int J Dermatol. 2003; 42(10):761–78.

36. Orchard T. Extraintestinal complications of inflammatory bowel disease. Curr Gastroenterol Rep. 2003;5:512–7.

37. Bernstein CN, Blanchard JF, Rawsthorne P, Yu N. The prevalence of extraintestinal diseases in inflammatory bowel disease: a population-based study. Am J Gastroenterol. 2001;96:1116–22.

38. Cury DB, Moss AC. Ocular manifestations in a community-based cohort of patients with inflammatory bowel disease. Inflamm Bowel Dis. 2010;16(8): 1393–6.

39. Yilmaz S, Aydemir E, Maden A, Unsal B. The prevalence of ocular involvement in patients with inflammatory bowel disease. Int J Colorectal Dis. 2007;22(9):1027–30.

40. Read RW. Uveitis: advances in understanding of pathogenesis and treatment. Curr Rheumatol Rep. 2006;8:260–6.

41. Rönnblom A, Holmström T, Tanghöj H, Rorsman F, Sjöberg D. Appearance of hepatobiliary diseases in a population based cohort with inflammatory bowel diseases (ICURE). J Gastroenterol Hepatol. 2015;16.

42. Charatcharoenwitthaya P, Lindor KD. Primary sclerosing cholangitis: diagnosis and management. Curr Gastroenterol Rep. 2006;8:75–82.

43. Silveira MG, Lindor KD. Clinical features and management of primary sclerosing cholangitis. World J Gastroenterol. 2008;14(21):3338–49.

44. Ito K, Mitchell DG, Outwater EK, et al. Primary sclerosing cholangitis: MR imaging features. AJR Am J Roentgenol. 1999;172(6):1527–33.

45. Lindor KD, Jorgensen RA, Anderson ML, Gores GJ, Hofmann AF, LaRusso NF. Ursodeoxycholic acid and methotrexate for primary sclerosing cholangitis: a pilot study. Am J Gastroenterol. 1996;91:511–5.

46. Parente F, Pastore L, Bargiggia S, Cucino C, Greco S, Molteni M, Ardizzone S, Porro GB, Sampietro GM, Giorgi R, Moretti R, Gallus S. Incidence and risk factors for gallstones in patients with inflammatory bowel disease: a large case-control study. Hepatology. 2007;45(5):1267–74.

47. Bernstein CN, Leslie WD, Leboff MS. AGA technical review on osteoporosis in gastrointestinal diseases. Gastroenterology. 2003;124:795–841.

48. American College of Rheumatology ad hoc Committee on Glucocoritcoid-Induced Osteoporosis. Recommendations for the prevention and treatment of glucocorticoid-induced osteoporosis: 2001 update. Arthritis Rheum. 2001;44:1496–503.

49. Munkholm P. Review article: the incidence and prevalence of colorectal cancer in inflammatory bowel disease. Aliment Pharmacol Ther. 2003;18 Suppl 2:1–5.

50. Freeman HJ. Colorectal cancer risk in Crohn's disease. World J Gastroenterol. 2008;14(12):1810–1.

51. Ullman TA, Itzkowitz SH. Intestinal inflammation and cancer. Gastroenterology. 2011;140(6):1807–16. doi:10.1053/j.gastro.2011.01.057.

52. Bernstein CN, Blanchard JF, Kliewer E, Wajda A. Cancer risk in patients with inflammatory bowel disease: a population-based study. Cancer. 2001;91(4): 854–62.

Radiological Follow-Up of Inflammatory Bowel Diseases

Giuseppe Lo Re, Dario Picone,
Federica Vernuccio, Fabrizio Rabita,
Gianfranco Cocorullo, Sergio Salerno,
Massimo Galia, and Massimo Midiri

15.1 Introduction

Inflammatory bowel diseases (IBD) are chronic gastrointestinal diseases that typically affect the young working-age population. Patients with IBD, both asymptomatic and symptomatic, often develop complications during their clinical course. This is particularly true in patients with Crohn's disease (CD) and biological signs of inflammation, despite being asymptomatic. In addition, it seems clear that the absence of symptoms does not imply an absence of inflammation.

For all the above mentioned reasons, patients should be followed up and objectively evaluated.

IBD are idiopathic diseases characterized by periods of remission and frequent exacerbations [1]. To appreciate the impact of disease progression, it is necessary to understand the natural history of IBD. In CD patients, the cumulative relapse rate during the first 10 years of disease is

reported to be 90% and the cumulative probability of surgery 38% [2]. High unemployment rates of 35–39% have been identified in IBD subjects from the USA, the Netherlands, and Sweden [3–5]. Recently, many authors affirmed that the therapeutic goal in IBD should be to change the course of the disease, and this can be reached not just achieving a clinical remission but mainly obtaining the so-called mucosal healing. For this reason, an accurate assessment of the severity of mucosal inflammation is necessary to optimize treatment [6, 7].

The gold standard for evaluating the inflammation of the intestine is endoscopy with multiple biopsies [8]. However, this is an invasive and expensive exam and requires sedation.

Moreover, direct observation of the affected mucosa or evaluation of the full extent of inflamed areas may be compromised by using endoscopy, either from inaccessibility given by fibrostenotic or edematous narrowings that limit progression or by proximal disease that skips the distal ileum or involves the more proximal small bowel [9].

Another key point is that treatment targets in Crohn's disease are evolving beyond symptoms, and this evolution requires the adoption of monitoring strategies that can readily and reliably detect the presence of complications and extraintestinal disease, can be repeated at specified intervals, and are cost-effective.

For these reasons, in gastroenterological practice, clinical scores, serum markers of

G. Lo Re (✉) • D. Picone • F. Vernuccio • F. Rabita
S. Salerno • M. Galia • M. Midiri
DIBIMED, Department of Biopathology and Medical
Biotechnology, University Hospital P. Giaccone –
University of Palermo, Palermo, Italy
e-mail: giuseppe.lore12@gmail.com;
massimo.midiri@unipa.it

G. Cocorullo
Department of General Surgery, Urgency and Organ
Transplantation, University Hospital P. Giaccone –
University of Palermo, Palermo, Italy

© Springer International Publishing Switzerland 2016
G. Lo Re, M. Midiri (eds.), *Crohn's Disease: Radiological Features and Clinical-Surgical Correlations*,
DOI 10.1007/978-3-319-23066-5_15

inflammation, and cross-sectional imaging techniques are widely used.

In patients with IBD, active disease, progressive course with cumulative intestinal damage, development of complications, the presence of extraintestinal manifestations, and treatment of adverse effects may result in disability. The young age of onset and the propensity to develop complications have consequences for the long-term prognosis and impact on future disability and quality of life. For these reasons, the disability evaluation in patients with IBD should be mandatory during the follow-up since it is an objective determination and differs from subjective assessments such as quality of life.

The Crohn's Disease Activity Index (CDAI) is a research tool used by clinicians to quantify the symptoms of patients with CD. Clinical trials of CD often use formal grading systems to describe disease severity. Two commonly used systems are the Crohn's Disease Activity Index (CDAI) and the Harvey-Bradshaw Index (HBI) [10], which is a simplified derivative of the CDAI. The HBI has been shown to correlate with the CDAI [11].

According to the American College of Gastroenterology, it may be more practical for clinical practice to take on mind the following definitions [12]:

- Asymptomatic remission (CDAI <150) – Patients who are asymptomatic either spontaneously or after medical or surgical intervention. Patients requiring steroids to remain asymptomatic are not considered to be in remission but are referred to as being "steroid dependent."
- Mild to moderate Crohn's disease (CDAI 150–220) – Ambulatory patients able to tolerate an oral diet without dehydration, toxicity, abdominal tenderness, mass, obstruction, or >10 % weight loss.

A new tool to assess disability in IBD has been recently developed [13]: this novel scoring system was designed for the International Classification of Functioning IBD-Disability Index (ICF IBD-DI), and it was validated as an instrument highly suitable for measuring IBD-related disability for both CD and UC. During its validation, this score proved to be sufficiently sensitive to detect disability in patients with IBD [14]. The ICF IBD-DI consists of 19 items divided into 28 parts covering the 5 domains of Overall Health, Body Function, Body Structures, Activity Participation and Environmental Factors [15]. The IBD-DI was specifically designed to exclude the use of any questions that examine patients' subjective coping and feelings. Moreover, age at diagnosis, sex, phenotype, perianal disease, prior surgery, steroid use, and disease duration do not influence the IBD-DI, but active use of biological agents significantly reduce disability.

15.2   Cross-Sectional Imaging Techniques in the Follow-Up of IBD

Although endoscopy remains the gold standard for assessing CD activity, it suffers from several limitations, as invasiveness, need for sedation, inability to assess extramural disease, and inadequate visualization of small bowel. Imaging techniques are therefore gaining importance in a complementary role, especially to evaluate the cumulative intestinal damage. Imaging of the small bowel has changed in recent years, but the imaging goals are primarily to determine the extent of small bowel involvement, assess complications, and define candidates for surgery.

Multiple imaging modalities have been used in IBD, divided into conventional and cross-sectional ones. Among the first ones, the small bowel follow-through (SBFT) has been the most commonly used to evaluate small bowel, and its use was justified before the introduction of cross-sectional modalities [16]. The SBFT demonstrates mucosal detail, length of small bowel involvement, and luminal diameter. However, one of the main features that is important for the clinician in the follow-up is to evaluate extraluminal disease, such as the presence of abscesses, in order to start biological therapy and assess response to it. Extramural complications including internal fistulas may be identified through SBTF [17], but other extramural complications such as abscess are not reliably demonstrated compared with other modalities [16, 18]. SBFT is a long-lasting examination, does not reliably exclude the presence of early disease, and exposes to high radiation dose.

On the other hand, cross-sectional techniques have advanced the ability to diagnose, classify, and monitor IBD and their extramural complications reducing or avoiding the radiation exposure, and this is particularly important since most of the patients are young and exams are repeated at specified intervals to monitor therapy.

In patients who have already been diagnosed with IBD, cross-sectional techniques have a role in evaluating response to therapy and disease activity and monitor progression and intestinal or extraintestinal complications of the disease, thus suggesting the appropriate therapy [16].

15.2.1 Intestinal Ultrasound

Transabdominal intestinal ultrasound (IUS) is a widespread, cheap, noninvasive, risk-free procedure, which is useful both in the diagnosis and management of patients with IBD [16].

Ultrasonography may show the transformation of the intestinal wall from normal to pathological state in inflammatory disease.

IUS for IBD mainly requires high-frequency (5–17 MHz) linear array probes to increase spatial resolution and to allow adequate assessment of bowel diameter and of the recognizable 5-layer wall pattern [19].

IUS is performed without sedation and just with 4 h fasting before the examination. The use of oral and/or IV contrast agents may increase diagnostic accuracy, though their use remains controversial. Recent studies [20, 21] on patients with CD proved the usefulness of small intestine contrast US to assess changes caused by anti-inflammatory treatment, through an evaluation before and after it, and its relationship with the clinical and biological response; however, these studies did not relate the changes to endoscopy but to clinical evaluation as CDAI.

Color or power Doppler imaging of the vascularity of thickened wall segments has been proved useful in the distinction between remission and active disease, as normal bowel wall does not show much vascularity [16]. In CD, the vascularization is involved: the estimation of "vessel density" seems to be a reliable semiquantitative score for disease activity [22]. As demonstrated by Bolondi et al. [23], in active IBD there is an increase in portal flow velocity and reduction of the resistance index of superior mesenteric artery.

The implementation of US with the intravenous administration of contrast medium (contrast-enhanced ultrasound, CEUS) has been widely used for the diagnosis, but mainly for the follow-up and the grading of CD due to its high diagnostic accuracy, comparable with CT or MR [24]. Elastography has been described recently in patients with IBD, but studies so far are lacking [25].

> **Keep in Mind**
> (i) CT should not be routinely used in the follow-up of IBD, because of radiation exposure and similar diagnostic accuracy compared to US and MR in the follow-up.
> (ii) CT has a high spatial resolution, and it is useful to evaluate extramural involvement, as abscesses, and in emergency situations thanks to its high velocity in performing examination.

15.2.2 Computed Tomography

CT examination by either CT enterography (CTE) or CT enteroclysis has become a widely used technique for SB investigation.

A good correlation has been shown between CT enteroclysis and histopathology results in regard to inflammatory changes [26]. However, CT enteroclysis is more invasive than CTE

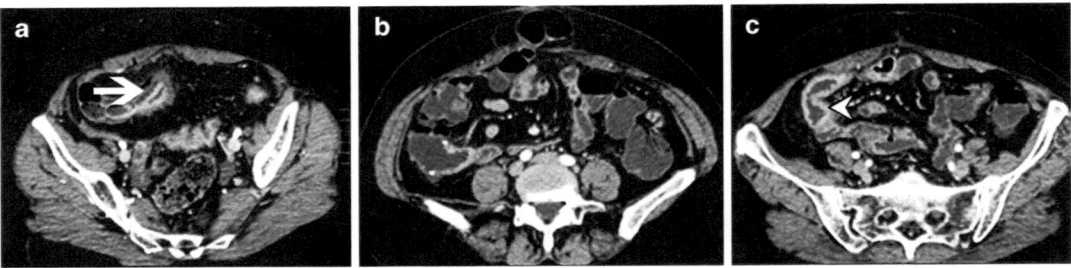

Fig. 15.1 Axial CT images show stratified bowel wall thickening (*arrow*) with surrounding creeping fat before surgery on (**a**) and after surgery in (**b**) and (**c**). After ileal resection (**b**), it can be still detected a mild stratified bowel wall thickening of the neo ileum terminal (*arrowhead* in **c**)

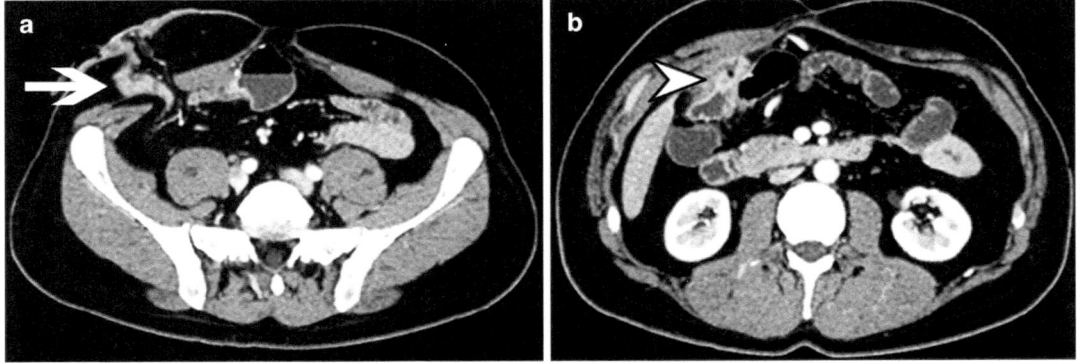

Fig. 15.2 (**a**, **b**) Patient with Crohn's disease who was submitted to ileostomy in the right side (*arrow* in **a**) with recurrence of the disease in the preterminal ileum and perivisceral abscess (*arrowhead* in **b**)

with a similar diagnostic accuracy, and for these reasons, it is rarely performed especially in children [27].

Compared to MR, CT enterography is more readily available, has a shorter image acquisition time, provides slightly better image quality, is available for patients with implanted MR-sensitive devices, and costs less than MR enterography [28].

Although the radiation dose associated with CTE can be minimized with the use of automatic exposure control, MR enterography is preferred for younger patients who are likely to undergo multiple lifetime scans, as a follow-up for asymptomatic adults, and when there is the possibility of low-grade obstruction or contraindications for CT, including pregnancy and contrast allergy [28].

For the above considerations, CTE is mainly preferred for acute emergency situations, because, thanks to its high spatial resolution, it allows to accurately assess potential complications of IBD that require surgical management, such as perforation, peritonitis, postoperative leaks, abscess, severe strictures/obstruction, and fistulas (Figs 15.1 and 15.2) [16]. This is particularly true in patients with low subcutaneous fat in whom MR does not allow an adequate assessment due to its lower spatial resolution. Furthermore, CTE is useful to evaluate the presence of any extraintestinal involvement of the disease, and it remains an examination of choice for abscess drainage, to assess its extension and select the most appropriate access route.

In the evaluation of response to therapy (Fig. 15.3), when comparing responders with nonresponders, only the presence of "comb sign" on the index CT is predictive of radiologic response [29].

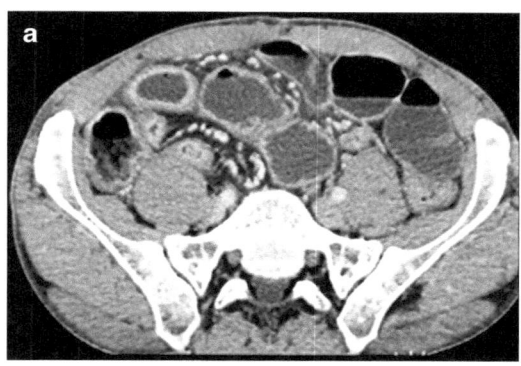
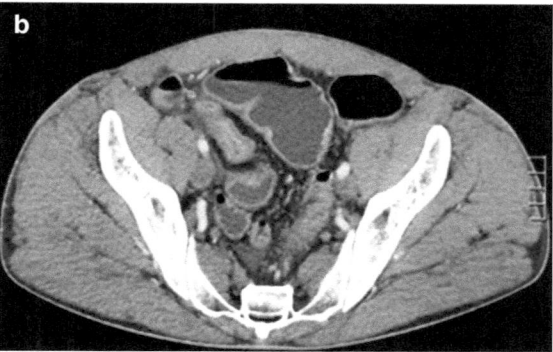
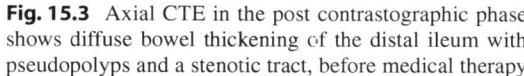

Fig. 15.3 Axial CTE in the post contrastographic phase shows diffuse bowel thickening of the distal ileum with pseudopolyps and a stenotic tract, before medical therapy (a); (b) shows the same patient after medical therapy with marked reduction of the wall bowel enhancement and of the mesenteric involvement

---

Keep in Mind

(i) Using fecal calprotectin, PCR, and US of the intestinal loops, it is possible to identify patients at high risk of IBD to be submitted as soon as possible to an endoscopic and histological evaluation of the gastrointestinal tract.

(ii) The simultaneous negativity of these 3 test allows to exclude, with a high degree of probability, the risk of being affected by IBD.

15.2.3 Magnetic Resonance Enterography

Magnetic resonance enterography (MRE) provides useful information in the study of IBD, mainly CD. In children, due its simplicity and the lack of radiation exposure, MRE is the preferred technique in the follow-up of IBD [16]. However, problems such as imaging artifacts due to bowel peristalsis and motion or poor cooperation of the child may be responsible of poor quality images [16].

Through the MR images, it is possible to identify the main features of the disease such as the involvement of the bowel wall, and in particular of the mucosa and submucosa, and the involvement of the near structures (comb sign, mesentery, nodes). In particular, MRE allows the detection of ulcers, inflammatory pseudopolyps, stenosis, adhesions, and fistulas. These signs usually allow to make the diagnosis of CD with good confidence [16, 30, 31].

Evaluation of CD through diffusion weighted imaging (DWI) is a more and more growing field since DWI yields high qualitative information. Inflammation of the bowel wall causes restricted diffusion shown as increased signal intensity and decreased ADC values [32].

Hence, MRE allows to differentiate among the three forms of CD: inflammatory, stricturing (stenosing), and penetrating disease. Regarding stricturing CD, thanks to motion sequences, MRE allows the differential diagnosis of functional and organic strictures: these latter can be identified by observing decreased peristalsis (frozen bowel sign) using cine balanced steady-state free precession (cine BSSFP) images [33].

MRI has been shown to be the best imaging technique to differentiate active inflammation from fibrosis [16]. For active disease, the sensitivity and specificity of MRE are estimated as 87.5% and 79.3% compared to 100% and 62.1% for CTE, while for fibrosis, the sensitivity and specificity of MRE are 57.1% and 82.1% compared to 42.3% and 67.9% of CTE, respectively [34].

MRE may also be used to monitor response to therapy in patients with CD. According to the ECCO/ESGAR guidelines, MRI is accurate for therapeutic monitoring in colonic Crohn's disease, while the accuracy of other modalities is not well defined [28]. In recent study [35], in patients with active CD and ulcers in at least one ileocolonic segment who underwent ileocolonoscopy and MR enterography at baseline and 12 weeks after therapy, MRE proved to have a high accuracy in detecting ulcer healing and endoscopic remission using ileocolonoscopy as a reference standard.

Moreover, through MR, it is possible to detect extraluminal findings and complications of IBD [36].

Comparing MRE with endoscopic findings, some authors derived the Magnetic Resonance Index of Activity (MaRIA) score to assess disease activity [37]. This score derives from the evaluation of many imaging MR findings as the relative contrast enhancement and wall thickness of bowel wall and the presence of edema and ulcerations. Moreover, it proved to be a valid, responsive, and reliable instrument for the assessment of therapeutic response.

Compared to laboratory tests and endoscopy, MRE shows a fair agreement between disease activity identified on endoscopy, and elevation in inflammatory markers is associated with enterography disease activity [36]. Moreover, there is a significant correlation between disease activity on enterography and histology from surgically resected bowel as well as Crohn's disease activity index (CDAI) score [38–41].

Finally, MRE allows to detect any "systemic" abnormality related to IBD, as the presence of gallstones, which can be detected also on US, and seronegative spondyloarthropathies, in particular ankylosing spondylitis (SpA) (if the entire spine is involved) or sacroiliitis (if only the sacroiliac joint is involved).

MRI may have a role in the diagnosis of SpA and sacroiliitis: active inflammatory lesions such as bone marrow edema/osteitis, synovitis, and enthesitis, and capsulitis associated with SpA can be detected by MRI. Also structural damage such as sclerosis, erosions, fat deposition, and ankylosis can be detected by MRI. Furthermore, MRI plays a key role in the early diagnosis of sacroiliitis; for this reason, in 2009, the ASAS (Assessment of SpondyloArthritis international Society) group published new criteria for the classification of axial spondyloarthropathy, based on sacroiliitis on MRI in patients without structural damage [42]. As demonstrated by Leclerc-Jacob et al. [43], sacroiliitis is mainly depicted on thin coronal slices acquired 3 min after contrast agent injection: in these conditions, contrast agent may enhance inflammatory bone marrow localized near subchondral bone or the articular surface.

Finally, considering that CD may lead to important disabilities and that there is recognized increased cancer risk in patients with IBD, MRE may play a pivotal role in the follow-up of the disease. Most cancers in patients with CD are small bowel adenocarcinomas, which are usually located in the jejunum and the terminal ileum, and they can be detected on MRE [44] mainly as thickening of the terminal ileum, usually extending from the ileocecal valve, with luminal narrowing and stranding of the surrounding mesenteric fat, and restricted signal on DWI. Compared to de novo adenocarcinoma, in CD it is particularly located in bypassed loops or in vicinity of chronic fistula. However, active CD shows increased signal too, so that this technique might not be appropriate to differentiate between active disease and tumor using just DWI and apparent diffusion coefficient, though it may be useful to detect cancer in patient with quiescent or inactive CD.

Key Points
  (i) MRE offers excellent imaging of transmural and perienteric lesions in IBD.
 (ii) Being x-ray-free, it allows to monitor IBD and response to therapy in IBD also considering that nowadays the diagnosis of CD is more often done with MRE than US or CT, mainly in pediatric patients.
(iii) Affected loops are easily detected through DWI sequences as loops with high signal that are easily recognized since they light up like a "bulb lamp."

also in the early stage before clinical symptoms.

(iv) MRI is the imaging modality of choice for the evaluation of perianal disease, fistula, and adjacent abscesses.

(v) MRI is accurate for therapeutic monitoring in colonic Crohn's disease.

15.3 Diagnosis of Colonic Complications in IBD

The Vienna classification of CD distinguishes three patient subgroups according to disease behaviour: penetrating, stricturing, and inflammatory. It is mandatory for the clinician and the surgeon to have an accurate assessment of any penetrating or stricturing complication occurring during the follow-up of patients with IBD because surgical management is mainly reserved for complications including strictures, adhesions and bowel obstructions, fistula, and perianal disease.

15.3.1 Penetrating Complications

Penetrating disease may be defined as the occurrence of intra-abdominal or perianal fistulas and/or abscesses.

According to the ECCO/ESGAR guidelines, morphologic demonstration of penetrating complication may be obtained through US, CT, and MRI; sensitivity and specificity of these techniques in the detection of penetrating disease are reported in Table 15.1 [28].

Fistulas usually occur in the advanced stage of the disease, when there is a transmural extension.

They are abnormal communications between two epithelial surfaces or between an epithelial surface and the skin. According to the involved loops, we can distinguish ileocecal, enteroenteral, and enterocolic fistulas; furthermore, leaks that go through to the skin are called enterocutaneous fistulas, but other organs can be involved in fistulas, such as the bladder, vagina, and anus.

Fistulas usually appear at US evaluation as hypoechoic, duct-like peri-intestinal lesions with lumen diameter <2 cm; at CT examination as linear enhancing tracts with or without communication with adjacent structures, tethering bowel loops; and at MRI hyperintense on T1-weighted images and hyperintense on T2-weighted images [16].

Inflammatory lesions in IBD may extend beyond intestinal wall leading to abscesses. These are seen at US examination as thick walled, hypoechoic, peri-intestinal round-like lesions; at CT exam as a ring-enhancing fluid collection, with or without air, and with well-defined borders; and at MR as an isolated collection of high-signal-intensity areas on the T2-weighted image, especially in ischioanal fossa [16].

15.3.2 Stricturing Complications

The most common complication of IBD, mainly CD, is obstruction, and it may arise from swelling and the formation of scar tissue. The result is thickening of the bowel wall and a narrowed intestinal passage. These narrowed areas are called strictures.

On US, strictures are defined as lumen diameter <1 cm with prestenotic distention defined as lumen diameter >2.5 cm; at CTE examination,

Table 15.1 Sensitivity and specificity of US, CT, and MR in the detection of fistulas and abscesses

	US	CT	MR
Fistulizing complications	Sensitivity 71–87 % Specificity 90–100 %	Sensitivity 68 % Specificity 91 %	Sensitivity 71–100 % Specificity 92–100 %
Abscesses	Sensitivity 81–100 % Specificity 92–94 %	Sensitivity 86–100 % Specificity 95–100 %	Sensitivity 75–86 % Specificity 91–93 %

Table 15.2 Sensitivity and specificity of US, CT, and MR in the detection of strictures

	US	CT	MR
Small bowel strictures	Sensitivity 75 % Specificity 93 %	Sensitivity 85–93 % Specificity 100 %	—
Colonic strictures	Sensitivity 100 % Specificity 90 %	—	Sensitivity 75–100 % Specificity 91–100 %

radiologists can identify mural stratification due to intramural edema and strictures, but they can be false positive due to an inadequate bowel distension; MRE is fundamental since it can distinguish between functional and organic strictures through CINE-MR.

According to the ECCO/ESGAR guidelines, contrast enema or cross-sectional imaging can be used to diagnose and assess colonic strictures, and accuracy is improved with colonic distension.

Sensitivity and specificity of US, CT, and MR in the detection of strictures are reported in Table 15.2 [28].

Pelvic MRI using T2-weighted images and contrast-enhanced T1-weighted images is the imaging modality of choice for the evaluation of perianal disease, fistula, and adjacent abscesses; it is superior to anal endosonography, CT, or surgical evaluation for showing disease extent [45, 46]. Extra-enteric complications may be visualized on MRE with less dependency on bowel distension as required for optimal CT imaging, an important technical advantage of MRE.

References

1. Escher JC, Taminiau JAJM. Treatment of inflammatory bowel disease in childhood. Inflamm Bowel Dis. 2003;9(1):34–58.
2. Solberg IC, Vatn MH, Hoie O, et al. Clinical course in Crohn's disease: results of a Norwegian population based ten-year follow-up study. Clin Gastroenterol Hepatol. 2007;5:1430–8.
3. Feagan BG, Bala M, Yan S, Olson A, Hanauer S. Unemployment and disability in patients with moderately to severely active Crohn's disease. J Clin Gastroenterol. 2005;39:390–5.
4. Boonen A, Dagnelie PC, Feleus A, Hesselink MA, Muris JW, Stockbrügger RW, et al. The impact of inflammatory bowel disease on labor force participation: results of a population sampled case-control study. Inflamm Bowel Dis. 2002;8:382–9.
5. Blomqvist P, Ekbom A. Inflammatory bowel diseases: health care and costs in Sweden in 1994. Scand J Gastroenterol. 1997;32:1134–9.
6. Chiou E, Nurko S. Functional abdominal pain and irritable bowel syndrome in children and adolescents. Therapy. 2011;8:315–31.
7. Walker LS, Beck J, Anderson J. Functional abdominal separation anxiety: helping the child return to school. Pediatr Ann. 2009;38:267–71.
8. Fefferman DS, Farrell RJ. Endoscopy in inflammatory bowel disease: indications, surveillance, and use in clinical practice. Clin Gastroenterol Hepatol. 2005;3:11–24.
9. Van Assche G, Herrmann KA, Louis E, Everett SM, Colombel JF, Rahier JF, Vanbeckevoort D, Meunier P, Tolan D, Ernst O, Rutgeerts P, Vermeire S, Aerden I, Oortwijn A, Ochsenkühn T. Effects of infliximab therapy on transmural lesions as assessed by magnetic resonance enteroclysis in patients with ileal Crohn's disease. J Crohns Colitis. 2013;7:950–7.
10. Harvey RF, Bradshaw JM. A simple index of Crohn's-disease activity. Lancet. 1980;1:514.
11. Vermeire S, Schreiber S, Sandborn WJ, et al. Correlation between the Crohn's disease activity and Harvey-Bradshaw indices in assessing Crohn's disease severity. Clin Gastroenterol Hepatol. 2010;8:357.
12. Lichtenstein GR, Hanauer SB, Sandborn WJ. Practice Parameters Committee of American College of Gastroenterology. Management of Crohn's disease in adults. Am J Gastroenterol. 2009;104:465.
13. Allen PB, Kamm MA, Peyrin-Biroulet L, Studd C, McDowell C, Allen BC, et al. Development and validation of a patient-reported disability measurement tool for patients with inflammatory bowel disease. Aliment Pharmacol Ther. 2013;37:438–44.
14. Leong RW, Huang T, Ko Y, Jeon A, Chang J, Kohler F, Kariyawasam V. Prospective validation study of the international classification of functioning, disability and health score in Crohn's disease and ulcerative colitis. J Crohns Colitis. 2014;8:1237–45.
15. Peyrin-Biroulet L, Cieza A, Sandborn WJ, Coenen M, Chowers Y, Hibi T, et al. International Programme to Develop New Indexes for Crohn's Disease (IPNIC) group. Development of the first disability index for inflammatory bowel disease based on the international classification of functioning, disability and health. Gut. 2012;61:241–7.
16. Athanasakos A, Mazioti A, Economopoulos N, Kontopoulou C, Stathis G, Filippiadis D, Spyridopoulos T, Alexopoulou E. Inflammatory bowel disease-the role of cross-sectional imaging

techniques in the investigation of the small bowel. Insights Imaging. 2015;6:73–83.

17. Maconi G, Sampietro GM, Parente F, Pompili G, Russo A, Cristaldi M, et al. Contrast radiology, computed tomography and ultrasonography in detecting internal fistulas and intra-abdominal abscesses in Crohn's disease: a prospective comparative study. Am J Gastroenterol. 2003;98:1545–55.

18. Lee SS, Kim AY, Yang SK, Chung JW, Kim SY, Park SH, et al. Crohn disease of the small bowel: comparison of CT enterography, MR enterography, and small-bowel follow-through as diagnostic techniques. Radiology. 2009;251:751–61.

19. Strobel D, Goertz RS, Bernatik T. Diagnostics in inflammatory bowel disease ultrasound. World J Gastroenterol. 2011;17:3192–7.

20. Quaia E, Migaleddu V, Baratella E, Pizzolato R, Rossi A, Grotto M, et al. The diagnostic value of small bowel wall vascularity after sulfur hexafluoride-filled microbubble injection in patients with Crohn's disease. Correlation with the therapeutic effectiveness of specific anti-inflammatory treatment. Eur J Radiol. 2009;69:438–44.

21. Paredes JM, Ripolles T, Cortes X, Martinez MJ, Barrachina M, Gomez F, et al. Abdominal sonographic changes after antibody to tumor necrosis factor (anti-TNF) alpha therapy in Crohn's Disease. Dig Dis Sci. 2010;55:404–10.

22. Bodily KD, Fletcher JG, Sclem CA, Johnson CD, Fidler JL, Barlow JM, et al. Crohn Disease: mural attenuation and thickness at contrast-enhanced CT enterography–correlation with endoscopic and histologic findings of inflammation. Radiology. 2006;238(2):505–16.

23. Bolondi L, Gaiani S, Brignola C, Campieri M, Rigamonti A, Zironi G, Gionchetti P, Belloli C, Miglioli M, Barbara L. Changes in splanchnic hemodynamics in inflammatory bowel disease. Noninvasive assessment by Doppler ultrasound flowmetry. Scand J Gastroenterol. 1992;27(6):501–7.

24. Ripollés T, Martínez-Pérez MJ, Blanc E, Delgado F, Vizuete J, Paredes JM, Vilar J. Contrast-enhanced ultrasound (CEUS) in Crohn's disease: technique, image interpretation and clinical applications. Insights Imaging. 2011;2:639–52.

25. Allgayer H, Braden B, Dietrich CF. Transabdominal ultrasound in inflammatory bowel disease. Conventional and recently developed techniques– update. Med Ultrason. 2011;13:302–13.

26. Chiorean MV, Sandrasegaran K, Saxena R, Maglinte DD, Nakeeb A, Johnson CS. Correlation of CT enteroclysis with surgical pathology in Crohn's disease. Am J Gastroenterol. 2007;102:2541–50.

27. Wold PB, Fletcher JG, Johnson CD, Sandborn WJ. Assessment of small bowel Crohn disease: noninvasive peroral CT enterography compared with other imaging methods and endoscopy— feasibility study. Radiology. 2003;229:275–81.

28. Panes J, Bouhnik Y, Reinisch W, Stoker J, Taylor SA, Baumgart DC, Danese S, Halligan S, Marincek B, Matos C, Peyrin-Biroulet L, Rimola J, Rogler G, van Assche G, Ardizzone S, Ba-Ssalamah A, Bali MA, Bellini D, Biancone L, Castiglione F, Ehehalt R, Grassi R, Kucharzik T, Maccioni F, Maconi G, Magro F, Martín-Comín J, Morana G, Pendsé D, Sebastian S, Signore A, Tolan D, Tielbeek JA, Weishaupt D, Wiarda B, Laghi A. Imaging techniques for assessment of inflammatory bowel disease: joint ECCO and ESGAR evidence-based consensus guidelines. J Crohns Colitis. 2013;7:556–85.

29. Bruining DH, Loftus Jr EV, Ehman EC, Siddiki HA, Nguyen DL, Fidler JL, et al. Computed tomography enterography detects intestinal wall changes and effects of treatment in patients with Crohn's disease. Clin Gastroenterol Hepatol. 2011;9:679–683.e1.

30. Ordás I, Rimola J, Rodríguez S, et al. Accuracy of magnetic resonance enterography in assessing response to therapy and mucosal healing in patients with Crohn's disease. Gastroenterology. 2014;146: 374–82.e1.

31. Chalian M, Ozturk A, Oliva-Hemker M, Pryde S, Huisman TA. MR enterography findings of inflammatory bowel disease in pediatric patients. AJR Am J Roentgenol. 2011;196:W810–6.

32. Oto A, Kayhan A, Williams JT, Fan X, Yun L, Arkani S, Rubin DT. Active Crohn's disease in the small bowel: evaluation by diffusion weighted imaging and quantitative dynamic contrast enhanced MR imaging. J Magn Reson Imaging. 2011;33(3):615–24.

33. Guglielmo FF, Mitchell DG, O'Kane PL, Deshmukh SP, Roth CG, Burach I, Burns A, Dulka S, Parker L. Erratum to: identifying decreased peristalsis of abnormal small bowel segments in Crohn's disease using cine MR enterography: the frozen bowel sign. Abdom Imaging. 2015;40:1138–49.

34. Quencer KB, Nimkin K, Mino-Kenudson M, Gee MS. Detecting active inflammation and fibrosis in pediatric Crohn's disease: prospective evaluation of MR-E and CT-E. Abdom Imaging. 2013;38:705–13.

35. Friedrich C, Fajfar A, Pawlik M, et al. Magnetic resonance enterography with and without biphasic contrast agent enema compared to conventional ileocolonoscopy in patients with Crohn's disease. Inflamm Bowel Dis. 2012;18:1842.

36. Patel NS, Pola S, Muralimohan R, Zou GY, Santillan C, Patel D, Levesque BG, Sandborn WJ. Outcomes of computed tomography and magnetic resonance enterography in clinical practice of inflammatory bowel disease. Dig Dis Sci. 2014;59(4):838–49.

37. Rimola J, Ordás I, Rodriguez S, García-Bosch O, Aceituno M, Llach J, Ayuso C, Ricart E, Panés J. Magnetic resonance imaging for evaluation of Crohn's disease: validation of parameters of severity and quantitative index of activity. Inflamm Bowel Dis. 2011;17:1759–68.

38. Zappa M, Stefanescu C, Cazals-Hatem D, et al. Which magnetic resonance imaging findings accurately evaluate inflammation in small bowel Crohn's disease? A retrospective comparison with surgical pathologic analysis. Inflamm Bowel Dis. 2011;17:984–93.

39. Messaris E, Chandolias N, Grand D, Pricolo V. Role of magnetic resonance enterography in the management of Crohn disease. Arch Surg. 2010;145:471–5.

40. Ha CY, Kumar N, Raptis CA, et al. Magnetic resonance enterography: safe and effective imaging for stricturing Crohn's disease. Dig Dis Sci. 2011;56: 2906–13.

41. Grieser C, Denecke T, Steffen IG, et al. Magnetic resonance enteroclysis in patients with Crohn's disease: fat saturated T2- weighted sequences for evaluation of inflammatory activity. J Crohns Colitis. 2012;6:294–301.

42. Rudwaleit M, Jurik AG, Hermann KG, et al. Defining active sacroiliitis on magnetic resonance imaging (MRI) for classification of axial spondyloarthritis: a consensual approach by the ASAS/OMERACT MRI group. Ann Rheum Dis. 2009;68:1520–7.

43. Leclerc-Jacob S, Lux G, Rat AC, Laurent V, Blum A, Chary-Valckenaere I, Peyrin-Biroulet L, Loeuille D. The prevalence of inflammatory sacroiliitis assessed on magnetic resonance imaging of inflammatory bowel disease: a retrospective study performed on 186 patients. Aliment Pharmacol Ther. 2014;39:957–62.

44. Placé V, Hristova L, Dray X, Lavergne-Slove A, Boudiaf M, Soyer P. Ileal adenocarcinoma in Crohn's disease: magnetic resonance enterography features. Clin Imaging. 2012;36:24–8.

45. Sahni VA, Ahmad R, Burling D. Which method is best for imaging of perianal fistula? Abdom Imaging. 2008;33:26–30.

46. Schwartz DA, Wiersema MJ, Dudiak KM, Fletcher JG, Clain JE, Tremaine WJ, Zinsmeister AR, Norton ID, Boardman LA, Devine RM, Wolff BG, Young-Fadok TM, Diehl NN, Pemberton JH, Sandborn WJ. A comparison of endoscopic ultrasound, magnetic resonance imaging, and exam under anesthesia for evaluation of Crohn's perianal fistulas. Gastroenterology. 2001;121: 1064–72.

Surgery and Crohn's Disease

Gianfranco Cocorullo, Tommaso Fontana,
Nicolò Falco, Roberta Tutino, Antonino Agrusa,
Gregorio Scerrino, and Gaspars Gulotta

16.1 Introduction

It is known that the treatment of Crohn's disease (CD) absolutely needs a multidisciplinary approach with an important relationship between gastroenterologist and surgeon.

CD, in fact, is a chronic inflammatory bowel disease interesting all segments of alimentary tract showing extreme variability of clinical presentations [1, 2]. Medical therapy when ineffective will give way to surgical treatment, and the last one isn't possible without adequate pharmacological support.

Synthetically, it's possible to affirm that gastroenterologist treats CD and the surgeon its complications.

16.2 Presurgery

Before evaluating surgical treatment of CD, it's important to focalize the three different patterns of the affection: inflammatory, stenosing, and fistulizing appearance [3–5].

The inflammatory one is characterized by mucosal edema; symptoms are fever, diarrhea, anemia, asthenia, abdominal pain, weight loss, and electrolyte imbalance.

The clinical presentation arises from a chronic evolution to very acute presentations that lead patients to kidney failure due to dehydration. Moreover it's known that reiteration of inflammatory facts can evolve to fibrosis and stenosis.

The stenosing presentation causes a significant reduction of caliber of bowel lumen due to edema or fibrosis. It is characterized by clinical history of transitory bowel obstruction with abdominal pain, vomit, and malnutrition due to reduction in food intake. The late evolution shows an acute bowel obstruction with abdominal distension and air-fluid levels.

The fistulizing presentation depends on anatomical site and fistula typology. It is possible to find entero-enteric or enterocutaneous fistulas but also the bladder can be involved, causing urinary symptomatology. Obviously the fistulizing pattern can determine localized or diffuse peritonitis due to free perforation.

An important tool in CD severity evaluation is the Crohn's Disease Activity Index (CDAI) [6]; the clinical stadiation, instead, is referred to the Vienna or Montreal classification [7].

As previously announced, surgery treats complications. These are distinguished in local and systemic [8].

G. Cocorullo (✉) • T. Fontana • N. Falco • R. Tutino
A. Agrusa • G. Scerrino • G. Gulotta
Department of surgical oncological and oral sciences,
University Hospital P. Giaccone, University of
Palermo, Palermo, Italy
e-mail: gianfranco.cocorullo@unipa.it

© Springer International Publishing Switzerland 2016
G. Lo Re, M. Midiri (eds.), *Crohn's Disease: Radiological Features and Clinical-Surgical Correlations*,
DOI 10.1007/978-3-319-23066-5_16

Local complications increase with the disease duration (from 19 % in the first year, till 60 % after 8 years) and include: internal or external fistulae, obstruction, perforation, bleeding, and abscess. Fistulas and abscesses are more frequent in fistulizing colonic localizations, while obstruction is the most frequent complication of stenosing ileal forms. Perineal findings, at last, are secondary to a colonic involvement and will be treated in another chapter.

Systemic complications, instead, include cutaneous, ocular and joint involvement, as well as gallstones formation due to alteration of the absorption of bile salts [9].

16.3 The Detection of Complications and the Surgical Planning

Surgery is mostly involved in the management of local complications [8].

Clinical history, laboratoristic analysis, and radiological findings determine the choice of a surgical treatment.

In the diagnostic assessment (see related chapters), the nature, the localization, the extension, and the type of injury have to be determined [10].

The surgical treatment can be required in emergency (see previous chapter) for acute presentations, but it must be planned whenever it's possible.

So, it is important to improve both local and general patient conditions in order to minimize any postoperative complications. The use of anti-inflammatory drugs and the drainage of abdominal collections together with bowel rest and the administration of parenteral nutrition can improve nutritional and immunological conditions of the patient and so his performance status [11].

16.4 Surgery

Since the CD can involve each tract of gastrointestinal tract, even its complications can occur in different localizations.

16.4.1 Esophagus

In the esophagus, it's possible to find an ulcerated mucosa or strictures; these conditions are usually treated with medical therapy, while surgery is infrequent.

16.4.2 Stomach and Duodenum

Gastroduodenal involvement is rare, and related complications are obstruction, perforation, fistula, and hemorrhage. The first attempt of treatment has to be conservative medical therapy, and surgery should be avoided when possible. However, in strictures, gastrojejunostomy and strictureplasty are the treatments of choice; even postoperative complications are frequent. Fistulas need a wedge resection of gastroduodenal orifice and a resection of the involved bowel tract.

16.4.3 Small Bowel

Generally, small bowel strictures are the most frequent indications of surgical treatment; however intraoperative previously undiagnosed findings can be encountered, such as the presence of fistulas or abscesses. The surgical management of fistulas is provided by the resection of the involved bowel and the closure of the secondary orifices.

The procedure of choice for the treatment of strictures is segmental resection and anastomosis in single time. Until a few decades ago, surgeons considered necessary to remove the lesions with a wide margin of macroscopically healthy gut. Today it is followed the concept of preserving as much bowel as possible, due to the high incidence of postoperative recurrences and the detection of possible regressions of mild lesions [12, 13]. Thus, when multiple stenotic tracts coexist or in already resected patients, strictureplasty becomes the treatment of choice [14].

Heineke-Mikulicz technique is used for short strictures, Finney technique is chosen for long ones (>10 cm), while Michelassi technique is performed for large stenotic tracts (Fig. 16.1).

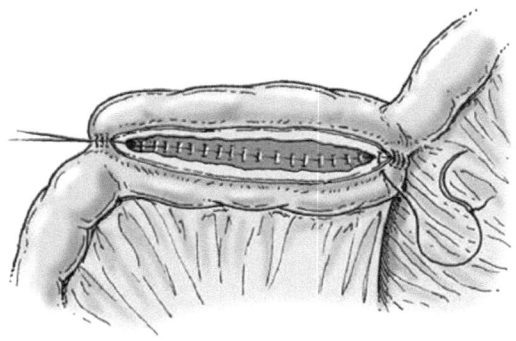

Fig. 16.1 Strictureplasty with a side-to-side anastomosis according to Michelassi

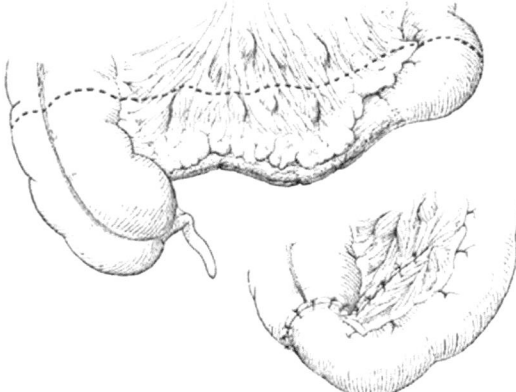

Fig. 16.2 End-to-end ileocolic anastomosis

These conservative surgical treatments have the aim of avoiding massive intestinal resections that can lead to the "short bowel syndrome" with fluid and electrolytes disturbance and malnutrition. Of course, strictureplasty has to be avoided in suspicious of malignancy or if morbid and bleeding mucosa is highlighted.

The obstructed tract often comprises the cecum and the terminal ileum; in these cases it becomes necessary an ileocecectomy [15] (Fig. 16.2).

16.4.4 Colon

Colonic involvements of CD rarely require surgical treatment, as, in these tracts, strictures occur less.

However, the solely colonic involvement can be treated with a colectomy with rectal preservation and an ileorectal anastomosis. A segmental colon resection can be an option. In this regard, Fazio recommends to perform a right hemicolectomy for involvement of ileocolonic or right side colon, a total or subtotal colectomy if the disease involves at least one-half of the colon, and a sigmoid colectomy or an anterior resection if only this area is affected [16]. Hartmann's procedure can be an alternative to the restoration of bowel transit.

It is still debated whenever to perform a total colectomy or a limited resection of strictures; total colectomies seem to encounter lower recurrence, even segmental colectomies will have a better functional outcome [17].

However, when the colon is entirely pathological and there is an involvement of the rectum or anus, a proctocolectomy with ileostomy should be realized. Distal ligation can be performed without the need for vascular isolation. Restorative proctocolectomy should be avoided, even in an apparent healthy small bowel.

16.5 The Role of Minimally Invasive Surgery in CD

Today the minimally invasive surgery finds an important role in the treatment of almost all surgical pathologies, including CD.

Laparoscopic surgery provides several advantages that have to be considered when planning and selecting the preferable approach for patients.

These advantages include:

- Faster postoperative course adding an inferior surgical stress
- Reduced postoperative pain
- Earlier hospital discharge
- Early recovery of preoperative performance status
- Better cosmetic outcome
- Lesser blood loss
- Lesser occurrence of peritoneal contamination

A meta-analysis was produced in order to analyze the advantages of laparoscopic approach compared to open surgery for ileocecal resection in CD [22]. In a review that collected data from 20 studies, it is shown that laparoscopy is a valid alternative to open surgery. An analysis, performed on 783 patients, 338 (43.2 %) of whom underwent laparoscopic ileocecal resection, shows longer operative time for the laparoscopic approach; in terms of intraoperative bleeding and complications, laparoscopic and open group were fairly consistent, while postoperative hospital stay was significantly shorter in the laparoscopic-treated patients as the recovery of bowel sounds occurs earlier; finally, complications were comparable. Therefore, laparoscopic resection offers substantial advantages in terms of postoperative recovery and hospital stay [18–23].

These results confirmed the safety of the procedure, so the laparoscopic surgical approach to CD can be an important option.

However, CD laparoscopic surgery suffers for the presence of a reduced tactile feedback that could hinder the identification of strictures. Moreover, the mesenterial thickening in the suffering tracts can make it difficult the resection.

In this case to exteriorize the tracts to be resected and to perform the resection trough the minilaparotomy can be an option to overcome these problems and to perform manual anastomosis. In these cases a L-L anastomosis is preferable to consent a large anastomotic lumen which prevents stenosing relapses.

The use of staplers in CD is described and utilized, even if mechanical anastomosis in thicken bowel walls should be avoided. Moreover it is possible to put over some discharging stitches (Fig. 16.3).

Laparoscopy should be preferable in young patients that probably will be submitted to other intervention in the next years; in fact, the reduced adhesions formation provided by the less bowel manipulation can make easy next access. Older patients can benefit from the less invasive approach in reducing the postoperative sequelae and thus in early recovery.

Of course, a very important factor is the surgeon's skill in laparoscopy and in CD treatment.

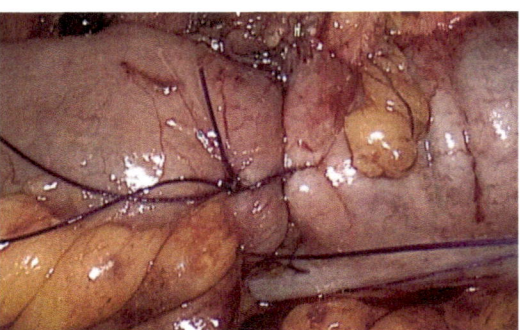

Fig. 16.3 Mechanical bowel anastomosis with additional stiches

References

1. Kirsner JB. Inflammatory bowel disease. Clinical and therapeutic aspects. Dis Mon. 1991;37(11):669–746.
2. Simian D, Estay C, Lubascher J, et al. Inflammatory bowel disease. Experience in 316 patients. Rev Med Chil. 2014;142(8):1006–13. doi:10.4067/S0034-98872014000800008.
3. Nos P, Garrigues V, Bastida G, et al. Outcome of patients with nonstenotic, nonfistulizing Crohn's disease. Dig Dis Sci. 2004;49(11–12):1771–6.
4. Schirin-Sokhan R, Winograd R, Tischendorf S, et al. Assessment of inflammatory and fibrotic stenoses in patients with Crohn's disease using contrast-enhanced ultrasound and computerized algorithm: a pilot study. Digestion. 2011;83(4):263–8. doi:10.1159/000321389. Epub 2011 Jan 28.
5. Su YR, Shih IL, Tai HC, et al. Surgical management in enterovesical fistula in Crohn disease at a single medical center. Int Surg. 2014;99(2):120–5. doi:10.9738/INTSURG-D-13-00038.1.
6. Kim ES, Park KS, Cho KB, et al. Development of a Web-based, self-reporting symptom diary for Crohn's Disease, and its correlation with the Crohn's Disease Activity Index: Web-based, self-reporting symptom diary for Crohn's Disease. Crohns Colitis. 2014. pii: S1873-9946(14)00268-2. doi:10.1016/j.crohns.2014.09.003. [Epub ahead of print].
7. Veloso FT. How useful is the Vienna classification in clinical practice? See comment in PubMed commons below. Inflamm Bowel Dis. 2008;14 Suppl 2:S161. doi:10.1002/ibd.20616.
8. Marineaţă A, Rezuş E, Mihai C, et al. Extra intestinal manifestations and complications in inflammatory bowel disease. Rev Med Chir Soc Med Nat Iasi. 2014;118(2):279–88.
9. Sastangi J, Sutherland LR. Inflammatory bowel diseases. London: Elsevier Limited (Churchill Livingstone); 2003.
10. Spinelli A, Allocca M, Jovani M, et al. Review article: optimal preparation for surgery in Crohn's dis-

ease. Aliment Pharmacol Ther. 2014;40(9):1009–22. doi:10.1111/apt.12947. Epub 2014 Sep 10.

11. Li G, Ren J, Wang G, et al. Preoperative exclusive enteral nutrition reduces the postoperative septic complications of fistulizing Crohn's disease. See comment in PubMed Commons below. Eur J Clin Nutr. 2014;68(4):441–6. doi:10.1038/ejcn.2014.16. Epub 2014 Feb 19.

12. Althausen TL, Doig RK, Uyeyama K, et al. Digestion and absorption after massive resection of the small intestine. II. Recovery of the absorptive function as shown by intestinal absorption tests in two patients and a consideration of compensatory mechanisms. Gastroenterology. 1968;54((4):Suppl):788–90.

13. Botti F, Carrara A, Antonelli E, et al. The minimal bowel resection in Crohn's disease: analysis of prognostic factors on the surgical recurrence. Ann Ital Chir. 2003;74(6):627–33.

14. Strong SA. Surgical treatment of inflammatory bowel disease. Curr Opin Gastroenterol. 2002;18(4):441–6.

15. Vettoretto N, Gazzola L, Giovanetti M. Emergency laparoscopic ileocecal resection for Crohn's acute obstruction. JSLS. 2013;17(3):499–502. doi:10.4293/108680813X13693422521872.

16. Fazio V. Crohn's disease and indeterminate colitis. In Corman's colon and rectal surgery. 6th ed. Philadelphia: Lippincott Williams and Wilkins; 2013.

17. Malafosse M. Crohn's disease: current surgical treatment. Bull Acad Natl Med. 2007;191(6):1143–56; discussion 1157–8.

18. Colon Cancer Laparoscopic or Open Resection Study Group, Buunen M, Veldkamp R, et al. Survival after laparoscopic surgery versus open surgery for colon cancer: long-term outcome of a randomised clinical trial. 2009;10(1):44–52. Epub 2008 Dec 13.

19. Veldkamp R, Gholghesaei M, Bonjer HJ, et al. Laparoscopic resection of colon cancer: consensus of the European Association of Endoscopic Surgery (EAES). Surgical Endosopy and other International techniques. 2004; 18(8):1163–85.

20. Simon T, Orangio GR, Ambroze WL, et al. Factors associated with complications of open versus laparoscopic sigmoid resection for diverticulitis. JSLS J Soc Laparoendosc Surg. 2005; 9(1):63.

21. Sun J, Jiang T, Qiu Z, et al. Short-term and medium-term clinical outcomes of laparoscopic-assisted and open surgery for colorectal cancer: a single center retrospective case–control study. BMC Gastroenterol. 2011;11:85. Source.Department of General Surgery, Affiliated First People's Hospital, Shanghai Jiao Tong University, 100 Hai Ning Road, Shanghai, 200080, China

22. Tilney HS, Constantinides VA, Heriot AG, et al. Comparison of laparoscopic and open ileocecal resection for Crohn's disease: a meta-analysis. Surg Endosc. 2006;20(7):1036–44.

23. Tavernier M, Lebreton G, Alves A. Laparoscopic surgery for complex Crohn's disease. J Visc Surg. 2013;150(6):389–93. doi:10.1016/j.jvisc-surg.2013.09.004. Epub 2013 Oct.

Surgical Emergencies in Crohn's Disease

17

Gianfranco Cocorullo, Roberta Tutino, Nicolò Falco,
Tommaso Fontana, Giovanni Guercio,
Giuseppe Salamone, and Gaspare Gulotta

17.1 Introduction

Crohn's disease, as a chronic inflammatory disease of unknown etiology that can affect any part of the alimentary canal from the mouth to the anus, has a highly variable course and a very unpredictable evolution [1, 2].

Even surgery does not cure CD, it has however a relevant role in its treatment in combination to medical therapy during the large course of the disease; indeed almost each CD patient is submitted to a surgical intervention during his life.

Nowadays, surgery is considered the last treatment to use whenever medical therapy is insufficient to control symptoms; this choice involves an intervention on more serious patients with more surgical complications. Surgery finds in the Crohn's disease a main role in the management of the obstructive or septic complications; however, elective surgical treatments are proposed in patients with sub-occlusive presentation due to chronic fistulas or with high CD index (>220) with a terminal ileum-cecum disease [3].

Systematic guidelines on the management of acute presentation of CD are difficult to define due to the high number of possible clinical presentation. In fact, the grade of urgency, general conditions of patient, the offset or the recurrence of the disease, and the medical and surgical team experience are determinants on the treatment [3].

Laparoscopy is preferable to open surgery, except in complex cases or in recurrent resections. It shows lower morbidity rates and lower mortality, faster recovery of intestinal motility, lower admission times, lower adhesions formation, and lower rates of incisional hernias [3]. Moreover, laparoscopy consents in patients with presentation of "acute appendicitis" a complete exploration of the bowel consenting differential diagnosis.

Of course a specific surgical skill is required in advanced laparoscopy, especially in patients needing resection because of the frequent complexity of anatomic presentation.

Emergency surgery is still performed in up to 19 % of the cases, even if the multidisciplinary approach to CD reduced the emergency operation rate over the years [3].

Anyway, within complication group, occurrence of intestinal perforation unfortunately increases, and in 23.5 % of cases, it represents the onset of CD [4, 5].

17.2 Pseudoappendicitis

Acute symptoms of an ileocolic localization of CD can frequently simulate an acute appendicitis.

G. Cocorullo (✉) • R. Tutino • N. Falco • T. Fontana
G. Guercio • G. Salamone • G. Gulotta
Department of Surgical Oncological and
Stomatological Sciences, University Hospital
P. Giaccone, University of Palermo, Palermo, Italy
e-mail: gianfranco.cocorullo@unipa.it

Patients can show a sudden pain located in the right iliac fossa; Blumberg sign can be positive; the patient can present pyrexia, vomiting, and neutrophil leukocytosis [6]. This "pseudoappendicitis" can be caused by an acute terminal ileitis or granulomatous enteritis [7].

International guidelines recommend different medical or surgical approaches, in relation to the different presentations of the disease [8].

Differential diagnosis is difficult, and whenever diagnosis has not yet done, a careful medical history has to be collected, and in suspicious cases, instrumental examination including ultrasounds and CT (or MRI) must be done.

Undoubtable, most of these patients reach the operating room without a correct diagnosis, and even during surgery, diagnosis is not always done; histological findings finally allow to the correct framing.

If the CD is known, an acute abdominal pain in the right iliac fossa should be managed with medical therapy whenever possible (like patients presenting an abdominal abscess), or alternatively, by a drainage of fluid collections with or without small bowel resections. However, when ileocecal resection is needed, a side-to-side mechanical anastomosis is recommended if the wall thickness consents its performance [3].

If there is an intraoperative diagnosis of CD, surgeon should perform a peritoneal toilet avoiding resection and appendectomy; prophylactic appendectomy could expose the patient to the risk of a fistulization even if it is a low risk [9]. Otherwise, to perform appendectomy permits a histological diagnosis of the disease, even if an endoscopic postoperative diagnosis is possible too.

17.3 Acute Intestinal Obstruction

Acute intestinal obstruction is the most frequent complication of Crohn's disease.

In 35–54 % of cases, this complication is related to a terminal ileum localization that is the most frequent form; however, a digiunal (22–36 %) or colonic disease (5–17 %) can cause an occlusive presentation too [8].

If correct diagnosis is done, medical therapy should be the treatment of choice, except in patients with sepsis incoming [3].

Granulomatous enteritis can develop a scar thickening evolving in fibrosis and also in a tight stenosis with bowel obstruction that imposes a surgical resolution if medical therapy is not effective.

The resection of the terminal ileum and cecum is the most widespread intervention in these cases.

The right hemicolectomy or more extensive resections are often not needed and harmful, so these are not recommended [3].

Whenever the granulomatous enteritis leads to fistulas or abscesses, involving many small intestinal loops, an initial lateral ileostomy and a colonic mucosa fistula may be appropriate to perform, and a second look should be done later [10].

17.4 Perforation

Enteritis can evolve versus bowel perforation, too.

This presentation occurs in 1–3 % of patients with CD, and in this group, it is the first manifestation in 25 % of cases [11].

Spontaneous perforations occur more frequently in the small bowel resulting in acute peritonitis; the treatment in these cases is abdominal toilet and bowel resection with or without single-step anastomosis depending on performance status of the patient and on severity of peritonitis [12].

17.5 Granulomatous Pancolitis

The colon can be affected in whole or in the form of "skip lesions."

This presentation will require an urgent surgical treatment if patients develop acute anemia, hypoproteinemia, hyperthermia, and diffuse peritonitis.

In cases of healthy rectoanal region, a subtotal colectomy with terminal ileostomy, with or without a mucous fistula on the sigma, should be done [13].

Because of the significant risk of dehiscences, restoration with anastomosis should be avoided.

The restorative intervention has to be delayed for at least 6 months.

17.6 Abdominal Abscess

The abscess, a complication that occurs in approximately 25 % of patients, is defined as an inflammatory mass which originates from bowel perforation [14].

The perforation is promptly covered by fibrin on the surface of the loops; fibrin causes adhesions between the loops among which it develops the abscess cavity (Fig. 17.1). It can be associated with a fistula in the 40 % of cases, a severe stenosis (51 %), or to anastomotic recurrence [15].

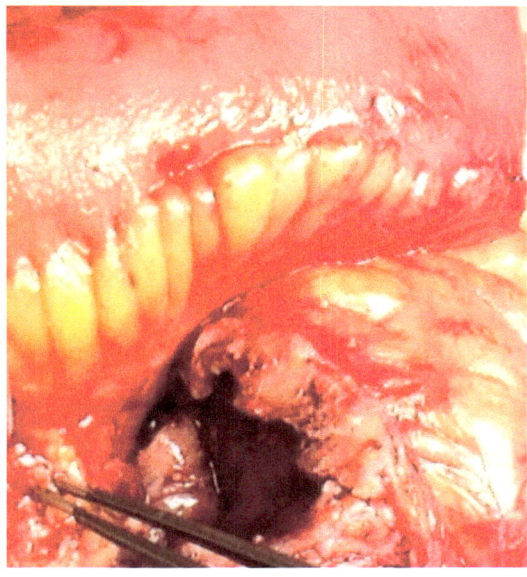

Fig. 17.1 Abdominal Abscess

Presentation can range from the complaint of subacute symptoms to a generalized sepsis that is showed in 28 % of patients [16].

Conservative therapy and interventional radiology drainage represent the first attempt of treatment; this choice allows to postpone the surgical act and, then, to perform a resection with one-step anastomosis [3].

The success of percutaneous drainage reported in literature varied from 65–96 %; failures are often related to the phenotype of the disease, the use of steroids, and the presence of compartmentalized abscess. If this treatment failed, patients require a surgical therapy with lysis of adhesions and surgical drainage. The risk of sepsis and anastomotic leakage could increase in not drained patient in whom biological immunosuppressive therapy is administered [17–21].

About whether to associate a resection or a temporary ileostomy, the "American Society of Colon and Rectal Surgeons" guidelines consider that for the surgical eradication of the abscess, a resection of diseased bowel is generally required, even if in presence of the risk of short bowel syndrome [18].

To avoid the resection of a large amount of bowel, the drainage and a temporary ileostomy without intestinal resections could be performed in urgency.

17.7 Hemorrhage

Intestinal hemorrhages represent a rare clinical presentation in Crohn's disease being the 1–3 % among all complications [22].

These originate by the erosion of a vessel, due to an ulceration of the bowel mucosa, and in 65 % of cases, the seat is represented by the small bowel [23].

Surgical interventions are often required. An attempt to control the bleeding by interventional endoscopy or interventional radiology should be done. Emergency surgery will be performed in patients with hemodynamic impairment or recurrent bleeding [24].

17.8   Severe Acute Colitis

Even for Crohn's disease, severe acute colitis can be defined based on the criteria of Truelove and Witts used for ulcerative colitis [25]. The criteria are enclosed in Table 17.1.

The abdominal X-ray depicts, in severe acute colitis, no colon distension.

The treatment of this complication should be conservative for 3–5 days; if medical therapy is ineffective, an emergency total colectomy will be performed, with ileostomy, and a mucous fistula in the sigma embedded in the lower part of the laparotomy [26].

Surgical therapy has to be applied to all patients not responding to medical therapy because, if perforation occurs, mortality reaches 40 % of cases [22].

This approach consents significant reduction of operative mortality rate (0.6 %), even if a high morbidity rate still remains, accounting up to 33 %. The reoperation rate, finally, is 14.6 % [27].

17.9   Toxic Megacolon

Toxic megacolon is a complication that occurs in 4–6 % of patients [22].

The definition used for ulcerative colitis according to the Truelove and Witts' criteria is used even for Crohn's disease [28]; criteria are showed in Table **17.2**.

Medical therapy should be attempted for a maximum of 3 days, if patient did not improve, a total colectomy in emergency have to be performed (Fig. 17.2).

Indeed, if there is a clinical improvement with medical therapy, the treatment strategy is to perform an elective total colectomy [29].

Table 17.1 Criteria of truelove and witts for severe acute colitis

1	>6 discharges per day with blood
2	Pyrexia (>37.5 ° C)
3	Tachycardia (>90 bpm)
4	Anemia (Hgb < 75 % of normal level)
5	Elevated erythrocyte sedimentation rate (>30 mm/h)

Table 17.2 Criteria of truelove and witts for toxic megacolon

1	>6 discharges per day with blood
2	Pyrexia (>37.5 ° C)
3	Tachycardia (>90 bpm)
4	Anemia requiring transfusion
5	Elevated erythrocyte sedimentation rate (>30 mm 1 h)
6	Colonic dilatation on X-ray of the abdomen >6 cm
7	Abdominal distension

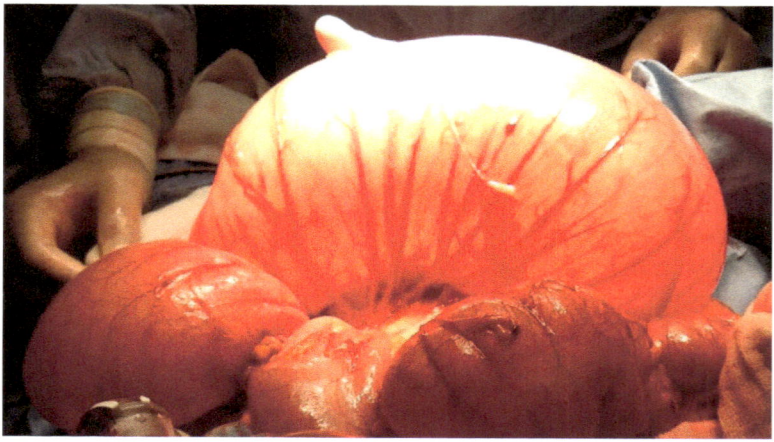

Fig. 17.2 Megacolon

References

1. Kirsner JB. Inflammatory bowel disease. Clinical and therapeutic aspects. Dis Mon. 1991;37(11):669–746.
2. Simian D, Estay C, Lubascher J, et al. Inflammatory bowel disease. Experience in 316 patients. Rev Med Chil. 2014;142(8):1006–13. doi:10.4067/S0034-98872014000800008.
3. Aratari A, Botti F, Carrara A, et al. Linee guida olelle macattia di crohn-acol (in colia borazione con siccr). www.acol.it/pratica-clinica-e-pubblicazioni/linee-guida.
4. Siassi M, Weiger A, Hohenberger W, et al. Changes in surgical therapy for Crohn's disease over 33 years: a prospective longitudinal study. Int J Colorectal Dis. 2007;22(3):319–24.
5. Latella G, Cocco A, Angelucci E, et al. Clinical course of Crohn's disease first diagnosed at surgery for acute abdomen. Dig Liver Dis. 2009;41(4):269–76.
6. Al-Mansour M, Watch L. Granulomatous stump appendicitis mimicking Crohn's disease. Am Surg. 2011;77(8):172–4.
7. Castillo Fernández AL, Paredes Esteban RM, Villar Pastor CM, et al. Appendectomy and Crohn's disease. See comment in PubMed Commons below. Cir Pediatr. 2013;26(1):5–8.
8. Lichtenstein GR, Hanauer SB, Sandborn WJ and the Practice Parameters Committee of the American College of Gastroenterology. Management of Crohn's disease in adults. Am J Gastroenterol. Advance online publication, doi:10.1038/ajg.2008.168. 6 Jan 2009.
9. Radford-Smith GL. What is the importance of appendectomy in the natural history of IBD? Inflamm Bowel Dis. 2008;14 Suppl 2:S72–4. doi:10.1002/ibd.20623.
10. Ueno F, Matsui T, Matsumoto T, et al. Evidence-based clinical practice guidelines for Crohn's disease, integrated with formal consensus of experts in Japan. J Gastroenterol. 2013;48(1):31–72.
11. Berg DF, Kaminski DL, Longo WE. Acute surgical emergencies in inflammatory bowel disease. Am J Surg. 2002;184:45–51.
12. Werbin N, Haddad R, Greenberg R, et al. Free perforation in Crohn's disease. Isr Med Assoc J. 2003;5(3):175–7.
13. Nakajima K, Nezu R, Hirota M, et al. The role of hand-assisted laparoscopic surgery in subtotal and total colectomy for Crohn's colitis. Surg Endosc. 2010;24(11):2713–7. doi:10.1007/s00464-010-1031-0. Epub 2010 Apr 7.
14. Ribeiro MB, Greenstein AJ, Yamazaki Y, et al. Intraabdominal abscess in regional enteritis. Ann Surg. 1991;213:32–6.
15. Yamaguchi A, Matsui T, Sakurai T, et al. The clinical characteristics and outcome of intraabdominal abscess in Crohn's disease. J Gastroenterol. 2004;39(5):441–8.
16. Jawhari A, Kamm MA, Ong C, et al. Intra-abdominal and pelvic abscess in Crohn's disease: results of non-invasive and surgical management. Br J Surg. 1998;85:367–71.
17. Dignass A, Van Assche G, Lindsay JO, et al. Travis SPL for the European Crohn's and Colitis Organisation (ECCO). The second European evidence-based consensus on the diagnosis and management of Crohn's disease: current management. J Crohns Colitis. 2010;4(1):28–62.
18. Strong SA, Koltun WA, Hyman NH, American Society of Colon and Rectal Surgeons: Practice Guidelines for Crohn's Disease, Buie WD and the Standards Practice Task Force of The American Society of Colon and Rectal Surgeons. Practice parameters for the surgical management of Crohn's disease. Dis Colon Rectum. 2007;50(11):1735–46.
19. Golfieri R, Cappelli A, Giampalma E, et al. CT-guided percutaneous pelvic abscess drainage in Crohn's disease. Tech Coloproctol. 2006;10(2):99–105.
20. Gervais DA, Hahn PF, O'Neill MJ, et al. Percutaneous abscess drainage in Crohn disease: technical success and short and long-term outcomes during 14 years. Radiology. 2002;222:645–51.
21. Luz Moreira A, Stocchi L, Tan E, et al. Outcomes of Crohn's disease presenting with abdominopelvic abscess. Dis Colon Rectum. 2009;52(5):906–12.
22. Berg DF, Kaminski DL, Longo WE. Acute surgical emergencies in inflammatory bowel disease. Am J Surg. 2002;184:45–51.
23. Cirocco WC, Reilly JC, Rusin LC. Life threatening hemorrhage and exsanguination from Crohn's disease. Dis Colon Rectum. 1995;38:85–95.
24. Driver CP, Anderson DN, Keenan RA. Massive intestinal bleeding in association with Crohn's disease. J R Coll Surg Edinb. 1996;41:152–4.
25. Truelove SC, Witts LF. Cortisone in ulcerative colitis: Final report on a therapeutic trial. BMJ. 1955;2:1041–8.
26. Carter MJ, Lobo AJ. Travis SPL, on behalf of the IBD Section of the British Society of Gastroenterology. Guidelines for the management of inflammatory bowel disease in adults. Gut 2004;53(Suppl V):v1–16
27. Alves A, Panis Y, Bouhnik Y, et al. Subtotal colectomy for severe acute colitis: a 20-year experience of a tertiary care center with an aggressive and early surgical policy. J Am Coll Surg. 2003;197(3):379–85.
28. Jones JH, Chapman M. Definition of megacolon in colitis. Gut. 1969;10:562–4.
29. Hanauer SB. Drug therapy: inflammatory bowel disease. N Engl J Med. 1996;334:841–8.

Gaspare Solina, Sara Renna,
and Ambrogio Orlando

18.1 Anatomy and Clinical Definitions

The perineum is a diamond-shaped anatomic region bounded anteriorly by the pubis, posteriorly by the end of last coccygeal vertebra and laterally by the ischial tuberosities. The perineum contains anteriorly the penis and the scrotum in males and the vulva in women and posteriorly the anus. Lesions of the anus and perianal region are localized by convention and independently by position of the patient (genucubital, gynecological, etc.) dividing the area into four quadrants and localizing the injury as if there was a clock with 12 o'clock (anterior perineum) corresponding to the scrotum in males or the vulva in females and 6 o'clock corresponding to the coccyx. Hence, all anal and perianal lesions on the left are between 12 o'clock, 3 o'clock and 6 o'clock, while the ones on the right are identified as being between 12 o'clock, 9 o'clock and 6 o'clock.

The anus is the external opening of the digestive system and continues proximally with the rectum through the anal canal.

The anal canal is lined by transition mucosa. More in the submucosa there is the hemorrhoidal venous plexus. More deeply there is the sphincter apparatus deputy to fecal continence. This sphincter apparatus consists of two concentric sphincter muscle layers, which are structurally different: the internal sphincter muscle, which is a muscle thickening in continuity with smooth muscle fibers of the rectum and the voluntary external sphincter muscle which is a continuation of the levator ani muscles.

The mucosal transit from the anal canal to rectum is lined by the pectinate line, a wavy line where the crypts of Morgagni lie. At the base of these crypts of Morgagni, in the antigravity position, there are the glands of Hermann and Desfosses that often involve also the fibers of the internal sphincter muscle.

The outside of the rectum is covered with adipose tissue that fills the ischiorectal space. It is bounded superiorly by the pelvic diaphragm that separates it from the pelvis-rectal space; this latter represents the pelvic preperitoneal part of the pouch of Douglas.

Therefore, a penetrating lesion of the anal canal may involve these perirectal spaces.

18.2 Types of Perianal Lesions

Perianal involvement in Crohn's disease may present with a variety of perianal lesions [1].

This variety is related to the different stages of the progression of the disease itself. Whether the origin is from the crypts of Morgagni (cryptogenic origin) or from Crohn's ulcer of the anal

G. Solina (✉)
UOC General Surgery, "V. Cervello" Hospital,
Azienda Ospedaliera "Ospedali Riuniti Villa
Sofia-Cervello", Palermo, Italy
e-mail: g.solina@villasofia.it

S. Renna • A. Orlando
UOC Internal Medicine, "V. Cervello" Hospital,
Azienda Ospedaliera "Ospedali Riuniti Villa
Sofia-Cervello", Palermo, Italy

© Springer International Publishing Switzerland 2016   159
G. Lo Re, M. Midiri (eds.), *Crohn's Disease: Radiological Features and Clinical-Surgical Correlations*,
DOI 10.1007/978-3-319-23066-5_18

canal, these lesions evolve penetrating in the submucosal layer, thus becoming septic and giving rise to an abscess. The natural evolution of the abscess is a fistula with the skin.

According to the fistula path, we can distinguish different types of perianal fistulae, including the rectovaginal fistula.

If the inflammatory process is extended and long-lasting, chronic inflammation may be responsible for anal stenosis and/or fecal incontinence and may lead to dysplasia or neoplasia.

The short-term goals in the treatment of perineal Crohn's disease are abscess drainage and reduction of symptoms.

The long-term goals are resolving fistula discharge, improvement in quality of life, fistula healing, preserving continence, and avoiding proctectomy with stoma.

18.2.1 Anal Ulcer and Fissure

Anal canal ulcer denotes an involvement of this region by Crohn's disease and is often associated with perianal fistula, being often its origin: in these cases, it is possible to find the entrance of the fistulous track on its undermined edge.

Anal ulcer is often confused with an anal fissure, but it may be placed either eccentrically around the anal canal in contrast to idiopathic fissure in ano which tends to lie in the midline and is not associated with the so-called sentinel skin tag.

Considering that this lesion has to be accounted as a Crohn's disease localization, surgical treatment is not indicated, while systemic and local drugs are required.

The anal ulcer and fissure are usually painless and spontaneously heal in more than 80 % of patients [2].

Operative intervention in unselected patients does not improve the outcome and should generally be avoided.

However, patients who have pain and who do not have macroscopic evidence of rectal inflammation or local sepsis, lateral sphincterotomy may achieve healing without subsequent incontinence in most patients. Fissurectomy is contraindicated [3].

18.2.2 Skin Tag

There are two types of skin tags:

- Large, edematous, hard, cyanotic skin tag and often tender or painful. Typically arising from a healed anal fissure or ulcer. Excision contraindicated due to problems with a high rate of postoperative complications, including poor wound healing
- "Elephant ear" tag is flat, broad, long (up to 2 cm) and narrow polypoid lesions (fibroepithelial polypoid tags), soft, painless. May cause perianal hygiene problems and can be safely excised (however, excision of these innocuous tags is rarely required) [2, 3]

18.2.3 Perianal Abscess

Potential anorectal spaces may become infected with an abscess, including intersphincteric, ischiorectal and supralevator or pelvic-rectal spaces. If fistula is present, the abscess is resultant of obstruction of a perianal fistula tract.

The symptoms are perianal pain, tenderness, swelling, and fever.

Perianal abscesses must be drained surgically. Superficial perianal abscesses may be associated with a low perianal fistula and can be treated with incision and drainage. Deep perianal abscesses may be associated with a complex perianal fistula and should be treated with incision and drainage and placement of a noncutting seton if the fistula can be identified or placement of a mushroom catheter if an associated fistula cannot be identified. The placement of setons, while allowing prolonged drainage of the abscess, in essence perpetuates a perianal fistula [2, 3].

18.2.4 Perianal Fistula

A fistula is a tract of pus and/or granulation tissue between two epithelial surfaces lined with a fibrous wall. Primary tracts are connections between the internal and external openings, while secondary tracts are blind extensions [2].

Surgical treatment of perianal fistulas differs depending upon the anatomic classification and the overall treatment; both medical and surgical depend upon the stage of anal and rectal disease.

The most commonly used anatomic classification is the St. Mark's Hospital [4] one, which distinguishes simple and complex fistulas; this classification is adopted by the ECCO guidelines [5] and accepted by the American Gastroenterological Association Clinical Practice Committee [2].

The presence of proctitis, defined as any ulceration and/or stricture in the rectum, or inflammation and/or stricture of the anal canal, is an important component for fistula assessment (Statement 4 IOIBD and European Society of Coloproctology Guidelines) [6].

Patients without macroscopic evidence of proctitis who have *simple fistulas* may be treated by laying open the fistula tract (fistulotomy) or by a complete fistula excision (fistulectomy). The use of a noncutting seton rather than fistulotomy in patients with low fistulas and proctitis is preferred.

A noncutting seton is a suture or drain that is threaded into the cutaneous orifice of a perianal fistula, through the fistula tract, and across the mucosal orifice of the fistula into the rectum and then out the anal canal. A noncutting seton maintains drainage of the fistula, thereby reducing the risk of perianal abscess formation.

In general, there is a trend toward greater healing rates following fistulotomy for simple fistulas in patients without macroscopic evidence of inflammation of the rectum when compared with patients with active proctocolitis [3].

Complex fistulas require a more conservative surgical approach. Indeed, we cure the fistula problem at the price of leaving the patient with fecal incontinence. The main objective is to reduce the risk of incontinence or proctectomy. The secondary objective is the healing and/or the elimination of recurrent disease.

In the complex fistulas, there are many steps of treatment.

In patients with complex fistula, the treatment is aimed at a cone-like excision of all the tissue in the ischiorectal fossa that contains the extrasphincteric part of the fistula with its eventual branches. The base of the cone is the perianal skin with one or more external fistulous tracks and the apex in the external side of the external sphincter muscle. This excision may be performed at one time or at multiple times if the extension of the removal would be too excessive and consequently too uncomfortable for patient's life and relationship. The residual cavity, in fact, heals by secondary intention and the healing time is proportional to the amount of removed tissue. If repeated removals are needed, the remaining fistulous branches are stabilized with extrasphincteric loose setons. When the removed parts heal, these residual fistulous branches are removed. Then a seton is put in the trans-sphincteric part of the fistula.

As in a tree, whose trunk is the trans-sphincteric part of the fistula and whose branches are the extrasphincteric parts, surgery consists in removing, at one or more times, all the branches, so that only the trunk, that corresponds as said to the trans-sphincteric part of the fistula, will remain (see Figs. 18.1 and 18.2).

Perianal disease is considered an exacerbation of CD or a resistance to the current treatment; hence, after reduction of the sepsis and downgrading of the disease, a biological therapy is needed (IG-IBD Statement 5D) [7].

The seton is left in place until at least the induction of the anti-TNF treatment period has

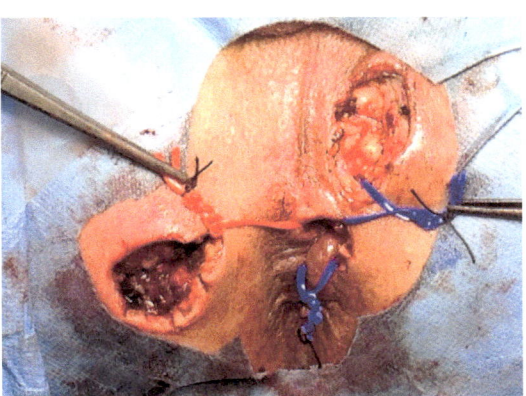

Fig. 18.1 Extra-sphinteric fistulectomy and setons placement

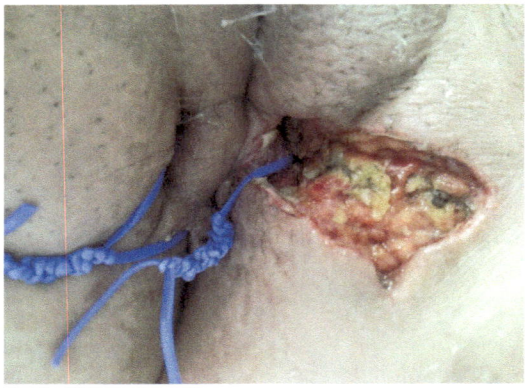

Fig. 18.2 Seton positioned only in the trans-sphinteric tract

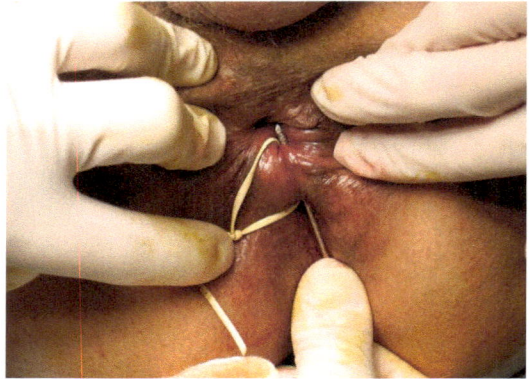

Fig. 18.3 Courettage to remove the seton

been completed. Then, the seton is removed (clearing the fistulous track) (see Fig. 18.3) and the fistula healed by the drug.

To date, this multidisciplinary approach represents the best management of complex perianal disease.

Indeed, the results of combined treatment lead to closure rate of the fistula of 78.5 % (11 out of 14) of patients who completed the surgical program after a mean follow-up of 18.8 months [8]. But in another study, the fistula closure rate was significantly lower (29 %, 14 out of 48) after a mean follow-up of 20 months [9]. In the only published abstract by Rizzello et al. [10], 100 patients were treated with adalimumab after a deep surgical perineum sanitization. A complete fistula closure was observed in 77 % of treated patients at 156 weeks.

In the only published controlled trial (ADAFI) planned on patients with perianal disease treated with biologics (± ciprofloxacin), the fistula closure rate at 24 weeks was 33 % (12 out of 36) in those treated with adalimumab and 53 % (18 out of 34) in those treated with adalimumab plus ciprofloxacin, but this difference was not significant ($p = 0.098$). Nevertheless in this trial, the number of patients with complex perianal disease was not specified; only about 20 % of patients were treated with seton placement presuming that the number of patients with complex perianal disease was low [11].

Finally, data from the retrospective study by El-Gazzaz et al., including more than 100 patients, the fistula closure rate, in those who completed the surgical program and started biologics, was 36.6 % (37 out of 101) after a mean follow-up of 3.2 years [12]. In the ADAFI trial and in the study by El-Gazzaz et al., the recurrence rate was not reported.

The large published series on perianal fistulizing CD treated with infliximab showed a long-term cumulative probability of recurrence of 16.6 %, 31.3 %, and 40 % at 1, 2, and 5 years, respectively. When considering only the subgroup of patients treated with maintenance infliximab treatment, the cumulative probability of recurrence was 12 % and 36.6 % at 1 and 5 years, respectively [13].

In the prebiological era, the cutting seton was used. An analysis in the St. Mark's Hospital of London showed that complex fistulas are treated obtaining healing in 55 out 79 fistulas (70 %). But this result has been obtained just using in 26 out 79 (33 %) fistulas the local conventional surgery (the study does not mention the incontinence rate) and in 21 out of 79 (38 %) treated with major surgery (defunctioning stoma, proctectomy)! [4].

The recurrence rate for "complex" fistulas managed with a cutting seton is reported to be 0–8 % with minor incontinence in 34–63 % and major incontinence reported in 2–26 % of patients [14, 15].

Cutting setons are also associated with significant morbidity related to discomfort from the seton [16].

In patients not responding or intolerant to biological therapy, a local biological therapy has been proposed. Evidences suggest that local injection of anti-TNF-α into the fistula tract may be beneficial. Two Italian groups described in pilot trials show local injections of both infliximab and adalimumab could improve fistula healing avoiding their systemic actions, but controlled and randomized trials are required to prove the value of this technique [17–20].

18.2.5 Rectovaginal Fistula

It is a particular type of fistula in ano, whose external opening is not on perianal skin but in the vagina. Rectovaginal fistula may be classified according to its track according to Parks classification in superficial, intersphincteric, trans-sphincteric, suprasphincteric and extrasphincteric fistulas.

This kind of fistula arises from penetrating ulceration of the anal canal or rectum into the vagina.

Surgical treatment of rectovaginal fistulas in patients with perianal Crohn's disease should only be attempted in the absence of active inflammation of the rectosigmoid colon.

Fistulotomy should rarely be used to treat low rectovaginal fistulas due to sphincter injury risk.

Placement of noncutting setons in this setting tends to enlarge the opening, making the fistula more symptomatic. An exception is when there is a rectovaginal septal abscess or inflammatory mass in addition to the fistulas.

Patients with rectovaginal fistulas may be treated by a number of other approaches, including primary closure, transanal advancement flap, sleeve advancement flap, and transvaginal advancement flap.

All the above-described techniques for fistulas have been used for this particular case but results were worse, while encouraging data were those using interposition of gracilis muscle [3].

18.2.6 Anorectal Stricture and Incontinence

Anorectal stricture may be short annular diaphragm-like strictures <2 cm in length or longer tubular strictures.

Anal or rectal strictures may arise as complications of ulceration of the anal canal or rectum, perianal abscesses, and complex perianal fistulas. They are often associated with ongoing proctitis.

Symptoms are typically those of urgency, incontinence, tenesmus, frequency, and difficulty with defecation. Some patients are asymptomatic.

The treatment is dilation: endoscopic and intraoperative during intervention for other associated lesions (gentle finger dilation to preserve sphincter function) and/or with specific devices like finger or bougie or Hegar's dilators at home. Repeat dilations are often required.

Some patients will require proctectomy [2, 3].

18.2.7 Anal Cancer

Cancer occurs rarely with an incidence rate of 0.2 per 1000 patient-years [21].

A systematic review of 34 case series and reports published in English language between 1950 and 2008 reports 61 cases of cancer, mainly in females (61 %). Females were significantly younger than males at the time of diagnosis of cancer (47 vs. 53 years, $P < 0.032$).

Females were noted to have the fistula for significantly shorter duration prior to cancer transformation when compared to males (8.3 vs. 16 years, $P = 0.0035$). The average duration of CD was 18 years for female versus 24 years for male (p 0.005).

Cancer was detected at the first visit and diagnosed with biopsy in only small number of patients (20 %). In 59 % of patients, the cancer was detected anywhere between 1 month and 2 years after the initial presentation. The average delay in diagnosis of carcinoma in fistula tract was 5.8 months (median 3 months).

Adenocarcinoma was the most common histology (59 %), followed by squamous cell carcinoma (31 %).

The most common presenting complaints were pain (39 %) and persistent fistula (25 %). An abscess was reported at the time of examination in 41 % of patients [22].

The treatment *is* the one reported by oncologic guidelines and the prognosis for these patients is poor [23].

18.3 Adjunctive techniques to fistula closure

The not entirely encouraging results of combined treatment pushed the research toward finding new therapies hoping in better results.

The presence of proctitis is a bad prognostic index due to the rate of not healing and/or relapse. Hence, in patients with proctitis, relapse or absence of healing with biological therapy, surgical sphincter-saving surgery can be associated to strengthen the biological drug.

These techniques have been borrowed from the treatment of cryptogenic fistulas and data for Crohn's fistulas are not enough.

Some of these techniques then are aimed at closing the internal orifice, others at closing the fistula although branched (liquids) and others at finding the best application in simple tracks. The various options can be combined. The best prerequisite for optimal results is the absence of sepsis and the presence of a single fistula track.

18.3.1 Surgical Techniques for the Closure of Internal Orifice

An *Mucosal Advancement Flap (MAF)* can be used as an alternative to noncutting setons or after stabilization of the fistula through the noncutting seton and the removal of sepsis, in patients with complex fistulas who *do not* have macroscopic evidence of rectal inflammation.

The concept of endorectal advancement flaps is to preserve the sphincter by closing off the primary opening by means of a mobilized flap.

An advancement flap consists of incising a flap of tissue (mucosa, submucosa, circular muscle) around the internal opening of a fistula, excising the internal opening of the fistula tract and pulling the flap down to cover the primary fistula opening. Thereby we close the high pressure end of the fistula tract but we untouch the sphincter complex. The excluded fistula segment is expected to dry out over time. It is more difficult to use this technique for anteriorly positioned internal orifices.

The guidelines provided by the American Society of Colon and Rectal Surgeons [24] in 2005 have established that an endorectal advancement flap should be the best option to treat a recurrent complex fistula.

In a systematic review of 35 studies with an average follow-up of 28.9 months, the success rate of MAF for Crohn's fistulas was 64 % (range 33.3–92.9 %). The incontinence rate was 9.4 % with a wide interstudy variability (range 0–28.6 %). Re-interventions were needed in almost 50 % of patients [25]. Data from Cleveland, after a mean follow-up of 7 years, report a healing rate of 68 %, but report also the opportunity, in case of failure, to repeat a second, and, if necessary a third flap. Hence, the healing rate in Crohn's diseases rises from 68 % to 89 % [26].

Ligation of the intersphincteric fistula tract (LIFT) is a surgical option in the management of trans-sphincteric fistulas when the tract has matured into a fibrotic tube with granulation tissue enabling ligation and transection.

The surgical approach consists of ligation of intersphincteric tract close to the internal opening and removal of intersphincteric tract, scraping out all granulation tissue in the rest of the fistulous tract and suturing of the defect at the external sphincter muscle [27, 28].

In a prospective study of 15 consecutive cases of *CD patients* with trans-sphincteric fistulas, none of them developed fecal incontinence, and LIFT site healing was seen in 67 % of patients with a follow-up of 12 months [29].

In a review of 18 studies, 592 patients were considered with trans-sphincteric fistula reported in 73.3 % of cases. The mean healing rate was 74.6 %. The mean healing time was 5.5 weeks, and the mean follow-up period was 42.3 weeks. No de novo incontinence developed secondary to the LIFT procedure [30].

18.3.2 Surgical Technique for Closure of the Fistulous Track

The aim is to facilitate the closure of the fistula tract using materials that serve as solid or semi-solid matrix to incorporate fibroblasts and tissue regeneration. Critic points: these materials are absorbed before scar tissue has formed, especially if there is sepsis. The semisolid material would have the advantage of filling also any associated ramifications or sinus.

18.3.2.1 Liquid or Semisolid Materials

Fibrin glue consists of fibrinogen and thrombin. Upon mixing, a fibrin clot is formed, which is thought to stimulate wound healing by inducing angiogenesis and fibroblast growth.

Initial studies of fibrin sealant for the management of anal fistulas were promising [31, 32]. Tyler et al. [33] reported also a prospective series of 89 patients with "complex" anal fistulas managed by obliteration of the fistula tract by fibrin glue. With at least 1 year of follow-up, 70.7 % of fistulas were healed. In contrast, a prospective series of 42 patients by Loungnarath et al. [34] reported that 31 % of fistulas were healed by use of fibrin sealant.

In a study of Johnson EK et al. [35], the success rate of plug vs. the fibrin glue was 87 % vs. 40 %. A meta-analysis found no significant difference between fibrin glue and conventional surgery with regard to recurrence and fecal incontinence rates [36] mainly between flap +/− fibrin glue showing worse outcomes after the combination of the two compared to flap repair alone [37]; thus, this material has not been used anymore.

As an alternative, it has been proposed the use of an injectable mixture consisting of *acellular porcine dermal matrix cross-linked* (Permacol©). The technique is the same as the glue one. Hammond TM et al. reported results of complex fistulas not related to IBD at 29 months: in 12 of 15 patients they healed [38].

It has been proposed the association of the flap with the mixture of Permacol© with a reported success after follow-up of only 6 months of 10 healings/11 patients including six IBD patients. The recurrence occurred in an IBD fistula [39].

18.3.2.2 Solid Materials

Bioprosthetic anal fistula plugs are more resistant to depolymerization, but they imply disadvantages in case of not previously detected secondary fistulous tracks (relapse).

Plugs, made of collagen, or *lyophilized porcine intestinal submucosa* (Surgisis© acellular biomaterial created from the endothelium of the porcine small bowel) or Gore-Tex©, are inserted via the internal fistula opening to fill the fistula tract and leave the sphincter apparatus untouched.

Plugs are put under general anesthesia. All fistula tracts and primary openings are identified using conventional fistula probe and/or hydrogen peroxide instillation. All tracts are irrigated with hydrogen peroxide; however, the tracts are not curetted to avoid enlarging or damaging the fistula tract. The plug is pulled tip-first into the internal opening until resistance is encountered. The excess plug material is trimmed flush with the mucosa, and the plug is buried into the primary opening using a figure-of-eight 2–0 vicryl, which is inserted deep to the internal sphincter muscle. The plug is trimmed at skin level at the secondary opening. Care is taken not to occlude the secondary opening to allow drainage of material and to avoid a closed system. At the end of the procedure, the plug is completely buried within the fistula tract. In the case of multiple separate fistulas, this is repeated for each fistula tract. In the event of an excessively large-diameter fistula, the tract is "matured" using setons and 10 % topical metronidazole, for a period of 6–8 weeks, before anal fistula plug insertion. This narrows the diameter of the fistula tracts to dimensions that are amenable to "plugging."

Success rates in retrospective cohorts and one open-label study with a median follow-up of 6–15 months varied between 24 % and 88 %. Patients with multiple fistula tracts had a significantly higher failure rate [6].

In a prospective study with porcine intestinal submucosa anal fistula plug on complex Crohn's anorectal fistula, 80 % of patients were healed [40], but in later studies, data were opposite with low healing rate (33 %) [41].

One of the studies reported that failure was caused by dislodgement of the plug in 22 % of the cases [42].

It is commercially available a type of Surgisis© modified with a "button" that should be fixed in the internal opening at the plane of the internal sphincter (Biodesign© Anal Fistula Plug with biologic button) [43].

The Gore Bio-A Fistula Plug© is made from a *synthetic bioabsorbable polyglycolide-trimethylene carbonate copolymer* and comprises a *disk* attached to six tubes. The Bio-A© Fistula Plug is designed to prevent unexpected migration or extrusion. Its round disk has been designed to cover the internal opening sufficiently to prevent passage of the plug down the track. It virtually prevents plug dislodgement. Furthermore, the disk and the submucosal covering should offer a double barrier to the passage of feces through the track.

The tracks are curetted and then irrigated with hydrogen peroxide. A small submucosal pocket is created around the internal opening to allow the disk of the device to be accommodated. The submucosal pocket is then closed with 3–0 absorbable stitch. The disk is included in the suture to prevent plug migration, and the protruding tubes were trimmed 2–3 mm beyond the surface of the perianal skin.

In a prospective study on 11 cryptoglandular fistulae, the success was reported in 72.7 % (8/11) of patients, but the follow-up was short and healing evaluation not performed through MR [44].

These data are better than the ones published by Portilla et al. [45]: in their study, the successful closure was observed in 3 of 19 patients (15.8 %), but in only 3 patients, setons had been previously placed and the treatment of sepsis may be responsible of the different healing rates.

Lastly, the study by Buchberg B et al. is also interesting, in which Cook Plug© is retrospectively compared to Gore Plug©. The overall procedural success rate in the Gore group was 6 of 11 (54.5 %) versus 2 of 16 (12.5 %) in the Cook group. A total of 19/27 (70 %) procedures failed to resolve the

fistulas. The reasons for failure were plug dislodgement in two attempts (10.5 %) and persistent drainage in 17 attempts (89.5 %) [46].

Data show varying success rates for fistula closure, which may be due to the heterogeneity of the studies regarding fistula origin (Crohn's vs. cryptoglandular) and follow-up.

In general, plugs may offer a valid first-line option for surgical treatment; measures to prevent dislodgement and perioperative antibiotics may increase success and safety, although costs can be a major concern [7].

In conclusion, there are very few randomized controlled trials comparing the various modalities of surgery for fistula in ano. Newer operations like the anal fistula plug and the LIFT procedure need to be evaluated by randomized clinical trials [55].

18.3.3 Other Techniques for Local Therapy

Mesenchymal stem cells seem to have promising applications in perianal CD. They are non-hematopoietic precursors of connective tissue cells with anti-inflammatory and tissue-regenerative properties, extracted from subdermal adipose tissue obtained through liposuction. They may be injected into the rectal mucosa around fistula opening and into fistula tract with fibrin glue [47, 48].

García-Olmo et al. [48] reported a phase II study in which adipose-derived stem cells in fibrin glue vs. fibrin glue alone were administered in 49 patients (14 affected by CD): fistula healing was observed in 16 % of the patients who received only fibrin glue vs. 71 % of the patients who received stem cells plus fibrin glue ($p < 0.001$). In another phase II study [49], complete fistula healing was observed in 27/33 patients (82 %) by 8 weeks after ASC injection.

An Italian study, employing autologous bone marrow-derived mesenchymal stromal cells, confirmed that this novel approach represents a feasible, safe, and beneficial therapy in refractory CD [50].

A recent multicenter open-label, single-arm clinical trial was conducted at six Spanish hospitals. Twenty-four CD patients with complex fistulas were treated intralesionally with 20–40 millions of expanded allogenic adipose-derived stem cells: 69 % of patients showed a reduction in the number of draining fistulas at week 24, while 56 % achieved complete closure of the treated fistula, and only *6/24 patients (30%)* obtained complete closure of all existing fistula tracts [51].

However, double-blind randomized placebo-controlled trials are needed to draw any conclusions on this therapeutic modality [6, 52].

In those patients with extensive and severe sepsis, mainly in the case of early relapse and conspicuous leakage of pus, it may be necessary to have a *diverting temporary stoma*. The rationale for fecal diversion is to reduce fecal flow across the fistula tract by reducing flow through the rectum, allowing the rectal mucosa to heal and the fistula to close. These procedures are now only rarely performed after a number of studies showed that most patients who undergo placement of a temporary diverting ileostomy or colostomy for perianal Crohn's disease never have intestinal continuity restored [4].

Complex fistulas associated with uncontrollable and recurrent sepsis and/or anal stenosis and/or incontinence are candidate, as last option, to perform *proctectomy* with a permanent stoma [52].

This proctectomy rates for patients with perianal Crohn's disease managed conservatively range from 10 % to 18 % [3].

Proctectomy does not always eradicate problems, as up to 40 % of patients experience delayed healing of a perineal wound and/or a persistent perineal sinus [53]. In these cases, it is possible to do a gracilis muscle transposition associated to proctectomy or to treat the residual sinus after previous proctectomy. In a single retrospective study including 18 CD patients, gracilis transposition was successful for complex fistulas in 64 % and for persistent nonhealing perineal sinuses in 50 % of the cases with maintained efficacy (90 % upon 10 months median follow-up) [54].

Bibliography

1. Hughes LE. Clinical classification of perianal Crohn's disease. Dis Colon Rectum. 1992;35:928–32.
2. Sandborn JW, Fazio WV, Feagan GB, Hanauer BC, American Gastroenterological Association Clinical Practice Committee. AGA technical review on perianal Crohn's disease. Gastroenterology. 2003;125:1508–30.
3. American Gastroenterological Association Clinical Practice Committee. American gastroenterological association medical position statement: perianal Crohn's disease. Gastroenterology. 2003;125:1503–7.
4. Bell SJ, Williams AB, Wiesel P, Wilkinson K, Cohen RC, Kamm MA. The clinical course of fistulating Crohn's disease. Aliment Pharmacol Ther. 2003;17:1145–51.
5. Caprilli R, Gassull MA, Escher JC, Moser G, Munkholm P, Forbes A, Hommes DW, Lochs H, Angelucci E, Cocco A, Vucelic B, Hildebrand H, Kolacek S, Riis L, Lukas M, de Franchis R, Hamilton M, Jantschek G, Michetti P, O'Morain C, Anwar MM, Freitas JL, Mouzas IA, Baert F, Mitchell R, Hawkey CJ, European Crohn's and Colitis Organisation (ECCO). European evidence based consensus on the diagnosis and management of Crohn's disease: special situations. Gut. 2006;55(Supplement 1):i36–58.
6. Gecse KB, Bemelman W, Kamm MA, Stoker J, Khanna R, Ng SC, Panés J, van Assche G, Liu Z, Hart A, Levesque BG, D'Haens G, World Gastroenterology Organization, International Organisation for Inflammatory Bowel Diseases IOIBD, European Society of Coloproctology and Robarts Clinical Trials. A global consensus on the classification, diagnosis and multidisciplinary treatment of perianal fistulising Crohn's disease. Gut. 2014;63:1381–92.
7. Orlando A, Armuzzi A, Papi C, Annese V, Ardizzone S, Biancone L, Bortoli A, Castiglione F, D'Incà R, Gionchetti P, Kohn A, Poggioli G, Rizzello F, Vecchi M, Cottone M. The Italian Society of Gastroenterology (SIGE) and the Italian Group for the study of Inflammatory Bowel Disease(IG-IBD) Clinical Practice Guidelines: the use of tumor necrosis factor-alpha antagonist therapy in inflammatory bowel disease. Dig Liver Dis. 2011;43(1):1–20.
8. Sciaudone G, Di Stazio C, Limongelli P, Guadagni I, Pellino G, Riegler G, Coscione P, Selvaggi F. Treatment of complex perianal fistulas in Crohn disease: infliximab, surgery or combined approach. Can J Surg. 2010;53(5):299–304.
9. Antakia R, Shorthouse AJ, Robinson K, Lobo AJ. Combined modality treatment for complex fistulating perianal Crohn's disease. Colorectal Dis. 2013;15(2):210–6.
10. Rizzello F, Calabrese C, Calafiore A, Laureti S, Poggioli G, Campieri M, Gionchetti P. Adalimumab in the treatment of perianal Crohn's disease: short and

long term results in a Single Tertiary Center AGA Abstract Sa. 2014;S-358.

11. Dewint P, Hansen BE, Verhey E, Oldenburg B, Hommes DW, Pierik M, Ponsioen CI, van Dullemen HM, Russel M, van Bodegraven AA, van der Woude CJ. Adalimumab combined with ciprofloxacin is superior to adalimumab monotherapy in perianal fistula closure in Crohn's disease: a randomised, double-blind, placebo controlled trial (ADAFI). Gut. 2014;63(2):292–9.

12. El-Gazzaz G, Hull T, Church JM. Biological immuno-modulators improve the healing rate in surgically treated perianal Crohn's fistulas. Colorectal Dis. 2012;14(10):1217–23.

13. Bouguen G, Siproudhis L, Gizard E, Wallenhorst T, Billioud V, Bretagne JF, Bigard MA, Peyrin-Biroulet L. Long-term outcome of perianal fistulizing Crohn's disease treated with infliximab. Clin Gastroenterol Hepatol. 2013;11(8):975–81.

14. Garcia-Aguilar J, Belmonte C, Wong WD, Goldberg SM, Madoff RD. Cutting seton vs. two-stage seton fistulotomy in the surgical management of high anal fistula. Br J Surg. 1998;85:243–5.

15. Hamalainen KP, Sainio AP. Cutting seton for anal fistulas: high risk of minor control defects. Dis Colon Rectum. 1997;40:1443–6.

16. Ellis NC, Rostas JW, Greiner FG. Outcomes with bio-prosthetic plugs for management of anal fistulas. Dis Colon Rectum. 2010;53:798–802.

17. Poggioli G, Laureti S, Pierangeli F, Rizzello F, Ugolini F, Gionchetti P, Campieri M. Local injection of Infliximab for the treatment of perianal Crohn's disease. Dis Colon Rectum. 2005;48:768–74.

18. Poggioli G, Laureti S, Pierangeli F, Bazzi P, Coscia M, Gentilini L, Gionchetti P, Rizzello F. Local injection of adalimumab for perianal Crohn's disease: better than infliximab? Inflamm Bowel Dis. 2010;16: 1631.

19. Tonelli F, Giudici F, Asteria CR. Effectiveness and safety of local adalimumab injection in patients with fistulizing perianal Cohn's disease: a pilot study. Dis Colon Rectum. 2012;55:870–5.

20. Asteria CR, Ficari F, Bagnoli S, Milla M, Tonelli F. Treatment of perianal fistulas in Crohn's disease by local injection of antibody to TNF-alpha accounts for a favourable clinical response in selected cases: a pilot study. Scand J Gastroenterol. 2006;41: 1064–72.

21. Laukoetter MG, Mennigen R, Hannig CM, Osada N, Rijcken E, Vowinkel T, Krieglstein CF, Senninger N, Anthoni C, Bruewer M. Intestinal cancer risk in Cohn's disease: a meta-analysis. J Gastrointest Surg. 2011;15:576–83.

22. Thomas M, Bienkowski R, Vandermeer TJ, Trostle D, Cagir B. Malignant transformation in perianal fistulas of Cohn's disease: a systematic review of literature. J Gastrointest Surg. 2010;14:66–73.

23. Beaugerie L, Itzkowitz SH. Cancers complicating inflammatory bowel disease. N Engl J Med. 2015; 372(15):1441–52.

24. Whiteford MH, Kilkenny III M, Hyman N, Buie WD, Cohen J, Orsay C, Dunn G, Perry WB, Ellis CN, Rakinic J, Gregorcyk S, Shellito P, Nelson R, Tjandra JJ, Newstead G. Practice parameters for the treatment of perianal abscess and fistula-in-ano. Dis Colon Rectum. 2005;48:1337–42.

25. Soltani A, Kaiser AM. Endorectal advancement flap for cryptoglandular or Cohn's fistula-in-ano. Dis Colon Rectum. 2010;53:486–95.

26. Jarrar A, Church J. Advancement flap repair: a good option for complex anorectal fistulas. Dis Colon Rectum. 2011;54(12):1537–41.

27. Rojanasakul A, Pattanaarun J, Sahakitrungruang C, Tantiphlachiva K. Total anal sphincter saving technique for fistula-in-ano; the ligation of intersphincteric fistula tract. J Med Assoc Thai. 2007;90(3): 581–6.

28. Rojanasakul A. LIFT procedure: a simplified technique for fistula-in- ano. Tech Coloproctol. 2009;13: 237–40.

29. Gingold DS, Murrell ZA, Fleshner PR. A prospective evaluation of the ligation of the intersphincteric tract procedure for complex anal fistula in patients with Crohn's disease. Ann Surg. 2014;260:1057–61.

30. Vergara-Fernandez O, Espino-Urbina LA. Ligation of intersphincteric fistula tract: what is the evidence in a review? World J Gastroenterol. 2013;19(40): 6805–13.

31. Cintron JR, Park JJ, Orsay CP, Pearl RK, Nelson RL, Sone JH, Song R, Abcarian H. Repair of fistulas-in-ano using fibrin adhesive: long-term follow-up. Dis Colon Rectum. 2000;43(7):944–9.

32. Sentovich SM. Fibrin glue for all anal fistulas. J Gastrointest Surg. 2001;5:158–61.

33. Tyler KM, Aarons CB, Sentovich SM. Successful sphincter-sparing surgery for all anal fistulas. Dis Colon Rectum. 2007;50:1535–9.

34. Loungnarath R, Dietz DW, Mutch MG, Birnbaum EH, Kodner IJ, Fleshman JW. Fibrin glue treatment of complex anal fistulas has a low success rate. Dis Colon Rectum. 2004;47:432–6.

35. Johnson EK, Gaw JU, Armstrong DN. Efficacy of anal fistula plug vs. fibrin glue in closure of anorectal fistulas. Dis Colon Rectum. 2006;49(3):371–6.

36. Cirocchi R, Santoro A, Trastulli S, Farinella E, Di Rocco G, Vendettuali D, Giannotti D, Redler A, Coccetta M, Gullà N, Boselli C, Avenia N, Sciannameo F, Basoli A. Meta-analysis of fibrin glue versus surgery for treatment of fistula-in-ano. Ann Ital Chir. 2010;81:349–56.

37. Ellis CN, Clark S. Fibrin glue as an adjunct to flap repair of anal fistulas: a randomized, controlled study. Dis Colon Rectum. 2006;49(11):1736–40.

38. Hammond TM, Porrett TR, Scott SM, Williams NS, Lunniss PJ. Management of idiopathic anal fistula using cross-linked collagen: a prospective phase 1 study. Colorectal Dis. 2011;13(1):94–104.

39. Sileri P, Franceschilli L, Del Vecchio Blanco G, Stolfi VM, Angelucci GP, Gaspari AL. Porcine dermal collagen matrix injection may enhance flap repair

surgery for complex anal fistula. Int J Colorectal Dis. 2011;26(3):345–9.

40. O'Connor L, Champagne BJ, Ferguson MA, Orangio GR, Schertzer ME, Armstrong DN. Efficacy of anal fistula plug in closure of Crohn's anorectal fistulas. Dis Colon Rectum. 2006;49:1569–73.

41. Owen G, Keshava A, Stewart P, Patterson J, Chapuis P, Bokey E, Rickard M. Plugs unplugged. Anal fistula plug: the Concord experience. ANZ J Surg. 2010;80:341–3.

42. Thekkinkattil DK, Botterill I, Ambrose NS, Lundby L, Sagar PM, Buntzen S, Finan PJ. Efficacy of the anal fistula plug in complex anorectal fistulae. Colorectal Dis. 2009;11:584–7.

43. Köckerling F, von Rosen T, Jacob D. Modified plug repair with limited sphincter sparing fistulectomy in the treatment of complex anal fistulas. Front Surg. 2014;1:17. www.frontiersin.org.

44. Ratto C, Litta F, Parello A, Donisi L, Zaccone G, De Simone V. Gore Bio-A Fistula Plug: a new sphincter-sparing procedure for complex anal fistula. Colorectal Dis. 2012;14:e264–9.

45. de la Portilla F, Rada R, Jiménez-Rodríguez R, Díaz-Pavón JM, Sánchez-Gil JM. Evaluation of a new synthetic plug in the treatment of anal fistulas: results of a pilot study. Dis Colon Rectum. 2011;54(11):1419–22.

46. Buchberg B, Masoomi H, Choi J, Bergman H, Mills S, Stamos MJ. A tale of two (anal fistula) plug: is there a difference in short-term outcomes? Ann Surg. 2010;76:1150–3.

47. García-Olmo D, García-Arranz M, Herreros D, Pascual I, Peiro C, Rodríguez-Montes JA. A phase I clinical trial of the treatment of Crohn's fistula by adipose mesenchymal stem cell transplantation. Dis Colon Rectum. 2005;48:1416–23.

48. Garcia-Olmo D, Herreros D, Pascual I, Pascual JA, Del-Valle E, Zorrilla J, De-La-Quintana P, Garcia-Arranz M, Pascual M. Expanded adipose-derived stem cells for the treatment of complex perianal fistula: a phase II clinical trial. Dis Colon Rectum. 2009;52:79–86.

49. Lee WY, Park KJ, Cho YB, Yoon SN, Song KH, Kim DS, Jung SH, Kim M, Yoo HW, Kim I, Ha H, Yu CS. Autologous adipose tissue-derived stem cells treatment demonstrated favorable and sustainable therapeutic effect for Cohn's fistula. Stem Cells. 2013;31:2575–81.

50. Ciccocioppo R, Bernardo ME, Sgarella A, Maccario R, Avanzini MA, Ubezio C, Minelli A, Alvisi C, Vanoli A, Calliada F, Dionigi P, Perotti C, Locatelli F, Corazza GR. Autologous bone marrow-derived mesenchymal stromal cells in the treatment of fistulising Crohn's disease. Gut. 2011;60:788–98.

51. de la Portilla F, Alba F, García-Olmo D, Herrerías JM, González FX, Galindo A. Expanded allogeneic adipose-derived stem cells (eASCs) for the treatment of complex perianal fistula in Crohn's disease: results from a multicenter phase I/IIa clinical trial. Int J Colorectal Dis. 2013;28:313–23.

52. Marzo M, Felice C, Pugliese D, Andrisani G, Mocci G, Armuzzi A, Guidi L. Management of perianal fistulas in Crohn's disease: an up-to-date review. World J Gastroenterol. 2015;21(5):1394–403.

53. Yamamoto T, Bain IM, Allan RN, Keighley MR. Persistent perineal sinus after proctocolectomy for Crohn's disease. Dis Colon Rectum. 1999;42: 96–101.

54. Maeda Y, Heyckendorff-Diebold T, Tei TM, Lundby L, Buntzen S. Gracilis muscle transposition for complex fistula and persistent nonhealing sinus in perianal Crohn's disease. Inflamm Bowel Dis. 2011;17: 583–9.

55. Jacob TJ, Perakath B, Keighley MR. Surgical intervention for anorectal fistula. Cochrane Database Syst Rev. 2010;(5):CD006319.

Index

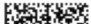